MILADY'S AESTHETICIAN SERIES

A Comprehensive Guide to Equipment

SUSANNE SCHMALING, L.E.

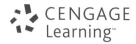

CENGAGE
Learning™

Australia • Brazil • Japan • Korea • Mexico • Singapore • Spain • United Kingdom • United States

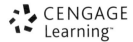

Milady's Aesthetician Series: A Comprehensive Guide to Equipment
Susanne Schmaling, L.E.

Vice President, Milady: Dawn Gerrain

Publisher: Erin O'Connor

Acquisitions Editor: Martine Edwards

Associate Product Manager:
  Anne Orgren

Editorial Assistant: Mike Spring

Director of Beauty Industry Relations:
  Sandra Bruce

Senior Marketing Manager:
  Gerard McAvey

Marketing Specialist: Erica Conley

Marketing Coordinator: Nicole Riggi

Production Director: Wendy Troeger

Senior Content Project Manager:
  Nina Tucciarelli

Art Director: Joy Kocsis

© 2009 Delmar, Cengage Learning

ALL RIGHTS RESERVED. No part of this work covered by the copyright herein may be reproduced, transmitted, stored, or used in any form or by any means graphic, electronic, or mechanical, including but not limited to photocopying, recording, scanning, digitizing, taping, Web distribution, information networks, or information storage and retrieval systems, except as permitted under Section 107 or 108 of the 1976 United States Copyright Act, without the prior written permission of the publisher.

For product information and technology assistance, contact us at
Professional & Career Group Customer Support, 1-800-648-7450

For permission to use material from this text or product, submit all requests
online at **cengage.com/permissions**
Further permissions questions can be e-mailed to
permissionrequest@cengage.com

Library of Congress Control Number: 2008928872

ISBN-13: 978-1-4180-5078-8

ISBN-10: 1-4180-5078-4

Delmar
5 Maxwell Drive
Clifton Park, NY 12065-2919
USA

Cengage Learning products are represented in Canada by Nelson Education, Ltd.

For your lifelong learning solutions, visit **delmar.cengage.com**

Visit our corporate website at **cengage.com**

Notice to the Reader

Publisher does not warrant or guarantee any of the products described herein or perform any independent analysis in connection with any of the product information contained herein. Publisher does not assume, and expressly disclaims, any obligation to obtain and include information other than that provided to it by the manufacturer. The reader is expressly warned to consider and adopt all safety precautions that might be indicated by the activities described herein and to avoid all potential hazards. By following the instructions contained herein, the reader willingly assumes all risks in connection with such instructions. The publisher makes no representations or warranties of any kind, including but not limited to, the warranties of fitness for particular purpose or merchantability, nor are any such representations implied with respect to the material set forth herein, and the publisher takes no responsibility with respect to such material. The publisher shall not be liable for any special, consequential, or exemplary damages resulting, in whole or part, from the readers' use of, or reliance upon, this material.

Printed in United States of America
1 2 3 4 5 XX 10 09 08

MILADY'S AESTHETICIAN SERIES

A Comprehensive Guide to Equipment

Dedication

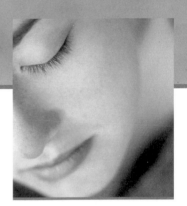

This book is dedicated to in loving memory to Erika Miller, the first person to support and believe in me; and to Paula Dean whose teaching was invaluable, and to Joyce Robinson, who first brought me information that started me on this path. Without my best friend, my husband, this would not be possible, and without the support and encouragement of my family through the hard times, I would not have been able to do this; and to my brother, I kept the faith.

v

Contents

■ **Chapter 5**

55 Skin Analysis Equipment: Woods Lamp and Skin Scanner

Preface

■ WHY THIS BOOK WAS WRITTEN

Working in the esthetics field has been a true pleasure for me. I love this profession, and it is a large part of who I am. Throughout my experience of owning a day spa and working as an esthetician, esthetics educator, and product representative, I have come across some very disturbing trends in this industry. It looks like we are one of those professions still open to the "snake oil salesman." So to help all estheticians, spa owners, and others in the esthetics profession make smart, independent decisions, I wrote this book.

It was important for me to get the most up-to-date scientific information on all of the esthetic equipment currently available to estheticians. I found that task more difficult than I ever imagined. Much of the technology is proprietary to certain manufacturers, and some did not want to disclose information. Based on that initial roadblock, I went back to basics, looking at the science behind the technology and how skin physiology works. Much of the equipment we use is proven in our clinics and treatment rooms to have a benefit, but has no independent scientific studies to prove it works on everyone. It is important for this book to be an objective and unbiased look at what equipment the esthetician can use. Some may not agree with everything they find here, and I encourage them to communicate their point of view backed up by research we can use.

There are new machines being released to our industry every day. New state laws are being implemented on the use of these machines and are impacting the esthetics profession. I have tried to give as much technical knowledge as possible, and many of these new machines will not be included in this review. I hope the basic guidelines will help you determine what to purchase. Always keep in mind, however, that estheticians' best tools are their hands. We are the experts on maintaining healthy skin, and the work we do can have an impact on clients physically, emotionally, mentally, and sometimes even spiritually. Never forget how important you are.

■ HOW TO USE THIS BOOK

This book is divided into seven sections. Section 1 will give you a general overview of why esthetic equipment is important, how to decide what equipment to purchase, good business practices, general guidelines, and rules. You will find a helpful Appendix that outlines the rules of each state. Please note that many of the states with no machine scope of practice have either no regulation at all or only recently implemented a scope of practice. You also will find included information on what machines work with different skin conditions and types.

Section 2 gives you an overview of the treatment room basics. These include the magnifying lamp, skin analysis equipment, treatment beds and chairs, wax heaters, and the steamer.

Section 3 covers optional equipment that is nice to have but generally is not mandatory for a practice. This section includes the hot cabinet, brush machine, UV sanitizer, vacuum spray machine, Lucas spray, and infrared heat lamp.

Section 4 talks about electrotherapy equipment that has been used for many years in the esthetic industry and can really make a difference. Electrotherapy is one of the most misunderstood areas, so we start with a brief introduction to electricity, to which all of us were introduced in our primary education. The equipment covered in this section is high-frequency, galvanic current, microcurrent, and electrical desiccation.

Section 5 covers advanced technological equipment. This is where the need for more scientific clarity is needed. Some of the equipment is very promising, such as microdermabrasion; other equipment, such as oxygen therapy, cannot be scientifically proven to function as claimed. Ultrasound is also included in this chapter; it is one of the most controversial pieces of equipment.

Section 6 gives you a general idea of the medical machines that are being used today. Whether you are in a medical office or practicing in a spa, you must have an idea of what procedures your clients may be receiving. If you are working in a medical spa or clinic, it is important for each manufacturer to train you specifically. This section will give you a general overview.

Section 7 introduces you to the machines used for body work. This section includes basic information that allows you to start your decision-making process as well as perform some basic treatments.

Throughout the chapters' you will also find a section to record information about your specific piece of equipment and the treatment protocols you use. This will prove helpful in the treatment room and will allow quick access to your information.

I hope you will find the information in this book informative. Remember: technology changes all the time, and science is continually moving forward. Learn the basics, and continually improve yourself with advanced education, and you will be a great success.

About the Author

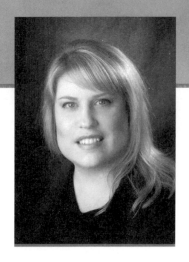

Susanne Schmaling is a licensed esthetician, nail technician, licensed esthetic instructor. and CEO of the Pacific Institute of Esthetics, based in Northwest Oregon. She currently teaches advanced cosmetology seminars for teachers, cosmetologists, massage therapists, and business owners. Her career includes extensive experience in esthetics, spa body therapies, makeup, and nail technology. She also created and operated an award-winning day spa for several years. She has presented seminars at various conferences including the International Esthetics, Cosmetics, and Spa Conference in Las Vegas.

Acknowledgements

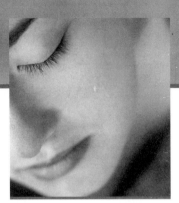

The author would like to thank Milady, a part of Cengage Learning, for the opportunity to write this book. She would also like to thank Martine Edwards and Anne Orgren for their help, along with the following people:

Danielle Tsolkis at Silhouet-Tone LTD, Joseph Bambach at Dermawave, Shannon Britt at Ageless Aesthetics, Pat Lam at Skin Care Consultants, Franck Lutz at Equipro Beauty Equipment, Peter Lebovitz at Canfield Scientific, Alan Bennett at The FDA, Moritex USA, Renee Harvey R.N., and all of the manufacturers that allowed us to use their photos.

Photo Credits

Chapter 1:

Figure 1-1: Image copyright Galina Barskaya, 2008. Used under license from Shutterstock.com. Figure 1-2: Image copyright Zsolt Nyulaszi, 2008. Used under license from Shutterstock.com. Figure 1-3: Image copyright Frank Herzog, 2008. Used under license from Shutterstock.com. Figure 1-5: From Milady's Aesthetician Series: Advanced Face and Body Treatments for the Spa, 1st edition by Hill. 2008. Reprinted with permission of Delmar Learning, a division of Cengage Learning: www.cengagerights.com. Fax 800 730-2215. Figure 1-7: From Milady's Aesthetician Series: Peels and Peeling Agents, 1st edition by Hill. 2006. Reprinted with permission of Delmar Learning, a division of Cengage Learning: www.cengagerights.com. Fax 800 730-2215. Figure 1-8: From Milady's Standard Comprehensive Training for Estheticians, 1st edition, by Milady/Hinds/Miller/Lees. 2003. Reprinted with permission of Delmar Learning, a division of Cengage Learning: http://www.cengagerights.com. Fax 800 730-2215. Figure 1-11: Image copyright Elena Ray, 2008. Used under license from Shutterstock.com. Figure 1-12: Image copyright Absolut, 2008. Used under license from Shutterstock.com.

Chapter 2:

Figures 2-1, 2-7, and 2-9: From Milady's Standard, Fundamentals for Esthetician, 9th edition by Gerson. 2004. Reprinted with permission of Delmar Learning, a division of Cengage Learning: www.cengagerights.com. Fax 800 730-2215. Figure 2-2: Image copyright DW Photos, 2008. Used under license from Shutterstock.com. Figure 2-3: Image copyright Alexander Orlov, 2008. Used under license from Shutterstock.com. Figures 2-4 and 2-5: Image copyright Jerko Grubisic, 2008. Used under license from Shutterstock.com.

Chapter 3:

Figure 3-1: Image copyright Rena Schild, 2008. Used under license from Shutterstock.com. Figure 3-2: Image copyright Rena Jansa, 2008. Used under license from Shutterstock.com. Figure 3-3: permission granted by Underwriters Laboratories. Figure 3-4: http://ec.europa.eu/comm/enterprise, European Communities, 1995-2008. Figure 3-5: Image copyright Mircea Bezergheanu, 2008. Used under license from Shutterstock.com. Figures 3-6 and 3-7: Image copyright Leah-Anne Thompson, 2008. Used under license from Shutterstock.com.

Chapter 4:

Figures 4-1 and 4-7a through 4-7g: From Milady's Standard, Fundamentals for Esthetician, 9th edition by Gerson. 2004. Reprinted with permission of Delmar Learning, a division of Cengage Learning: www.cengagerights.com. Fax 800 730-2215. Figures 4-2 and 4-5: Courtesy of Silhouet-Tone Ltd. Figure 4-3: From Milady's Standard Comprehensive Training for Estheticians, 1st edition, by Milady/Hinds/Miller/Lees. 2003. Reprinted with permission of Delmar Learning, a division of Cengage Learning: http://www.cengagerights.com. Fax 800 730-2215.

Chapter 5:

Figure 5-1: Courtesy of Silhouet-Tone Ltd. Figures 5-2 and 5-8: From Milady's Standard Comprehensive Training for Estheticians, 1st edition, by Milady/Hinds/Miller/Lees. 2003. Reprinted with permission of Delmar Learning, a division of Cengage Learning: http://www.cengagerights.com. Fax 800 730-2215. Figure 5-3: Courtesy of Equipro. Figures 5-4 and 5-6: Illustrated based on source photographs from Moritex USA, Inc. Figure 5-5: Moritex USA, Inc. 2007. Figure 5-7: Photograph Courtesy of Canfield Imaging Systems.

Chapter 6:

Figures 6-1, 6-3, and 6-5: Courtesy of Silhouet-Tone Ltd. Figures 6-2, 6-4, 6-6, and 6-7: Courtesy of Equipro. Figures 6-9a through 6-9k: From Milady's Standard Comprehensive Training for Estheticians, 1st edition, by Milady/Hinds/Miller/Lees. 2003. Reprinted with permission of Delmar Learning, a division of Cengage Learning: http://www.cengagerights.com. Fax 800 730-2215.

Chapter 7:
Figure 7-1: Courtesy of Silhouet-Tone Ltd. Figures 7-2, 7-4, and 7-5: Courtesy of Ellisons. Figure 7-3: Courtesy of Ellisons, PhD Safewax. Figures 7-6a through 7-6m: Courtesy of Rob Werfel, photographer. Figure 7-7: From Milady's Aesthetician Series: Advanced Hair Removal, 1st edition by Hill. 2007. Reprinted with permission of Delmar Learning, a division of Cengage Learning: www.cengagerights.com. Fax 800 730-2215.

Chapter 8:
Figure 8-2: Courtesy of Silhouet-Tone Ltd. Figures 8-3 and 8-4a through Figure 8-4k: From Milady's Standard Comprehensive Training for Estheticians, 1st edition, by Milady/Hinds/Miller/Lees. 2003. Reprinted with permission of Delmar Learning, a division of Cengage Learning: http://www.cengagerights.com. Fax 800 730-2215.

Chapter 9:
Figure 9-1: Courtesy of Equipro. Figure 9-2: From Milady's Standard Comprehensive Training for Estheticians, 1st edition, by Milady/Hinds/Miller/Lees. 2003. Reprinted with permission of Delmar Learning, a division of Cengage Learning: http://www.cengagerights.com. Fax 800 730-2215. Figures 9-3a through 9-3d: Courtesy of Rob Werfel, photographer.

Chapter 10:
Figure 10-1: Courtesy of Silhouet-Tone Ltd. Figure 10-2: Courtesy of Pacific Bioscience Laboratories. Figure 10-6: From Milady's Standard Comprehensive Training for Estheticians, 1st edition, by Milady/Hinds/Miller/Lees. 2003. Reprinted with permission of Delmar Learning, a division of Cengage Learning: http://www.cengagerights.com. Fax 800 730-2215.

Chapter 11:
Figures 11-1 and 11-3: Image copyright Tischenko Irina, 2008. Used under license from Shutterstock.com. Figures 11-2 and 11-10: From Skin Care, Beyond the Basics, 3rd edition by Lees. 2007. Reprinted with permission of Delmar Learning, a division of Cengage Learning: www.cengagerights.com. Fax 800 730-2215. Figures 11-4 and 11-5: Image copyright Sebastian Kaulitzki, 2008. Used under license from Shutterstock.com. Figure 11-7: Image copyright Muriel Lasure, 2008. Used under license from Shutterstock.com. Figure 11-9: Used under license from Shutterstock.com. Figure 11-11: Image copyright Angelo Gilardelli, 2008. Used under license from Shutterstock.com. Figures 11-12, 11-13, and 11-14: Courtesy of Equipro. Figure 11-6: Image copyright Mariusz Szachowski, 2008. Used under license from Shutterstock.com. Figure 11-15: Ultronics UL-12 Ultrasonic Cleaning System.

Chapter 12:

Figure 12-1: Courtesy of Silhouet-Tone Ltd. Figures 12-2, 12-3, and 12-4: Oxford Designers & Illustrators. Figure 12-5: From Professional Beauty Therapy: The Official Guide to Level 3, Third Edition, by Nordmann. 2007. Reprinted with permission of Cengage Learning. Figures 12-7 and 12-8: From Milady's Standard, Fundamentals for Esthetician, 9th edition by Gerson. 2004. Reprinted with permission of Delmar Learning, a division of Cengage Learning: www.cengagerights.com. Fax 800 730-2215.
Chapter 13:
Figure 13-1: Courtesy of Equipro. Figures 13-5a through 13-5g: Courtesy of Rob Werfel, photographer.
Chapter 14:
Figure 14-1: Courtesy of Ellisons.
Chapter 15:
Figures 15-1 and 15-3: From Milady's Standard, Fundamentals for Esthetician, 9th edition by Gerson. 2004. Reprinted with permission of Delmar Learning, a division of Cengage Learning: www.cengagerights.com. Fax 800 730-2215. Figures 15-2, and 15-4: Courtesy of Equipro.
Chapter 16:
Figures 16-1 and 16-3: Courtesy of Amber Products. Figures 16-2, 16-4, and 16-5: From Milady's Aesthetician Series: Advanced Face and Body Treatments for the Spa, 1st edition by Hill. 2008. Reprinted with permission of Delmar Learning, a division of Cengage Learning: www.cengagerights.com. Fax 800 730-2215. Figures 16-8, 16-9, 16-10, 16-11, 16-12, and 16-13: From Milady's Standard, Fundamentals for Esthetician, 9th edition by Gerson. 2004. Reprinted with permission of Delmar Learning, a division of Cengage Learning: www.cengagerights.com. Fax 800 730-2215.
Chapter 17:
Figures 17-1, 17-2, 17-6, 17-7, and 17-11: From Milady's Standard, Fundamentals for Esthetician, 9th edition by Gerson. 2004. Reprinted with permission of Delmar Learning, a division of Cengage Learning: www.cengagerights.com. Fax 800 730-2215. Figures 17-3, 17-4, and 17-9: From Milady's Standard Comprehensive Training for Estheticians, 1st edition, by Milady/Hinds/Miller/Lees. 2003. Reprinted with permission of Delmar Learning, a division of Cengage Learning: http://www.cengagerights.com. Fax 800 730-2215. Figure 17-12: Image copyright Tatiana Popova, 2008. Used under license from Shutterstock.com. Figure 17-13: Image copyright David Asch, 2008. Used under license from Shutterstock.com.
Chapter 18:
Figure 18-1: Courtesy of Silhouet-Tone Ltd. Figures 18-2 and 18-6: From Milady's Standard Comprehensive Training for Estheticians, 1st

edition, by Milady/Hinds/Miller/Lees. 2003. Reprinted with permission of Delmar Learning, a division of Cengage Learning: http://www.cengagerights.com. Fax 800 730-2215. Figures 18-3 and 18-4: Oxford Designers & Illustrators. Figure 18-5: SORISA.CO.UK. Figures 18-15, 18-16, 18-17, 18-18, 18-19, and 18-20: Courtesy of Rob Werfel, photographer.

Chapter 19:

Figures 19-1 and 19-7: Courtesy of Silhouet-Tone Ltd. Figure 19-2: SORISA.CO.UK. Figure 19-3: From Milady's Standard Comprehensive Training for Estheticians, 1st edition, by Milady/Hinds/Miller/Lees. 2003. Reprinted with permission of Delmar Learning, a division of Cengage Learning: http://www.cengagerights.com. Fax 800 730-2215. Figures 19-4 and 19-5: From Milady's Standard, Fundamentals for Esthetician, 9th edition by Gerson. 2004. Reprinted with permission of Delmar Learning, a division of Cengage Learning: www.cengagerights.com. Fax 800 730-2215. Figures 19-10, 19-11, 19-12, 19-13, 19-14, 19-16, and 19-17: Courtesy of Rob Werfel, photographer. Figures 19-15, 19-18, and 19-19: Oxford Designers & Illustrators.

Chapter 20:

Figures 20-1 and 20-19: Courtesy of Ageless Aesthetics. Figures 20-2 and 20-5: Image copyright Sebastian Kaulitzki, 2008. Used under license from Shutterstock.com. Figures 20-3 and 20-4: From Milady's Standard Comprehensive Training for Estheticians, 1st edition, by Milady/Hinds/Miller/Lees. 2003. Reprinted with permission of Delmar Learning, a division of Cengage Learning: http://www.cengagerights.com. Fax 800 730-2215. Figures 20-6 and 20-7: Courtesy of Arasys Perfector, LLC. Figure 20-8: Courtesy of Bio-Therapeutic, Inc. Figure 20-10: Image copyright Wheatley, 2008. Used under license from Shutterstock.com. Figure 20-11: Image copyright Max Blain, 2008. Used under license from Shutterstock.com. Figure 20-12: Image copyright Benjamin Howell, 2008. Used under license from Shutterstock.com. Figure 20-13: Image copyright Jo Ann Snover, 2008. Used under license from Shutterstock.com. Figure 20-14: Image copyright Leah-Anne Thompson, 2008. Used under license from Shutterstock.com. Figures 20-16 and 20-17: Courtesy of Silhouet-Tone Ltd. Figure 20-15: Image copyright Ovidiu Iordachi, 2008. Used under license from Shutterstock.com.

Chapter 21:

Figures 21-1 and 21-2: Courtesy of Bio-Therapeutic, Inc.

Chapter 22:

Figure 22-1: Image copyright Terekhov Igor, 2008. Used under license from Shutterstock.com. Figure 22-3: Image copyright Kevin Renes, 2008. Used under license from Shutterstock.com. Figures 22-6 and 22-7: From Milady's Standard, Fundamentals for Esthetician, 9th edition by

Gerson. 2004. Reprinted with permission of Delmar Learning, a division of Cengage Learning: www.cengagerights.com. Fax 800 730-2215. Figure 22-8: Image copyright ArturKo, 2008. Used under license from Shutterstock.com.

Chapter 23:

Figures 23-1 and 23-2: Courtesy of Dermawave. Figure 23-4: Illustrated based on source figure from Silhouet-Tone Ltd.

Chapter 24:

Figure 24-1: Courtesy of Silhouet-Tone Ltd. Figure 24-3: From Milady's Aesthetician Series: Advanced Face and Body Treatments for the Spa, 1st edition by Hill. 2008. Reprinted with permission of Delmar Learning, a division of Cengage Learning: www.cengagerights.com. Fax 800 730-2215.

Chapter 25:

Figure 25-1: Courtesy of Aesthetic Solutions. Figures 25-2 and 25-3: Courtesy of Altair Instruments. Figures 25-5 and 25-14: From Hill. Milady's Aesthetician Series: Microdermabrasion, 1E. 2006 Delmar Learning, a part of Cengage Learning, Inc. Reproduced by permission. www.cengage.com/permissions.

Chapter 26:

Figures 26-1 and 26-4a through 26-4c: Printed with kind permission by Skin Care Consultants. www.lamskin.com. Figure 26-2: Courtesy of Silhouet-Tone Ltd. Figure 26-3: Image copyright Dario Sabljak, 2008. Used under license from Shutterstock.com.

Chapter 27:

Figure 27-1: Image copyright Falk Kienas, 2008. Used under license from Shutterstock.com. Figures 27-3, 27-7, and 27-8: From Milady's Aesthetician Series: Advanced Hair Removal, 1st edition by Hill. 2007. Reprinted with permission of Delmar Learning, a division of Cengage Learning: www.cengagerights.com. Fax 800 730-2215. Figure 27-6: Image copyright Dragan Trifunovic, 2008. Used under license from Shutterstock.com. Figure 27-10: Image copyright Terekhov Igor, 2008. Used under license from Shutterstock.com.

Chapter 28:

Figure 28-1: Image copyright James Steidl, 2008. Used under license from Shutterstock.com. Figure 28-2: From Professional Beauty Therapy: The Official Guide to Level 3, Third Edition, by Nordmann. 2007. Reprinted with permission of Cengage Learning. Figures 28-3, 28-5, 28-6, and 28-9: Oxford Designers & Illustrators. Figure 28-7: Courtesy of Silhouet-Tone Ltd. Figure 28-4: Image copyright Dmitriy Shironosov, 2008. Used under license from Shutterstock.com. Figure 28-8: Courtesy of Bio-Therapeutic, Inc.

The Importance of
Esthetic Equipment

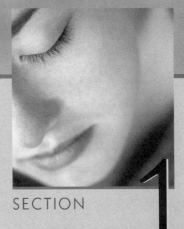

SECTION

1

The Importance of Esthetic Equipment

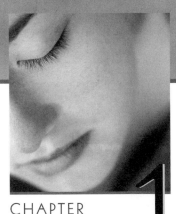

Many estheticians, spa owners, and other spa professionals wonder if esthetic equipment is really that important. The answer depends on many factors. Certain product manufacturers will tell you equipment is not important, but machine manufacturers will tell you it is. The answer lies somewhere in between. Estheticians cannot perform the best skin treatment without at least some equipment. For example, clients definitely need beds to lie on, and during a treatment, you must have warm towels to use. Of course the esthetician's greatest tool is his or her hands. Massage is the one of the reasons clients visit estheticians on a regular basis, and massage has been used for centuries to relieve pain and increase general well-being. All estheticians should strive for advanced education in massage.

Esthetic machines increase the level of effectiveness of many treatments, and so they have a long and varied history in the beauty industry. Salons as early as the 1930s were using equipment to improve the appearance of the skin.

■ HOW TO DECIDE WHAT MACHINE TO USE

Making a decision about what machines to use can be stressful and confusing. No one can use every **modality** on the market, so how do you choose? There are many factors to consider. The first step is to identify who your clients are.

The second step involves asking the right questions.

How Old Are Your Clients?

If you have a clientele of baby boomers wanting to fight skin aging, you will want to look at **microcurrent, Intense Pulsed Light (IPL), Light Emitting Diode (LED),** and **microdermabrasion** technology.

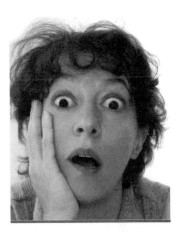

Figure 1-1 Buying equipment can be a challenging experience.

A younger clientele may only require a microdermabrasion machine and the most basic equipment, such as a steamer and wax pots.

What Is Their Household Income?

This will determine how much clients are willing to spend on your treatments. If your IPL machine costs $150 to $300 a treatment, can your market handle it? It is a large monthly lease to be locked into. Incomes of $50,000 or less may not have the disposable income to get multiple treatments. Higher income levels will, but they also can take advantage of esthetic medicine services.

What Are Their Buying Habits?

Are your clients infrequent spa visitors, or are they committed to multiple sessions to correct their skin? Will they follow a prescribed at-home protocol? If they really just want to be pampered, you may want to invest in some basic equipment, such as a steamer, **galvanic current,** magnifying lamp, and brush machine.

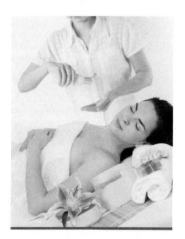

Figure 1-2 A holistic healing philosophy uses touch and natural products as the primary focus.

DECIDE YOUR PHILOSOPHY ON SKIN CARE

Holistic/Alternative Healing: Massage and stress reduction is the focus. Skin care products are **pH** balanced and **essential oil,** herbal, or **marine based.** The goal is to balance the skin with an emphasis on internal nutritional support and lifestyle education. Alternative therapies such as **ayurveda, aromatherapy, acupressure,** and **shiatsu** are also used.

Clinical care: Immediate-results driven, skin care products are focused on high levels of active cosmetic ingredients with advanced technology. The goal is to correct skin conditions or to provide preoperative and postoperative skin care. The esthetician may work in a medical setting or medical spa.

After you decide what skin care philosophy to focus on, you can determine which machines will fit with your intended treatment modality. If you are trying to balance holistic with clinical care, plan your equipment purchases accordingly. For example, if the majority of your clientele are 50 and up and concerned with aging, but they do not want plastic surgery, your investment could be in microdermabrasion, microcurrent, and LED technology. We list some some general guidelines to follow. Of course, there is no rule that states that you must purchase all of these machines; it is up to you to look at your budget and skill level.

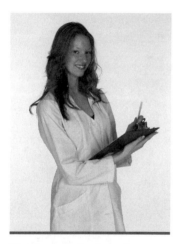

Figure 1-3 A clinical esthetician.

Holistic and Alternative Healing Philosophy

If you would like to use the holistic healing philosophy, you will need a steamer, **loupe** (magnifying lamp), hot cabinet, and treatment table.

To expand your practice you may want to purchase Lucas spray, a Woods lamp, UV sterilizer, paraffin heater, and rotary brush machine.

Clinical Care Philosophy

If you choose the clinical care philosophy you will need a steamer, loupe, Woods lamp, galvanic current, high frequency, rotary brush, vacuum/spray, hot cabinet, UV sterilizer, treatment table, and microdermabrasion. To expand your practice, an LED light system, microcurrent toning, IPL, and advanced skin analysis equipment may be useful.

Balancing Both Philosophies

If you would like to use both philosophies, it is very important to really know who you are treating. It is possible to try to do too much. Most clients have no idea what machines we use; they just want results.

Once you have chosen the philosophy of your skin care practice, you will decide which machines to start with. It is always a good idea to start small and build your business, then increase what you are using.

■ FIND YOUR EQUIPMENT VENDOR

As important as creating a plan of how you would like your practice to look is which manufacturer to choose. This is not a decision to be made quickly. Do not buy just because of the price of the equipment; it can be tempting, but ultimately will cause you problems in the long run.

Questions to Ask the Vendor

There are many important questions to ask before committing to a purchase. Some of these are outlined below.

How long have you been in business?

Many companies have not been in business more than five years. Does this mean you should not buy from them? Absolutely not, but it is important to feel comfortable with them and to be aware that something may happen to the business in the future. This can also true for businesses

TIP If you are working in a medical setting, you will be under a physician's supervision and generally will use a laser modality for hair removal and skin rejuvenation. You may also use a medical microdermabrasion machine. A traditional facial treatment is rarely used in this environment.

around for a longer period of time. Businesses with longer track records have established reputations, which should allow you to get a broad range of opinions from others who have used their products.

Are you registered with the FDA, and if so, what is the registration number?

Manufacturers of medical devices must register with the FDA, regardless of device classification. Distributors or resellers do not have to be registered, and there is no classification for cosmetic purposes only. The FDA looks at the intended use of the machine. If it will impact the function of the body, it is considered a medical device.

Do you provide education with purchase?

Every piece of equipment that you have must come with some educational material on how to use it effectively. Even a steamer has specific usage guidelines from the manufacturer. If you are purchasing any advanced equipment—such as microdermabrasion, microcurrent, LED, or ultrasound—it is a requirement in some states that a certification of training be issued. Good education on the equipment you use is very important; do not purchase without it.

Do you have a technical support department that I can easily access?

You need to have an immediate contact in case something goes wrong. It may be something simple, but it is always good to have someone who can help you right away. A sales consultant is a good contact but not always available.

Is your equipment UL, CSA, CE, or ISO listed?

Make sure your equipment has a safety certification such as a UL listing or a CSA or ISO certification. UL and CSA approval indicates that the equipment has been tested for safety. ISO and CE marking indicates that it has been manufactured per international standards and that the manufacturer is tested twice a year.

What is the warranty?

It is important to get the details of the warranty. For example, are you required to use only the manufacturer's products to make the warranty valid? This does not mean you should not purchase the equipment, but it does mean that you must get an accurate picture of what the price per use is actually going to be, because you will have to use one supplier. Is the warranty only on certain parts? Does it cover wear and tear? Most do not. Ask to read the warranty document.

*Do you have a loaner unit for use if something goes wrong
with the machine?*

It is important to have a vendor or manufacturer provide a loaner while
your machine is being repaired. Time lost when your equipment is out
for repair is money lost. With basic equipment, it is rare to find a manufacturer who will give you a loaner, so look for very well-made machines.

Do you offer payment terms?

Some companies have payment terms that require you to put a certain
amount down, usually a third, and they will allow you to make monthly
payments over a 12- to 18-month period. This is generally secured with a
monthly credit card charge. This can be helpful if you do not qualify for a
lease. You will most likely have to come up with your own financing.

What is the best price you can get me for this equipment?

Many vendors have the ability to negotiate price. They will offer
discounts at various shows. These can be from 10% to a closeout dis-
count of 40% to 50% on older model equipment. Do not be afraid to ask
and negotiate.

*Do you have clinical studies that prove your
equipment works?*

Clinical studies are very controversial (see the guidelines given in Chapter 3 on clinical studies). In general only Class II and Class III equipment
will have FDA-approved studies. Most of what you see are *before* and
after pictures. Some of the problems inherent with this approach are that
no independent group has overseen the study, and that certain variables
may not have been controlled, such as the position of the camera in the
before picture and in the *after* picture, the actual treatment performed,
the at-home protocol used, and what the client has done on their own. It
is important to show that the equipment works, especially if it is an advanced technology with a high purchase price.

What efficacy information can you provide?

Most companies will provide you with information about their claims. If
they cannot, it is wise to look at other options.

Questions for You to Analyze

In addition to the preceding questions that you ask your vendor, there
are other questions you must ask yourself. Consider the answers you get
carefully, and use these to make a decision that works for your benefit.

Is your vendor cooperative with you on the phone?

The first impression of your business is very important for your client; it is just as important for the vendor you consider purchasing from. If you call and are treated rudely or dismissed, that is a good indicator that you may not want to work with this vendor, even if their equipment is the hot buy of the moment. After all, you are going to spend thousand of dollars, so the bottom line is this: make sure you are treated with respect before they know you are going to buy, because you are entering into a long-term relationship with this vendor.

Is it hard to get a timely response from your salesperson or the manufacturer?

Do you leave messages that are not returned? Do you e-mail your contact and never get a response? Can you get your questions answered? If you cannot, look closely at working with this vendor. Customer service is very important. It is also your responsibility to respond to your contacts in a timely manner to create a professional relationship. Do not inquire about a manufacturer's product line without at least confirming that you received the information when they call.

Will they give you clinical study information?

Do they claim to have proof that their equipment works but will not provide you with the actual data? It is important that they can back up their claims and are transparent about it.

Are they making impossible claims?

A good working knowledge and understanding of the scientific practice of skin care is needed to understand whether a technology can possibly work. Topics to pursue further are cell biology, anatomy and physiology, electrical theory, chemistry, and physics. It may sounds like a lot to learn, but in this book you will find chapters on much of this, including electrical and light and sound theory, as well as a brief overview of cell biology. The suggested reading guide also includes resources for you to use.

Is your vendor or manufacturer competing in your market?

Many manufacturers in large markets are opening their own spas using their equipment as the center of the business. This is different from a training center, because they will work directly with the public. If you are in the same market, it is important to look at how this will affect your business. Many estheticians use the same equipment, but it is different when the manufacturer is using it in the same market and making thousands of dollars from you as well. If they do not compete in your market, their practical experience with the equipment may add another layer of efficacy; you can test to verify the equipment works, and you can take advantage of in-depth training.

Will they allow you to try the equipment for a couple of days, or will they give a demonstration?

It is very important to see the equipment, feel the quality, see the actual treatment being done, and be able to use the equipment yourself. Many vendors will not allow you to keep the equipment to try due to liability issues, but their representative should be able to at least show you the equipment. If it is basic equipment you are looking for, such as steamers or brush machines, the best way to look at the quality of the machine is at an esthetics show.

What is the vendor's reputation in the industry?

This is very important. Not everyone will have the same opinion, but by networking with other professionals, you will get a feel for the overall impression that the company gives you.

Do you know anyone using their equipment?

It is a great resource to know others who have used or are currently using the equipment that you are looking to buy. Some companies will also supply a list of people you can contact who are currently using the equipment.

▪ SKIN ANALYSIS: THE RIGHT MACHINE FOR EACH SKIN

With any esthetic treatment, knowing your clients' skin is mandatory. Many books have been written on different systems and techniques, so this is where your advanced training is very important: learn skin biology, cosmetic chemistry, and diseases and disorders. In resources listed at the end of the book, you will see a list of educational material that can help you.

In esthetics school, most professionals were taught the four basic skin types related to **sebaceous secretions.** Now a fifth type, sensitive skin, has been added. Estheticians also must have knowledge of the **Rubin system,** the **Glogau classification of aging,** and **Fitzpatrick skin typing,** especially when working with physicians. The medical field approaches skin typing in a different manner, so you can see where the esthetician can be confused. Here is a relatively simple system that will incorporate the esthetic and medical typing that the esthetician must be familiar with.

Step 1: Determine Skin Type

This is important for many reasons. Without understanding how much sebaceous activity the skin has, you are likely to use a product that will not give you an optimal outcome. For example, using an emollient antiaging product on an oily skin is not the best choice. Determining the skin type is also the step that will make use of the magnifying lamp and Woods lamp.

The four skin types you will be looking at are normal, dry, combination, and oily. Each one must be approached differently.

Normal Skin

This is a rare skin type, and usually only a young client will have it.
Look and feel:

- This type is a skin that is in perfect balance.
- Pores are not large, and there will be normal sebaceous secretions seen under a Woods lamp. The key is that this skin is *balanced*.
- Texture is smooth and the skin has a good tone.
- There will be no special conditions associated with this skin type.
- Under a Woods lamp, skin will show an even blue florescence.

Ask:

- After cleansing, does your skin feel tight and dry? (The answer should be no.)

Dry Skin

Another term for *dry* is **alipidic,** or skin that has little or no sebaceous secretions.
Look and feel:

- Pores are fine, almost invisible.
- Texture is smooth and fine.
- Under a Woods lamp, skin will show a white florescence.

Ask:

- After cleansing, does your face feel uncomfortable? (The answer will be yes.)
- Do you find that a very emollient cream absorbs quickly? (The answer will be yes.)
- Do you feel like you can never get enough moisture? (Generally, the answer will be yes.)

Combination Skin

This is the most common type of skin, and it may have additional conditions that will determine which machine and products to use.

Look and feel:

- Pore size can range from small to large, but only through the center panel of the face, in what is known as the *T-Zone*.
- Texture can be rough in some areas and smooth in others.
- There will be conditions associated with this skin type.
- Under a Woods lamp, the skin will show small orange dots where sebum is being produced; you will also see areas of white florescence, which indicate the dry areas.

Ask:

- Do you generally feel tightness and dryness in some areas of the face and oiliness in others?

Oily Skin

This skin type usually has many conditions associated with it.

Look and feel:

- Pore size is large and visible throughout the face.
- Texture can be like an orange peel: rough and thick.
- Tone will have a shine with obvious oil.
- There are no areas of dryness, and the skin may be dehydrated.
- Under a Woods lamp, you will see small orange dots throughout the face.

Ask:

- Do you feel that you need to wash your face during the day?

Step 2: Determine Fitzpatrick Skin Type

Fitzpatrick skin types are used to determine a client's potential reaction to an advanced clinical treatment by estimating that client's genetic background and reaction to **ultraviolet (UV)** exposure. Skin typing is a useful tool to determine a client's tolerance and potential reaction to a facial treatment, especially skin resurfacing. It is also a guideline to recognizing a more sensitive skin, healing ability, and **keloid** scarring. Manufacturers also use this typing system when developing laser, IPL, and some LED machines. They calibrate programs in the machine to each different skin type. See Figure 1-4 for the Fitzpatrick skin type chart.

TIP As our population grows and merges, genetic skin typing is becoming increasingly difficult. It is more important to determine a client's reaction to UV sun exposure. Even if they do not tan or have current exposure, ask about childhood UV exposure and current reactions to any chemical or manual peels, cosmetic treatments, and any environmental irritants that they may have been exposed to.

Skin Type	UV Exposure	Characteristics	Possible Reactions
Skin Type I	Always burns, never tans; usually burns within 10-15 minutes	White, very fair, red or blond hair, blue eyes, freckles likely	Sensitivity to topical products, the environment, heat, cold, and wind
Skin Type II	Burns easily, tans minimally; usually burns within 30-40 minutes	Fair-skinned, blue, green, or hazel eyes, blond, dishwater blond, or red hair	Rarely develop post-inflammatory pigmentation, least defense against UV damage
Skin Type III	Sometimes burns, gradually tans; usually burns within 60-70 minutes	Cream-white, fair with any eye or hair color, very common coloring	
Skin Type IV	Rarely burns, gradually tans	Brown skin, brown eyes, Mediterranean, southern European, Hispanic	More susceptible to pigmentation problems and keloid scarring, greater defense against environmental & UV damage
Skin Type V	Tans	Dark brown skin, brown-black hair, brown eyes, Asian, Indian, some Africans	
Skin Type VI	Tans well	Black skin, black hair, brown-black eyes, Africans	

Figure 1-4 Fitzpatrick skin types and possible reactions.

Step 3: Determine Skin Conditions

Skin conditions are any disorders of the skin that will cause a client to seek professional help. Most of the treatments that we will use are focused on correction of the skin. In this list is terminology that we use in esthetics, and this terminology is mixed with medical terminology. Because we operate in both worlds, it is important to learn how to clinically document conditions as well as how to translate what these mean to the client. Some of the conditions listed are not considered conditions by the medical community; these are conditions estheticians primarily treat. You will use your magnifying loupe or your Woods lamp, but more advanced tools can be used as well. See Chapter 6 for more details, because there are several types of conditions to consider.

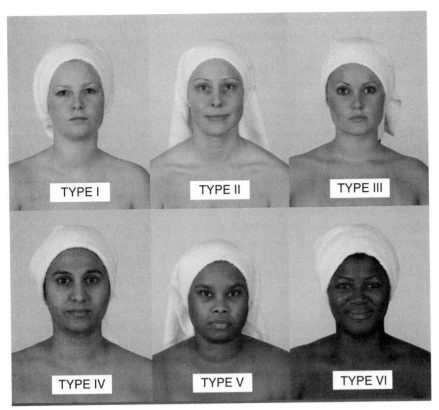

Figure 1-5 Fitzpatrick skin type examples.

Vascular Conditions

Vascular conditions are related to the **microcirculation** within the skin. They appear as redness or inflammation in various areas. Clients will visibly notice this and comment on it. These conditions include the following:

- **Telangiectasia:** cuperose, broken capillaries
- **Diffuse redness:** may indicate sensitive skin
- **Erythema:** abnormal redness of the skin due to capillary congestion
- **Rosacea, Stages I, II, III:** a chronic inflammatory disorder that affects the nose, forehead, and cheeks; it is characterized by congestion, flushing, telangiectasia, and marked nodular swelling of the tissues

Lipid System Conditions

These conditions are related to the amount of sebum secretion in the skin. Every skin type you see may have some of these common conditions, and clients are particularly sensitive to them due to the impact on their appearance; they want them corrected quickly.

TIP Rosacea is a medical disorder that requires the attention of a dermatologist. Do not work outside the esthetic **scope of practice** and try to treat this disorder.

TIP Acne grades III and IV should be treated by a dermatologist.

- **Comedones** (open and closed)
- **Acne** (**papules** and **pustules**) grades I, II, III, IV
- **Seborrhea**
- **Folliculitis** (ingrown hairs)
- **Milia** (whiteheads) and **cysts**
- **Scarred ostia** (scarred follicles)
- **Sebaceous hyperplasia**

Pigmentation Conditions

These conditions are related to the production of melanin in the skin. They can be caused by UV damage or influenced by hormones. Pigmentation conditions are complicated to treat.

- **Hyperpigmentation**
- **Hypopigmentation**
- **Solar Lentigines** (freckles)
- **Melasma** (pregnancy mask)
- **Postinflammatory pigmentation**

Aging Conditions

Aging conditions are what many advanced machines are targeted to correct, and they represent the largest group in the population at this time. The simplest system to use is the Rubin system, which will be referred to in this section.

- **Rubin classification system**
- **Glogau classification of aging**
- **Rhytids** (wrinkles)
- **Elastosis** (loss of elasticity)

Level	Characteristics	Explanations	Machines indicated for best use
Level One—minor aging	Pigmentation and rough, dull texture, thicker stratum corneum, few if any wrinkles	Minor sun damage	Microdermabrasion, micro-current, galvanic current, high frequency
Level Two—moderate aging	Irregular skin color, thick skin, pigmentation changes, actinic keratosis	Wrinkles found around eyes, naso-labial folds deepen, crinkling of skin, loss of elasticity	LED, microdermabrasion, microcurrrent
Level Three—severe aging	Thick leathery appearance, yellow tint and pebbly texture, open comedones	Wrinkled at rest, loss of elasticity	Lasers, IPL, LED, microdermabrasion

Figure 1-6 The Rubin chart of aging and equipment to use.

Damage	Description	Characteristics
Level One—mild	"No wrinkles"	Early photoaging • Mild pigmentary changes • No keratoses • Minimal wrinkles Patient age: 20s or 30s • Minimal or no makeup • Minimal acne scars
Level Two—moderate	"Wrinkles in motion"	Early to moderate photoaging • Early senile Lentigines are visible • Keratoses palpable but not visible • Parallel smile lines beginning to appear Patient age: 30s-40s • Some foundation usually worn • Mild acne scarring
Level Three—advanced	"Wrinkles at rest"	Advanced photoaging • Obvious dyschromia, telangiectasia • Visible keratoses • Wrinkles present even when not moving Patient age: 50s or older • Heavier foundation always worn • Acne scarring present that makeup does not always cover
Level Four—severe	"Only wrinkles"	Severe photoaging • Yellow/gray skin color • Prior skin malignancies • Wrinkles throughout; no normal skin Patient age: 60s-70s • Makeup cannot be worn because it cakes and cracks • Severe acne scarring

Figure 1-7 Glogau classification.

Keratinization Conditions

This relates to skin that has problems with **desquamation,** or dead cell turnover, of the **stratum corneum.**

- **Hyperkeratosis:** increased roughness in skin, referred to as *congested skin*

Skin Hydration Conditions

- **Dehydration:** appears white under a Woods lamp with a parchment-paper look
- **Hyperhydrosis:** overhydrated skin

Skin Sensitivity

- **Tactile sensitivity:** The client feels uncomfortable when certain fabrics or pressures are used on the skin. Towels can even feel uncomfortable.
- **Cosmetic sensitivity:** The client cannot tolerate certain cosmetics, usually those that contain fragrances and preservatives.
- **Environmental sensitivity:** The skin is irritated easily by sun and wind exposure.

	Allergies	Irritants
What causes the reaction?	The rejection of a particular substance by the immune system of the body.	A localized irritation caused by a chemical that burns or overexfoliates the skin.
Who has the reaction?	Only people who have a specific allergy to a particular substance.	Any person can have an irritant reaction if enough of the substance comes in contact with the skin.
Can you have the reaction the first time the skin is exposed to a product or chemical?	No.	Yes.
Can the entire body be affected by the reaction?	Yes.	Not usually.
Does the amount of chemical exposure affect the degree of reaction?	Not necessarily. Allergies can occur from a very small amount of exposure.	Yes.
Does the reaction usually occur quickly?	No.	Yes.

Figure 1-8 Allergies vs. irritants.

Step 4: Consider Lifestyle and Health

It is important for the client to fill out an intake form, shown in Figure 1-9, prior to the skin analysis. Medications, illnesses, and lifestyle habits such as smoking must be identified. It is also significant to note

TIP HIPAA stands for the Health Insurance Portability and Accountability Act. Title II provides privacy rules that dictate how protected health information (PHI) is used. PHI relates to all aspects of client care, including payment information.

CONFIDENTIAL SKIN HEALTH SURVEY

Name: Date:

Address:

Phone (H):   (C):   E-Mail:

Birthday: ____ / ____ / ____   How did you hear about us?

Is this your first facial treatment? YES NO	Do you have acne? YES NO
What improvements would you like to see in your skin?	Are you using (or have in the past): Azelex Differin Renova Retin A Tazarac Glycolic or alphahydroxy acids at home? Microdermabrasion? Accutane? If so, when & how long?
Are you currently under a physician's care for a skin condition or other problem? YES NO	Do you experience frequent blemishes? YES NO If so how frequently?
Are you pregnant? YES NO	Do you have any allergies to food, cosmetics or drugs? Please list:
Are you taking birth control or hormone replacement therapy? YES NO	Please list current medications:
Do you wear contact lenses? YES NO	What is your current skin care program?
Do you smoke? YES NO	Cleanser:
On a scale of 1 (low) – 10 (high) what is your stress level?	Toner:
Have you had skin cancer? YES NO	Moisturizer:
Please circle if you have the following:	Sunscreen:
	Special treatments:
Asthma Heart problems High/Low Blood Pressure Herpes Sinus Problems Diabetes Epilepsy Frequent Migraines Immune Disorders Metal pins or plates Thyroid disease Pacemaker Psoriasis	Have you had any of the following within the last 6 months? Cosmetic Surgery Laser Resurfacing Chemical Peels Botox Restylane or other fillers Microdermabrasion
Have you had permanent cosmetics done? YES NO	Have you had any waxing or electrolysis in the last week? YES NO

I understand that the services offered are not a substitute for medical care, and any information provided will be kept confidential.

SPA Policies: We require a 24 hour cancellation notice. We do not give cash refunds.	 _____ Client Signature

---

Figure 1-9 Confidential Client Intake Form.

that although we are not considered a medical profession, it is wise to comply with **HIPAA** rules for client confidentiality.

Now, we will put it all together using the skin analysis chart, shown in Figure 1-10.

Genetic Skin Type				Fitzpatrick Type
Oily	Combination	Normal	Dry	I, II, III, IV, V, VI Circle one

Skin Conditions

Vascular	Lipid System		Pigmentation	Keratin
Telengectasia	Comedones	Scarred Ostia	Hyperpigmentation	Hyperkeratosis
Diffuse Redness	Seborrhea	Sebaceous Hyperplasia	Hypopigmentation	Skin Hydration
Erythema	Folliculitis		Solar Lentigines	Dehydration
Rosacea	Milia		Melasma	Hyperhydrosis
	Acne I, II, III, IV			

Skin Sensitivity	Aging	Disease or Disorders
Cosmetic Sensitivity	Rubin Type	Rosacea
	Glogau Type	Eczema
Tactile Sensitivity	Rhytids	Psoriasis
	Elastosis	Lesions
Environmental Sensitivity		Skin cancer

Lifestyle
Products used at home _____

Smokes __yes__no   UV exposure __intermittent __frequently__tanning beds

Recent cosmetic procedures _____ Medications _____

Treatment Focus	Treatments Given
	Date Type Formula Notes

Figure 1-10 Client skin assessment.

Step 1: Interpret the health questionnaire with your client; focus on the conditions your client feels are most important.

Step 2: Identify the genetic skin type.

Step 3: Identify the Fitzpatrick skin type.

Step 4: Identify all skin conditions.

Step 5: Formulate a treatment plan based on client goals and equipment available.

For example: You have a client who is 45 years old, on thyroid medication and hormone replacement therapy, who does not smoke. She is concerned with hormonal breakout, loss of elasticity, and pigmentation problems.

Step 1: Cleanse the skin and perform a skin analysis with a loupe and a Woods lamp. Determine her genetic skin type. This client has combination skin.

Step 2: Identify Fitzpatrick type by looking at pigmentation of the skin and asking about previous burning from sun exposure. Refer to Figure 1-1 for the Fitzpatrick skin chart. This client is a Fitzpatrick type II.

Step 3: Determine conditions and degree of aging using the Glogau and Rubin scales. With this client you see hyperkeratinization, dehydration, deep pigmentation (noticed under the Woods lamp), and surface pigmentation. Aging using the Rubin scale is level 2, and elasticity is good.

If your philosophy is clinical care, you could use microdermabrasion and LED treatment; galvanic current can also be used to penetrate a melanin suppressant after a microdermabrasion treatment.

If your philosophy is holistic or alternative healing, you could use a brush machine for **manual exfoliation,** a steamer, and a paraffin wax heater; the esthetician will primarily need to rely on a good professional skin care line.

If you would like to blend the two philosophies, you could use a brush machine for a second cleansing, a steamer for enzyme exfoliation prior to microdermabrasion, and an LED light treatment.

The Esthetician's Options to Combat Aging

By now every esthetician has heard that the baby boomers are the largest aging population. Most estheticians are being asked about treatments to reverse the signs of aging that have seemingly appeared overnight on our clients' skin. What options are available to estheticians outside of

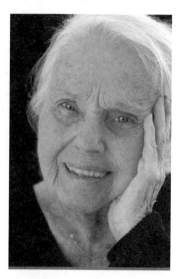

Figure 1-11 Intrinsic aging is based on genetic factors.

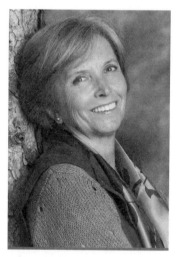

Figure 1-12 Extrinsic aging is visible in the 40s and 50s.

TIP It is important to avoid sensitizing ingredients such as alcohols, propylene glycol, tocopherol, and sulfate surfactants; do not overcleanse the skin.

working for a physician? First, we should look at the different aspects of aging: extrinsic and intrinsic.

Extrinsic aging is aging that is caused by environmental factors such as smoking, sun damage, diet, and lifestyle. Extrinsic aging is approximately 90% of the aging process. The theory is that free radicals created by stress, environmental exposure, and diet cause inflammation that leads to disease and aging.

Intrinsic aging is caused by genetic factors such as heredity, general physical health, and the natural aging process. The aging process is affected by how well our bodies repair **DNA,** a factor that can be both genetically and environmentally driven. See Figure 1-11 and Figure 1-12 for examples of extrinsic and intrinsic aging.

The signs of aging appear as more visible pores, increased dryness, rough skin texture, age spots, fine lines, wrinkles, blotchiness, and loss of elasticity. This number of visible conditions to treat can be quite daunting.

Strides are being made every day in science and technology that address many of these issues. Equipment and product usage are very important. A machine alone will not correct all visible signs of aging. Estheticians have an important role to play but are limited to certain technology.

The Esthetician's Options to Combat Acne

Acne is the physical change in the skin caused by disease of the sebaceous hair follicle, and it is as hard to treat as aging conditions. Acne can be found on the face, back, chest, and upper arms. There are several classifications of acne, and these can be divided into **inflammatory lesions**—such as cysts, papules, and pustules—and **noninflammatory lesions,** such as comedones and milia. The **pathogenic factors,** or causes of acne, are being extensively researched. They are thought to be hyperkeratinization, inflammation, hormones, enzymes, weak pore walls, or overproduction of sebum and bacteria (e.g., propionibacterium acnes).

5-alpha reductase is an enzyme that converts to **dihydrotestosterone (DHT),** which causes the sebum to become thick and promotes a follicular blockage. When hyperkeratinization or a buildup of dead cells occurs in the follicle, it causes a blockage that traps sebum and creates an anaerobic environment in which bacteria will grow. Anaerobic bacteria secrete the enzymes **lipase** and **hyaluronidase,** causing further inflammation that damages the tissue. This is a very simplified description of acne, but it should give you a general idea of the process.

Condition	Characteristics	Explanations	Machines indicated for best use
Type I Acne–congested skin, comedones	Thick rough texture, orange peel appearance, comedones, milia	Non-inflammatory extraction & exfoliation will help	Microdermabrasion, galvanic current, high frequency
Type II Acne–inflamed papules & pustules on more than ½ of face	Pustules, comedones, milia, papules may see a cyst	Inflammatory very sensitive skin–use a light touch extracting	Blue LED, microdermabrasion, galvanic current, high frequency, oxygen, IPL
Type III/IV Acne–very inflamed papules, pustules, cysts and scarring. Entire face inflamed	Pustules, cysts, papules, comedones, scarring, diffuse redness possible	Inflammatory very sensitive–must be under dermatologist care	Lasers, IPL, LED (photodynamic therapy), microdermabrasion

Figure 1-13 Equipment to use in the treatment of acne.

To treat this disease, it is important to look at the causes rather than the symptoms of acne. Equipment can help the management of acne, but a good professional product line is mandatory. In general the esthetician should treat acne as a sensitive skin condition with a focus on reducing hyperkeratinization, bacteria, and inflammation.

See Figure 1-13 for chart of equipment options used to treat acne.

REFERENCES

1. D'Angelo, J., Dean, P., Dietz, S., Hinds, C., Lees, M., Miller, E., & Zani, A. (2003). *Milady's Standard Comprehensive Training for Estheticians.* New York: Thomson Delmar Learning.
2. Simmons, J.V. (1989, 1995). *Science and the Beauty Business, The Beauty Salon and its Equipment* (2nd ed.). United Kingdom: Macmillan Press Ltd.
3. Lees, M. (2001). *Skin Care: Beyond the Basics.* New York: Thomson Delmar Learning.
4. Nordman, L. (2005). *Professional Beauty Therapy, The Official Guide to Level 3* (2nd ed.). London: Thomson Learning.
5. Root, L. CIDESCO (2004). *A Complete Guide to Microdermabrasion, Treatment, Technique, and Technology.* Arizona: Esthetician Education Resource.

6. Hill, Pamela RN (2006). *Peels and Peeling Agents*. New York: Thomson Delmar Learning.
7. Zouboulis, C. C., et al (2005, Feb). Experimental Dermatology 14(2):143–152
8. Del Rosso J. Q., & D.O. F.A.C.O.D., Goodman, M., MS (August 2003, Aug) Skin & Aging *11*(8):50–58.

WEBSITES

http://www.yglabs.com: Information on cosmetic ingredients, aging, and acne.

http://www.skincarephysicians.com: Information on all aspects of dermatology.

http://www.pubmed.gov: Information on the latest published studies.

http://www.skinandaging.com

Good Business Practices

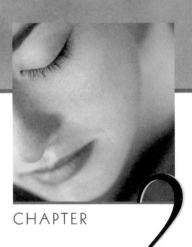

To make good business decisions regarding what equipment to purchase, you must follow careful planning guidelines. These include financial impact, insurance liability, and the ability to market your new treatments to your clientele. Here are some guidelines to follow.

■ LEASE VERSUS BUY

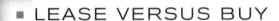

Leasing is one way of decreasing your initial capital expenditure, but it will immediately impact your cash flow. If your basic equipment purchases are less than $5,000, you may be better off purchasing your machines outright. If you are a start-up company, most leasing companies will not work with you, unless you have had three years of active business. If you are starting out with a financing package, you may be able to work with someone to put together a loan and leasing package.

There are many financing options available to new business owners, but none are without risk. Make sure that you shop carefully and work closely with a good financial advisor. The small business administration is a good place to start.

There are also tax implications involved in leasing or buying, so this is one decision in which professional advice will help you avoid future problems.

What Is Actual Cost?

The **actual cost** of your machine includes not only the actual price of the equipment but the cost per service, amount paid to the technician, and overhead costs. This is one of the most important considerations to explore carefully, because many vendors will have their own cost-per-service breakdown. Of course this only covers the cost of the materials used with that machine and possibly the cost of the machine divided

TIP Remember that although you will save capital expenditure at the start of your business, you will have a high monthly payment due when you lease. Make sure your monthly cash flow can handle the payment.

23

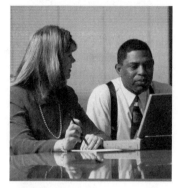

Figure 2-1 A professional business consultant can help you plan your equipment purchase.

by a specific price per service. This price may or may not be within your market **demographic**.

Here is a simple form to follow when determining actual costs:

1. What can you charge for this new service? Poll your current customers; look at the competition and your market demographic. For example, can your clients afford a $150 antiaging treatment with microdermabrasion and LED light in a series of six treatments with six separate payments?
2. What is the total price of the equipment—including shipping, possible interest, and products needed—to perform the service? Include the cost of training if it is not included in the purchase price, and break this down to a daily rate. Usually this will be your lease payment divided by the number of days you intend to have the machine in use.
3. Determine what the technician will be paid; or, if you are independent, determine how much money you need to make. Base this on the going compensation rate in your area, or you will not be able to attract qualified professionals.
4. Determine your overhead costs. What is the cost per hour to use your treatment room? Factor in the cost of insurance, support staff, linens, sundries, **support equipment,** rent, utilities, maintenance, and marketing materials. This is a variable cost but one you should have a general idea about for every service you perform.

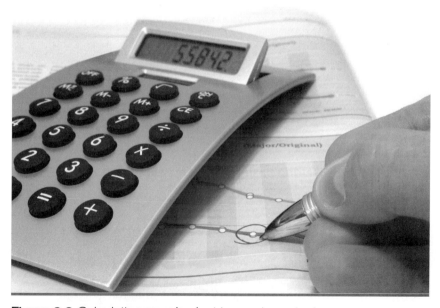

Figure 2-2 Calculating your budget is very important.

For example:

You want to purchase a microdermabrasion machine that costs $13,500.
You can charge $100 per service for your market.
You have a lease payment of $350 a month and plan on using the machine
*   24 days a month, and it costs $4.50 in supplies per treatment.*
You need to pay a rate of $50 per service to your esthetician to meet the
*   market demand. Your basic overhead costs are $13 per hour based*
*   on $117 a day.*

1. Daily machine cost: monthly lease payment ($350.00) / 24 days
   = $14.58 + $4.50 (cost of supplies). Total = $19.08
2. Daily total cost: technician rate ($50) + overhead rate ($13) + daily
   machine total ($19.08) = $82.08 total machine cost. Since you can
   only charge $100 per service, you will receive a profit of $17.92 per
   service.

If you want to increase your profit, you have several options:

- Raise your service price.
- Lower your variable costs.
- Increase the amount of time the machine is in service. Keep in mind
  it takes some time to build interest around a new service.
- Find a lower-priced machine to start with.

If you are purchasing a machine outright, you need to look at the **amortization** rate, divide that number by the total price and expected time in service, and break that down into a daily and hourly rate.

■ MARKET YOUR NEW EQUIPMENT

When you decide what machine to add to your practice, or if you are a start-up business, marketing and advertising will be vitally important. It also is one of the areas in which money can be wasted if it is spent without a plan. Before you finalize your machine purchase, put a marketing plan together.

The components of a marketing plan include the following:

- **Your unique selling position.** Who are you? What are you selling? Do you run a luxury day spa that seeks to impress upon the clientele a certain level of exclusivity? Your location and interior design also conveys this message. Is your focus medical instead of a relaxing spa environment? All of these things help determine your unique selling position (USP).
- **The benefits to the client.** Why should they buy your service? Remember: features are different from benefits. *Features* are what your service offers; for example, your microdermabrasion treatment

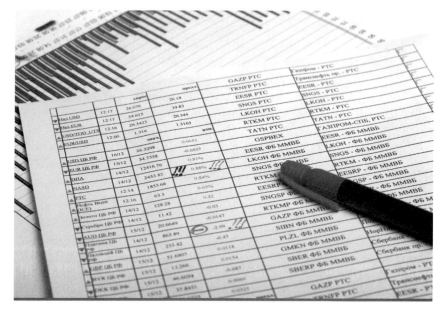

Figure 2-3 Creating a marketing plan will help assure success.

uses the latest techniques and products. *Benefits* are what your client can expect to see or feel from the service; for example, the client's skin will glow, it will feel soft and well hydrated, and fine lines and wrinkles will be reduced. Remember to always be honest with your client. Do not oversell what your equipment can really do.

- **Identify your target market**. For example, women aged 45 to 65 with a median income of $75,000, or women 18 to 24 with a median income of $35,000. You must identify your markets, and try to be as specific as possible. Good places to gather information are your local chamber of commerce, real estate agents, noncompeting businesses, and the government census bureau.

- **Define your marketing budget.** This will definitely help determine how you will be using different types of advertising media. A general rule for your budget is that it should be 10% of sales. This is a yearly total that can be roughly calculated using the formula in Figure 2-6.

- **The tools and techniques you will use to reach your clients.** Are you interested in direct mail, phonebook, and radio? Define what works in your market.

- **A specific timetable for the marketing program.** It is important to track the monthly return on your marketing program to judge how effective it is.

Marketing and advertising require persistence and commitment. They also force you to really identify what your business is about and

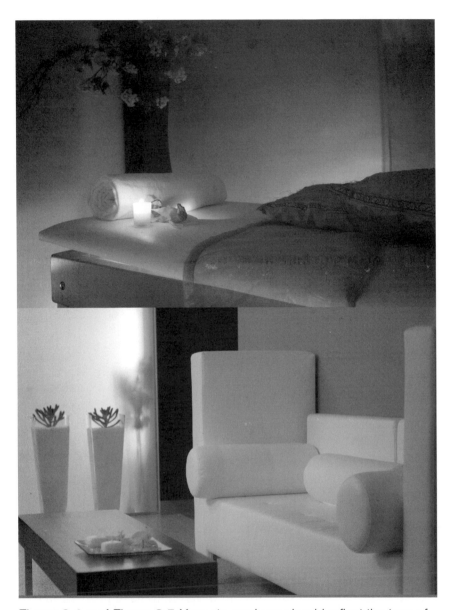

Figure 2-4 and Figure 2-5 Your atmosphere should reflect the type of clients your marketing is targeted for.

how to position it in your marketplace. There are many good reference books and classes that you can take on both subjects that will help you make informed decisions.

In the following example, the spa has a $13,500 microdermabrasion machine, charges $100 per service, performs 10 treatments per day, is open 24 days per month and has a COGS of $82.09. You can figure a monthly marketing budget using the following table.

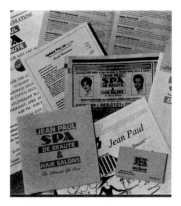

Figure 2-7 Brochures are a helpful marketing tool.

1.	Cost per service:	A
	Number of services per day:	B
	Total dollar intake per day:	C = (A * B)
	Total Revenue (D):	D = C * number of days open
2.	Net Revenue = D - COGS (daily total costs * number of days open)	N = D - COGS
	Marketing Budget (B) = 10% of Net Revenue	B = N * 10%
Example:	$13,500 Microdermabrasion machine	
	COGS = $82.09 per day * 24 days = $1,970.16	
	A = $100	
	B = 10 clients per day	
	C = 10 x $100	$1,000
	D = $1,000 * 24 days open	$24,000 Total Revenue
	N = $24,000 - COGS	$22,082.40 Net Revenue
	Marketing Budget (B) = 10% of $22,082.40	$2,208.24 Marketing Budget

Figure 2-6 Calculate approximate marketing costs.

■ DEMYSTIFYING INSURANCE

Insurance is one of the most complicated and important aspects of buying equipment. It is very important to have a general understanding of insurance and where to get accurate information.

The first place to start is to fully understand the scope of your practice as defined by your state insurance board. The insurer will sell you insurance regardless of whether you can actually use the equipment you have purchased. If there is a claim, and it is revealed that you are working outside your scope of practice, the claim will not be paid by your insurance policy.

Regardless of your liability, costs are involved with defending yourself against a lawsuit; it is imperative to have professional liability coverage as well as property coverage. If you are employed by a spa, salon, or **medi-spa,** you still need personal liability insurance, unless your employer specifically adds you to their liability insurance. It is also important to make sure that the modalities you are practicing are included under the policy. For example, if you are performing microcurrent treatments, your liability insurance should specifically state that you have coverage for that. It is also important to understand that even if you are covered under your employer, there

TIP If you are working in a medical setting, you must verify that you are included specifically under the doctor's medical malpractice insurance. Most medical malpractice policies do not cover nonmedical personnel who perform medical treatments. You will have to carry your own insurance, which includes *all* of the services that you will perform in the medical setting. Do not forget to add product liability to the policy.

New
Clinical Skin Care
With Susanne

Spa on the Pier

Experience the hottest new beauty treatment for smoother younger looking skin

Microdermabrasion

Proven safe and effective for
Fine lines and wrinkles
Sun damaged skin
Large pores – blackheads

$100
1 hour

Includes professional skin sensor analysis & facial
$585 FOR A SERIES OF 6 WITH ONE FREE

Make your appointment today

Call Susanne 503-741-0106 or 503-325-7271

Figure 2-8 In-spa marketing example.

is a limit to the amount of damages the policy will cover. You are only covered to that dollar limit.

Here is a general description of types of insurance.

General Liability Insurance   A form of insurance designed to protect practitioners from liability arising from accidents happening on the premises, such as someone slipping and falling in your treatment room. Even if you work for someone who has this insurance, your name must be specifically listed on the policy, or you can be personally sued as well.

Professional Liability and Malpractice Insurance   Professional liability and malpractice insurance is insurance on a professional practitioner that will defend suits instituted for malpractice and pay any damages set by a court, subject to the policy limits. For example, these policies will pay if you are sued after doing a microdermabrasion treatment because your client experiences complications. Make sure this policy covers all of the machines that you work with, and that these are

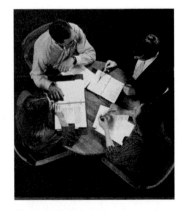

Figure 2-9 It is important to get sound advice when buying insurance.

clearly outlined in the policy. Most insurance will have a separate Laser Rider if you also perform laser treatments.

Claims Made Policy   A claims made policy is insurance that pays claims arising out of incidents that occur during the policy term, and the claim must be reported while coverage is active to be covered. If you have a claim and report it after the policy term, and you did not renew, the claim will not be covered.

Occurrence-Based Policy   If the policyholder did not renew the policy, but a claim came in for the covered period, then an occurrence-based policy would still cover that claim. For example, this type of policy would pay if you performed a pedicure, and a client filed a claim during the time the policy was active stating that you caused her to get an infection. Even though you are no longer paying for that policy, and you no longer even work for the same employer, an occurrence-based policy would pay the claim.

Product Liability Policy   A product liability policy pays if a client is injured in some way by a product you use. For example, you apply a numbing cream to a client before a laser hair-removal service, and she has an allergic reaction.

Rental and Fire Damage Liability Insurance   This insurance covers damage that the policyholder is liable for, which includes damage that the policyholder caused. For example, if your machine short circuits and causes a fire in a room that you are renting, this policy would pay for the damages.

Advertising Injury Liability   An advertising injury liability can arise out of **libel** or **slander,** violations of a client's right to privacy, misappropriation of advertising ideas, or infringement of copyright, title, or slogan committed in the course of advertising your services or products.

Malpractice Insurance   Malpractice insurance covers professional misconduct or lack of ordinary skill in the performance of a professional act that renders the practitioner liable for damages. *This policy will not cover you if you are working outside your scope of practice.* An example of malpractice would be performing a microdermabrasion treatment with no training and causing harm to your client.

Possible Liability

Once you understand the basic types of policies and what they cover, you need to look at your personal situation and the possible liability involved.

Here are some possible situations and the type of insurance needed to protect you and your business.

Employee Working for a Spa:

You are an *employee* working for a spa, not an independent contractor. You perform every modality in the scope of your licensing that the spa advertises. Your employer has listed you, and your current license, on their general liability insurance.

Type of Insurance You Need:

Professional liability and *malpractice insurance* (an *occurrence-based policy*) would be best for your situation. Many of these general liability policies can be provided at a reasonable rate through a trade association, and many employers will voluntarily cover you with this type of policy. Be sure to ask before you get hired, because this will impact what your true salary is.

Independent Contractor Leasing a Room in an Existing Business, or if you Have your Own Space:

You are self-employed and perform all services that are within your scope of practice, as well as being responsible for the condition of the space you are renting. You control all advertising, marketing, and the types of machines you use.

Type of Insurance You Need:

Professional liability and *malpractice insurance,* either a *claims made* or an *occurrence-based policy,* along with *product liability insurance, rental and fire damage liability,* and—if you are going to aggressively advertise—*advertising injury insurance.* Most landlords require you to have general liability insurance at the minimum. This is a good idea, even if you are in an existing spa that has an existing policy.

Employee Working in a Doctor's Office or in a Medi-Spa:

You are hired as an employee and will be performing medically-based treatments under the supervision of a doctor. These could include laser hair removal, laser skin rejuvenation, radio frequency treatments, and deep chemical peels.

Type of Insurance You Need:

Your liability is high. Most medical malpractice policies will not cover you, and doctors are a high-value target for litigious clients. For your situation, *professional liability* and *malpractice insurance,* a *claims made* or *occurrence-based policy,* along with *product liability insurance* and *general liability insurance,* would be a good idea. Many employers will purchase this for you in this type of environment. Find out before being hired; it will impact your true salary. Keep in mind that you are performing very invasive procedures for a doctor, so you must have insurance.

This is a general overview of how to protect you, but it is always important to get good professional advice before purchasing. Figure 2-10 provides a quick reference on different types of insurance and why you might need them.

How to Purchase Insurance

Now that you understand the basics of insurance, it is important to know how to purchase it. Many **trade associations** offer low-cost insurance with membership. This is a good place to start, but make sure the company that underwrites the insurance is not rated lower than A-. Rating agencies evaluate the financial strength of an insurer, and ratings range from F to A+, like a student might be graded. It is not a requirement that an insurer release its financial rating, so this is only one aspect of choosing insurance. The **A.M. Best Company** publishes an annual insurance report. See the list of references for the Web site. **Standard and Poor's** also offers a rating service; theirs is less comprehensive, but it will still give you valuable information.

All states also have insurance divisions through which insurance companies and insurance agents must be licensed. This is the second place to look before buying insurance. You need to find out if the insurance carrier is admitted, which means that they are accepted by the state insurance division and will be included in a guaranty association that will

Type	Description of Insurance	Reason
Independent Contractor	Professional liability, malpractice insurance with claims made or occurrence Possibly advertising injury	Higher liability due to being self-employed
Employee	Professional liability and malpractice insurance	Only if your employer will not add you to their policy
Employee of a Medical Spa	Professional liability and malpractice insurance, product liability and general liability	Higher liability due to type of services preformed Employer will possibly purchase for you

Figure 2-10 Chart of types of insurance.

cover the claims in case the insurer goes bankrupt. Each department of insurance also handles complaints, lists how many complaints are filed, and provides a summary of each insurer.

A good rule of thumb for the esthetic professional is to make sure your broker or insurance company truly understands this industry. If they do not know what microdermabrasion or spa services are, do not use them.

■ WARRANTIES AND DISPUTES

The type of **warranty** that you have on your equipment is very important. Equipment is usually a large capital expenditure and a major part of your service menu. You need to make sure that the equipment will be replaced or serviced after purchase. Every manufacturer has a specific warranty, and there is no mandated standard for our industry to follow. Congress did enact the **Magnuson-Moss Warranty Act of 1975** for consumer protection. Unfortunately, it does not apply to warranties on products sold for resale or for commercial purposes.

At a minimum, your warranty on basic equipment should be for a year on all parts and components. The more expensive the equipment, the longer the warranty should be, and it should include more. This is an area where your business consultant or lawyer can really help you look at the options and determine what is best for you.

What happens if you have a dispute with your vendor? For example, you purchase an esthetic machine that was very inexpensive and offered no warranty, and it malfunctions. Here are a few steps you can take:

1. **Contact the seller:** Note the date, time, and who you spoke with. Explain your situation clearly, and be precise about the outcome you would like. For example, you might say: "Mr. Vendor, on this date the steamer on my multifunction machine caught on fire, damaging the entire unit. I purchased this unit on this date, and it is clear the workmanship is inferior. I would like to return this machine for an immediate refund of my money." Hopefully, your vendor is an upstanding quality company and will handle it immediately. If not, move to step two.

2. **Write a letter:** Again, be precise and state clearly what you need. Also include the date and time of the first phone conversation, and the date that you expect a response from them. Send the letter registered mail so that you know the company received it. The **FTC** has a sample dispute letter for you to follow. See the Web site listing on the next page. If that does not work, proceed to step three.

3. **Make one more call:** Inform the business that you will be reporting the situation to your state attorney general's consumer protection

division, the Better Business Bureau, and the Federal Trade Commission. Not all of these organizations may deal with business-to-business complaints, but it is important to look at all your options. If this does not motivate your vendor, then proceed to step four.

4. **Dispute resolution:** At this point, you should consider filing a small claims suit, a mediation claim, or an arbitration claim. In step three, you contacted your state's attorney general and consumer protection agency; these are the contacts for further information in your state for taking your dispute to the next level.

This can be quite a frustrating process, one we hope you will never have to go through. Remember to check out your vendor in detail before purchasing. With careful and thoughtful decision making, you will avoid many pitfalls. Do not worry: everyone makes mistakes, but it is important to learn from them and know what your rights are.

REFERENCES

1. FTC. (1998). *FTC Facts for Consumers, Solving Consumer Problems.* USA: Federal Trade Commission, Bureau of Consumer Protection.
2. Lees, M. (2001). *Skin Care: Beyond the Basics.* New York: Thomson Delmar Learning.
3. Levinson, J. C., & Godin, S. (1994). *The Guerrilla Marketing Handbook.* New York: Houghton Mifflin Company.
4. Stevens, C. *Shopping for insurance*, New Jersey: Marine Agency Corporation.

WEB SITES

Federal Trade Association: http://www.ftc.gov
Small Business Administration: http://www.sba.gov
The Marine Agency: http://www.marineagency.com
The Hartford: http://www.sb.thehartford.com

Equipment Guidelines and Rules

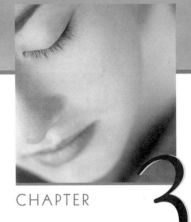

The esthetics industry is changing rapidly; unfortunately, the regulations that govern the use of certain machines are not keeping pace. This is an issue that will change the esthetician's scope of practice, which ultimately affects earning potential. In this chapter you will find the definitions of FDA Class I, II, and III medical devices, and you will learn what UL, CE, CSA, and ISO standards are.

CHAPTER 3

■ THE FDA

The **Food and Drug Administration**'s role as a regulatory body is often misunderstood in regard to equipment. The FDA's role is to regulate the firms that manufacture, repackage, relabel, and import medical devices. The department responsible for this is the Center for Devices and Radiological Health (CDRH). They classify devices based on the **intended use, indications for use,** and risk the device poses to the patient and the operator. Class I includes devices with the lowest risk, and Class III includes those with the greatest risk. All devices are subject to the General Control Guidelines, which comprise the baseline requirements of the **Food, Drug, and Cosmetic (FD&C) Act** that apply to all medical devices. The FDA is part of the executive branch, as shown in Figure 3-1.

After approval of classification, it is up to the state to determine if a device is within the scope of an esthetician's practice and to regulate that use. The FDA's classification does not expressly warrant any machine, so when you see a manufacturer that is FDA-registered, this is only one indication of the quality of the equipment.

Here Are the Classifications Currently Used:

Class I: Class I devices are subject to the least regulatory control, and **Class I Exempt** does not require **510k submission.** These devices present minimal potential for harm to the user and client and are often simpler in design than Class II or Class III devices, and the intended use

35

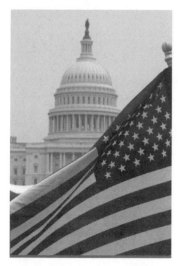

Figure 3-1 The FDA is part of the Health and Human Services Department in the executive branch.

is noninvasive. Class I devices are subject to the General Control Guidelines, which state that they must be manufactured under a **quality assurance program,** be suitable for the intended use, be adequately packaged and properly labeled, and have establishment registration and device listing forms on file with the FDA. Class I devices are not for use in sustaining or supporting life or preventing impairment of human life, and do not present an unreasonable risk of injury.

If a device falls into the generic category of Class I Exempt, a premarket notification and FDA clearance is not required before selling the device in the United States. The manufacturer of the device is required to register their business by filing FDA form 2891, the initial registration of the device, and also FDA form 2892, which lists the generic category or classification name of the device being registered.

Class II: Class II devices are those which may cause harm to the client, or in which general controls alone are insufficient to assure safety and effectiveness, and existing methods are available to provide such assurances. In addition to complying with general controls, Class II devices are also subject to special controls, such as specific labeling requirements, minimum performance standards, and post-market surveillance. Examples of Class II devices are IPL, lasers, and ultrasound.

Class III: Class III devices are considered prescriptive, and this is the most stringent regulatory category for devices. Class III devices are those for which insufficient information exists to assure safety and effectiveness solely through general or special controls.

Class III devices are usually those that support or sustain human life, are of substantial importance in preventing impairment of human health, or present a potentially unreasonable risk of illness or injury. Premarket approval is the required process of scientific review to ensure the safety and effectiveness of Class III devices, such as lasers.

What Is Considered a Medical Device?

What is considered a medical device by the FDA, and does that include our esthetic equipment? The FDA's definition follows:

The term "device" means an instrument, apparatus, implement, machine, contrivance, implant, in vitro reagent, or other similar or related article, including any component, part, or accessory, which is

recognized in the official National Formulary, or the United States Pharmacopeia, or any supplement to them, intended for use in the diagnosis of disease or other conditions, or in the cure, mitigation, treatment, or prevention of disease, in man or other animals, or intended to affect the structure or any function of the body of man, and which does not achieve its primary intended purposes through chemical action within or on the body of man and which is not dependent upon being metabolized for the achievement of its primary intended purposes.

For comparison, the definition of a cosmetic product is listed as follows: The term "cosmetic" means

Articles intended to be rubbed, poured, sprinkled, sprayed on, introduced into, or otherwise applied to the human body or any part thereof for cleansing, beautifying, promoting attractiveness, or altering the appearance, and articles intended for use as a component of any such articles; except that such term shall not include soap.

So what does this mean? The intent of the device is the first place to start. Does the device intend to treat any disease or condition? Treating a disease is outside of our scope of practice. The visible signs of aging are not considered a medical condition. Acne and rosacea are considered conditions, so if the device were primarily used for treatment of these conditions, it would be considered a medical device. Does the device affect the structure or function of the body without a chemical reaction?

Let us look at microdermabrasion. At the esthetic level, the device is not meant to treat any disease or condition, but it does affect the structure of the skin without a chemical reaction. This effect is mild, but does include removal of the stratum corneum. Under the FDA definition, microdermabrasion is considered a medical device and is currently Class I Exempt.

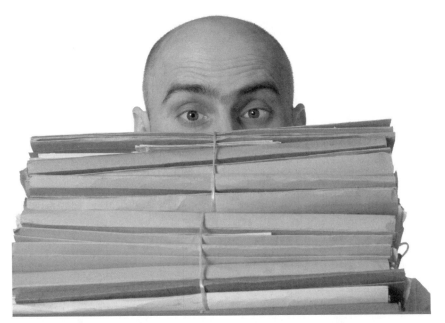

Figure 3-2 The regulatory process can feel overwhelming.

Most of the devices used in esthetics are cleared for marketing under the 510k provisions of the Food and Drug Act. Legally it is not an approval; the law allows a firm to claim its equipment is FDA-approved only if it has had a legal approval. Figure 3-2 shows how confusing the regulatory process can be.

Manufacturer Registration

All manufacturers of medical devices must register with the FDA. Those that do not have to register are distributors of esthetic devices. The definitions for exemption from registration are:

- A manufacturer of raw materials or components to be used in the manufacture or assembly of a device that would otherwise not be required to register under the provisions of this part.
- A manufacturer of devices to be used solely for veterinary purposes.
- A manufacturer of general purpose articles, such as chemical reagents or laboratory equipment, whose uses are generally known by persons trained in their use and which are not labeled or promoted for medical uses.
- Licensed practitioners—including physicians, dentists, and optometrists—who manufacture or otherwise alter devices solely for use in their practice.
- Pharmacies, surgical supply outlets, or other similar retail establishments making final delivery or sale to the ultimate user. This exemption also applies to a pharmacy or other similar retail establishment that purchases a device for subsequent distribution under its own name (e.g., a properly labeled health aid such as an elastic bandage or crutch, indicating "distributed by," or "manufactured for," followed by the name of the pharmacy).
- Individuals who manufacture, prepare, propagate, compound, or process devices solely for use in research, teaching, or analysis and do not introduce such devices into commercial distribution.
- Carriers by reason of their receipt, carriage, holding, or delivery of devices in the usual course of business as carriers.
- Persons who dispense devices to the ultimate consumer, or whose major responsibility is to render a service necessary to provide the consumer (i.e., patient, physician, layman, etc.) with a device or the benefits to be derived from the use of a device; for example, a hearing aid dispenser, optician, clinical laboratory, assembler of diagnostic x-ray systems, and personnel from a hospital, clinic, dental laboratory, or orthotic or prosthetic retail facility, whose primary responsibility to the ultimate consumer is to dispense or provide a service through the use of a previously manufactured device.

■ UL LISTING AND CE MARKING

Most are familiar with the UL mark on electrical appliances; this is also one of the marks that should be found on esthetic equipment. **Underwriters Laboratories (UL)** is an organization within the United States that develops safety standards and test procedures for consumer and business products. The UL mark is not an approval of the product, but rather a certification that the equipment tested met all of the standards set forth by Underwriters Laboratory. You can tell when a piece of equipment has been UL listed by the familiar trademark, shown in Figure 3-3. The company's file number will be listed on the label (usually a letter followed by six numbers). This number can be used on the UL Web site to locate a company's certificate.

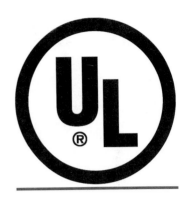

Figure 3-3 Always look for the UL mark.

UL Standards

Typical standards for a UL listing consider electrical safety, fire spread, and mechanical hazards. This is not a government-required listing and requires voluntary involvement by the manufacturers. It also does not guarantee that the equipment will perform in a certain way. Although it is a private company, many distributors will not buy an unlisted product, and it may be extremely difficult to get insurance coverage on a non–UL-listed product.

A manufacturer must demonstrate compliance with UL standards and must provide a program to ensure that those standards will be met with each unit produced. If a design is modified, it will need to be retested before the UL mark can be used. Inspections at the manufacturing locations are unannounced and are conducted several times per year.

UL listing not used only used in the United States. Canada and other countries have access to the certification as well. The label will state which countries the equipment has been listed in. The European analogue is the **CE mark**, which has more stringent regulations equal to our **FCC** Part 15 electronic requirements.

■ CE MARKING

The CE mark is a mandatory safety mark on equipment and products sold within the European Union (EU). The CE mark represents that the manufacturer or distributor of the equipment or product meets the

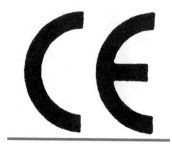

Figure 3-4 An example of the CE mark.

essential safety requirements of all EU participating countries. These directives concern the safety of machinery, low-voltage equipment, communication equipment, and consumer products. There are 25 requirements to be met for CE marking.

To obtain a CE marking, the equipment manufacturer must provide proof that the standards have been met. This can be done by in-company testing or independent testing agencies. The manufacturer then must file an EC-Declaration of Conformity, stating which standards the equipment complies with. Figure 3-4 shows a CE marking.

ISO LISTING

Every manufacturer has its own definition of quality. Without a standard that all manufacturers can refer to, customers are at the mercy of vendors and manufacturers. To deal with this issue, the **International Organization for Standardization (ISO)** was created. The ISO is a nonprofit organization in Geneva Switzerland with 140 member countries. In 1987, the ISO panel published a set of guidelines that businesses must comply with in order to qualify for quality certification. This certification is called ISO 9000, and it is issued by independent auditors.

ISO certification is not a legal requirement, but rather a standard that 140 countries agree to. It is so prevalent in European countries that many customers will refuse to do business with a noncertified company. This is a very relevant certification for customers in the United States as well, because the FDA does not certify the quality of manufacturing processes. The FDA has good manufacturing guidelines, and it will classify different devices, but it does not send in independent auditors to look for international standards.

A new standard that has been incorporated by the ISO is ISO 14000. This deals with international standards that incorporate environmental concerns in the ISO's manufacturing practices. It is wise to look for an ISO certification on any equipment you are purchasing. It is not a widely used certification in the esthetic industry, but some manufacturers are using it.

CLINICAL TESTING

Many claims are made by esthetic machine manufacturers. They cite clinical studies that prove their technology works. Understanding the basics of clinical research will help you decipher the information given.

Clinical trials, also known as *clinical research*, are research studies that use human volunteers to answer specific efficacy and safety questions about drugs, medical devices, and other biologics, such as vaccines. These are done in strictly controlled settings and are monitored by the regulatory body of the country the test is conducted in. In the United States, it is the FDA; in Europe, the European Medicines Agency; and in Japan, the Ministry of Health, Labor, and Welfare. In the United States, studies that are meant to intervene in a disease process must be approved by an ethics committee, the Institutional Review Board; for example, this committee must review clinical trials of new cancer treatments.

Different types of clinical studies fall into the experimental or observational categories. An **experimental study** is a study under the direct control of the investigator, which will allow for it to be randomized. An example of a **randomized controlled trial (RCT)** is a drug study with two groups of people in which one randomly chosen group is given a

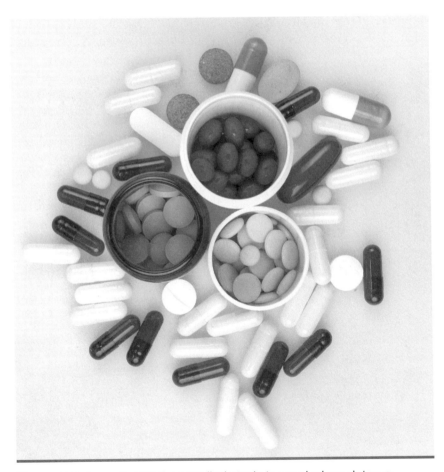

Figure 3-5 A randomized controlled study is used when doing a clinical drug study.

placebo and the other is given the drug being studied. This is considered the most effective type of study. Within this group is the randomized crossover clinical trial, which focuses on specific treatments for a condition after the main data are collected in the RCT. A clinical drug study is considered a randomized controlled study (see Figure 3-5).

The next is the **randomized controlled laboratory study.** This is an experimental study done strictly in a lab that facilitates basic research. These results are not always applicable to the clinical study, because they do not also consider the impact of the study on the group. An example would be the often-cited Cheng study on microcurrent effects on rat skin. See Figure 3-6 for an example.

Observational studies are not as controlled as experimental studies. The observational study provides weaker empirical evidence than the experimental study; it is based on clinical observation, which is subject to interpretation by the investigator. These studies can provide preliminary information that may lead to an experimental controlled study. Much of what we see in the esthetic industry is the observation study. The differ-

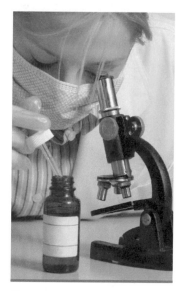

Figure 3-6 A randomized controlled laboratory study is done strictly in the lab.

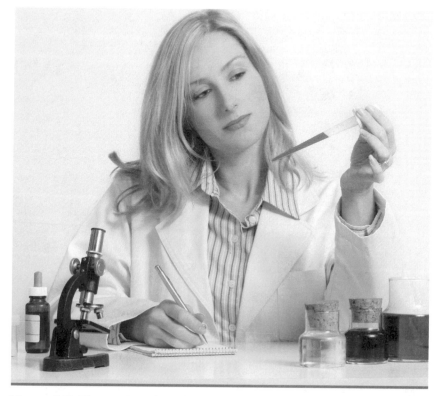

Figure 3-7 Observational studies are open to interpretation by those involved.

ent types of observational studies are the *cohort, case control, ecologic, cross-sectional, case series,* and *case report. Observational studies are open to interpretation* (see Figure 3-7).

Cohort (Incidence, Longitudinal) Study: An analytical, observational study based on data, usually primary, from a certain period for a group that has had the exposure of interest to determine the association between that exposure and an outcome. Cohort studies are susceptible to bias by lack of follow-up and the lack of control over risk assignment. Cohort studies are stronger than case control studies when well-executed, but they also are more expensive.

Case Control Study: A study, often based on secondary data, in which the group with the disease and a potential risk factor is compared to the control group (individuals without the disease) with the same risk factor. The common association measure for a case control study is the odds ratio. A common example would be the study of the risk factors of heart disease in different groups. Case control studies provide somewhat weak empirical evidence, even when properly executed.

Ecologic (Aggregate) Study: An observational study based on sum total secondary data. The sum total data on risk factors and disease prevalence from different population groups are compared to identify associations. For example, the lifespan of Asian populations is compared to that of western populations. Because all sum data are from the group level, relationships at the individual level cannot be empirically analyzed. This type of study provides weak empirical evidence.

Cross-Sectional (Prevalence) Study: A study of the relationship between diseases and other factors at one point in time in a defined population. Cross-sectional studies have less information on timing of exposure and include only prevalent cases. An example would be an area that has a prevalent cancer increase.

Case Series: An observational study of a series of cases, typically describing the symptoms, clinical course, and prognosis of a condition. A case series provides weak empirical evidence because of the lack of comparability, unless the findings are dramatically different from expectations. Case series are best used as a source of ideas for investigation by experimental studies. The case series could be regarded as clinicians talking to researchers, and it is the most common study type in clinical literature.

Case Report: A report of a single case that will typically describe the symptoms, a clinical course of treatment, and prognosis of that case.

Case reports provide little empirical evidence. They do describe how others have diagnosed and treated the condition and what the clinical outcome was. An example in the esthetics industry would be "before" and "after" pictures of improvement of the skin with a specific protocol cited as the treatment.

REFERENCES

1. Simmons, J. V. (1989, 1995). *Science and the Beauty Business, The Beauty Salon and its Equipment* (2nd ed.). United Kingdom: Macmillan Press Ltd.
2. Nordman, L. (2005). *Professional Beauty Therapy, The Official Guide to Level 3* (2nd ed.). London: Thomson Learning.
3. Code of Federal Regulations, Title 21, Volume 8, Revised as of April 1, 2006. From the U.S. Government Printing Office via GPO Access [CITE: 21CFR801.109] Pp. 20–21.
4. Pride, W., Hughes, R., Kapor, J. (2005). *Business*. Boston, MA: Houghton Mifflin Company.

WEB SITES

http://www.fda.gov

Treatment Room Basics

SECTION

2

Magnifying Lamp

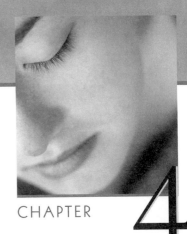

The magnifying lamp is an essential piece of esthetic equipment. Estheticians must use it to perform a correct skin analysis. It is also important to use it during extractions to avoid any damage to the skin, and it will help when doing facial waxing. It does not matter what type of skin care philosophy you have; a **magnifying lamp**—also called a **loupe**—is essential. A magnifying lamp is considered essential in a basic treatment room setup, which is shown in Figure 4-1.

CHAPTER 4

■ FUNCTIONS

A magnifying lamp is used to magnify the surface of the skin to facilitate accurate skin analysis and effective extraction, facial waxing, and other detail-oriented tasks (see Figure 4-2).

■ WHY IT WORKS

The magnifying lamp works by using a magnifying glass in a metal holder and a fluorescent light in a circular shape on the underside of the lamp head. It can come in several magnifications: 3×, 5×, and 10×. Most estheticians use a 5×. This means that the skin is illuminated 50× the normal view. The lens is very important, and it must be clear and free of distortions. Most magnifying lamps come on a movable stand and have an adjustable arm to raise or lower the lamp for the correct position, as shown in Figure 4-3.

■ HOW TO USE A MAGNIFYING LAMP

The magnifying lamp is very easy to use. After cleansing the skin and applying eye pads, place the lamp 1 to 2 inches from the face, depend-

TIP Magnifications scales are coded as follows: 3× is 30-times magnification, 5× is 50-times magnification, and 10× is 100-times magnification.

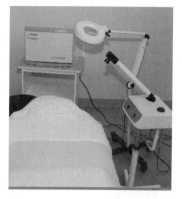

Figure 4-1 The magnifying lamp is an essential part of a treatment room setup.

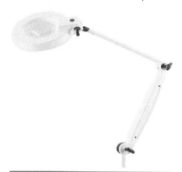

Figure 4-2 Silhouet-tone Cirrus magnifying lamp.

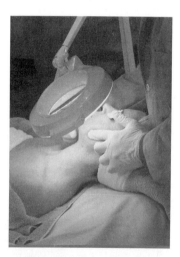

Figure 4-3 Demonstration of magnifying lamp.

ing on the strength of your magnification. Proceed with analysis or other activity; refer to Figure 4-4 for an illustration.

▪ HOW TO BUY

Magnifying lamps are a relatively inexpensive purchase but incur a lot of wear and tear. It is important to buy the best you can afford. The magnifying lamp can last up to 10 years if it is well-made and properly maintained. A very well-made magnifying lamp can cost up to $500. Some new models include both a Woods lamp and fluorescent lamp. Magnifying lamps can be purchased separately or in a multifunction machine, like the one shown in Figure 4-5.

Buy from a reputable manufacturer or from a vendor that has been in business for a long time. The spring that allows the lamp to move will wear out and need replacement (see Figure 4-6).

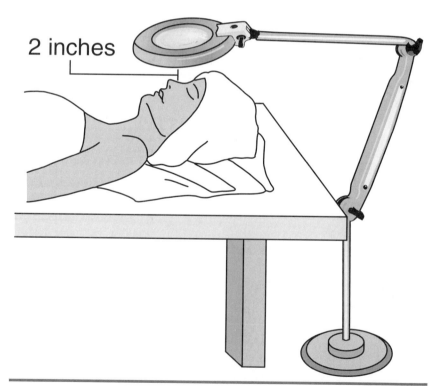

2 inches

Figure 4-4 Illustration of correct magnifying lamp distance.

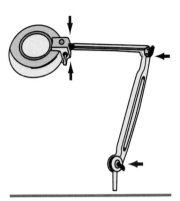

Figure 4-6 Illustration of areas that can become loose.

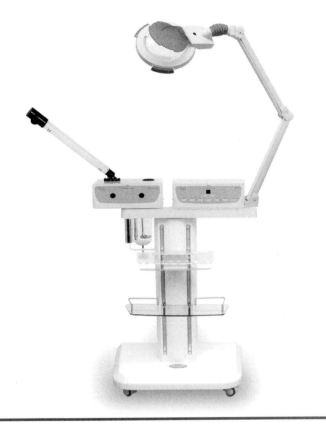

Figure 4-5 Cirrus system.

Because a lamp is a piece of electrical equipment, it is important to make sure your equipment has a safety certification such as a UL listing or a CSA, CE, or ISO certification. UL, CSA, and CE listings indicate that the equipment has been tested for safety. ISO indicates that it has been manufactured per international standards and that the manufacturer is tested twice a year.

Buyer's Checklist

- What is the price?
- Do you have an instruction manual or DVD?
- Is the machine UL listed, ISO certified, or CSA or CE tested?
- Does it come with a stand, or is the stand sold separately?
- Can I buy replacement parts?
- What is the warranty?

TIP Underwriters Laboratory is the U.S. organization responsible for testing products for consumer safety. Many international products are not UL certified, so Underwriters Laboratory has recently started an international section of certification. The alternative to UL listing is **CSA or CE certification.** The UL mark on a product tells you that the machine has been thoroughly tested and investigated by a team of product safety professionals.

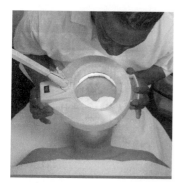

Figure 4-7a Performing a skin analysis.

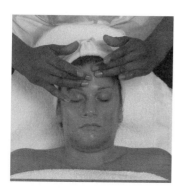

Figure 4-7b Feeling the texture of the skin.

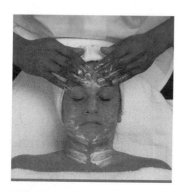

Figure 4-7c Cleansing the skin.

■ SAFETY

Magnifying lamps are very safe, but the following tips are important:

- When a machine is not well-maintained and a spring is loose, it is possible for the lamp fall on your client. Always be aware of how you are positioned when using the lamp. If you get too close, it can be very uncomfortable.
- It is important to have your client wear eye pads to avoid discomfort.
- If you need a closer look at the eye area, you can remove one eye pad, take a look, and then replace the pad. The idea is to do it quickly without making the client feel uncomfortable.

■ MAINTENANCE

Maintenance is one of the most important aspects of owning esthetic machines. Maintenance for a magnifying lamp is easy. Manufacturers will also have their own protocols, so be sure to follow their directions. In general, use these guidelines:

- Clean the glass and arms of your lamp every day. Product residue will be left on the lamp when touched during a service.
- Check the springs and adjuster knobs for the correct tension.
- Check the cord for breaks or anything that looks unusual.

■ DISINFECTION AND SANITIZATION

- Clean all debris and product residue off the lens with a clean cloth; do not use rough material that might scratch the lens.
- Clean all debris off of the lamp arm and stand.
- Use an EPA-registered high-level disinfectant spray daily, especially when using the lamp for extractions. Follow manufacturer instructions and your state requirements.

■ CONTRAINDICATIONS AND CAUTIONS

The magnifying lamp is the primary tool for determining many contraindications for other treatments. There are no contraindications for the use of the magnifying lamp.

■ PREPARATION FOR TREATMENT

- Have your client fill out a health assessment form.
- Check for contraindications.
- Have your client change into a treatment gown and remove all jewelry.
- Cleanse all makeup and debris from the skin.
- Cover client's eyes with eye pads.

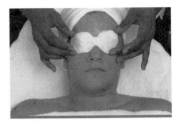

Figure 4-7d Covering the eyes.

■ PROTOCOLS

Listed below are protocols for use in your treatment room.

Basic Skin Analysis

Step 1: Have client fill out a client intake form (see Chapter 1).

Step 2: Position client appropriately and place eye pads over the client's eyes (see Figure 4-7d).

Step 3: Place magnifying lamp 1 to 2 inches from the face, look at the skin, and feel the texture of it (see Figure 4-7a and Figure 4-7b).

Step 4: Cleanse the skin (see Figure 4-7c).

Step 5: Replace eye pads and continue analysis and consultation. Ask questions about lifestyle and daily routine and clarify medications (see Figure 4-7e).

Step 6: Note all findings on the client skin analysis form (see Chapter 1 and Figure 4-7f).

Step 7: Choose correct treatment options, including which products to use (see Figure 4-7g).

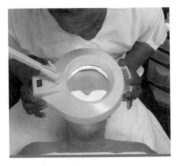

Figure 4-7e Ask questions during analysis.

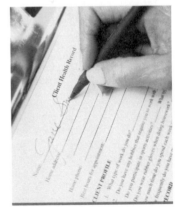

Figure 4-7f Note information on client's intake form.

Your Protocol:

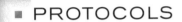

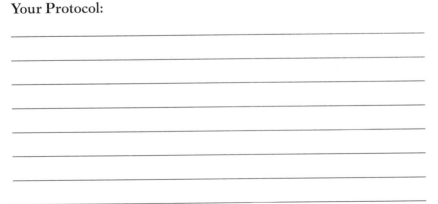

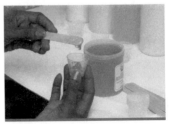

Figure 4-7g Choosing products for treatment.

■ YOUR EQUIPMENT INFORMATION

Manufacturer info:

Name/phone number: _____

Web site: _____

Date purchased: _____ Registration: _____

Warranty info: _____

Replacement part info: _____

TROUBLESHOOTING

The arm keeps slipping down when I position the lamp over a client's face.

Check the brackets that hold the arm up; make sure all screws are tight and that there is no damage to any springs, if any are on the arm. If that does not work, contact the manufacturer.

I am getting a blurred, distorted image when I look through the lens.

Clean the lens with an optical glass cleaner: regular glass cleaner can leave a residue. Check for cracks in the glass. The thickness may need to be reduced.

Q & A

Can I purchase replacement light bulbs anywhere, or do I have to buy from my manufacturer?

In general it is a good idea to get your bulb from your manufacturer; if that is not possible, make sure you purchase a fluorescent light that can fit in a drafting light, usually sold in an office supply store. Always remember to check the voltages to make sure they are compatible.

Is price the most important factor when choosing a magnifying lamp?

No. Look at the quality of the equipment and factor in how long you need to have the lamp last. If you do not mind replacing it in two years, you can purchase an inexpensive model.

REFERENCES

1. Lees, M. (2001). *Skin Care: Beyond the Basics.* New York: Thomson Delmar Learning.
2. Nordman, L. (2005). *Professional Beauty Therapy, The Official Guide to Level 3* (2nd ed.). London: Thomson Learning.
3. Simmons, J.V. (1989, 1995). *Science and the Beauty Business: The Beauty Salon and its Equipment* (2nd ed.). United Kingdom: Macmillan Press Ltd.
4. Tangelo, J., Dean, P., Dietz, S., Hinds, C., Lees, M., Miller, E., & Zani, A. (2003). *Milady's Standard Comprehensive Training for Estheticians.* New York: Thomson Delmar Learning.

Skin Analysis Equipment:
Woods Lamp and Skin Scanner

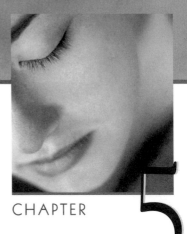

Skin analysis equipment is very important to have. It allows you to do a professional, in-depth skin analysis to recommend the right treatments and home care products. In this chapter we will cover the Woods lamp, skin scanner, new electronic skin imaging, and sensor systems.

CHAPTER 5

■ FUNCTIONS

Skin analysis provides an accurate view of skin types, skin conditions, fungi, bacterial disorders, moisture content, and pigmentation problems that are usually invisible to the naked eye. It offers an accurate and consistent view of a client's skin with a computerized analysis.

■ WHY IT WORKS: WOODS LAMP

The Woods lamp (see Figure 5-1) works by using a filtered blacklight viewed through a magnifying lens. It is best to have a Woods lamp that has two rows each of violet light. It is also very important to be able to control the light in the room. Used in the correct manner, the Woods lamp allows you to see pigment conditions, sebaceous secretions, dehydration, bacteria, fungus, and hyperkeratosis of the skin. Figure 5-2 shows a chart of Woods lamp indications.

The skin scanner is a Woods lamp in a stationary box; the client inserts his or her head into a tent to close out all light. The esthetician sits on the other side, and a two-way magnifying mirror lets both esthetician and client see the same effects on the skin. It is a wonderful tool to use to educate the client about the condition of his or her skin and the effects of sun damage. Figure 5-3 shows a skin scanner.

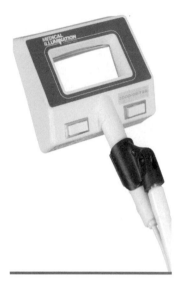

Figure 5-1 Silhouet-tone Woods lamp.

Skin	What You See
Normal to combination skin	Overall bluish cast
Dehydration to dryness	Color changes from bluish to violet to very deep purple in dehydrated or dry areas
Oiliness	Pinkish to orange dots in oily areas around the nose, chin, and forehead
Hyperpigmentation	Brownish to dark patches in cheeks, forehead, chin, etc., or where lesions have left marks
Hypopigmentation	White patches where pigmentation would normally show darker casts
Other skin disorders	Bright or neon yellow: • Bacteria such as herpes or fungi • Clients on a course of antibiotics or other drug therapy • Lipstick or other cosmetics

Figure 5-2 Woods lamp chart of indications.

Why It Works: Skin Sensor

A new breed of technology, typically called a **skin sensor,** is allowing estheticians to also analyze the elasticity of the skin and the sebum within it. An example of a skin sensor can be seen in Figure 5-5. This system can be combined with a video camera display and computer software that prints an analysis for your client. To measure elasticity in the skin, the sensor vibrates with an electrical **oscillation** frequency of approximately 50 kHz. The sensor head measures the change in frequency when the sensor is applied to the skin, and the oscillation frequency decreases. The frequency is then measured; the greater the change in frequency, the more elasticity in the skin. Figure 5-4 provides a visual on how this works.

Sebum measurement uses the concept of a **refractive index.** The sensor uses **photodiodes** to detect differences in how much reflection is received from the LED light. A greater reflection back to the photodiode indicates less sebum within the skin, and vice versa. Figure 5-6 shows a visual on how the sebum measurement works.

Another form of skin sensor is the **moisture meter.** This compact tool has been used by estheticians for years. This technology works by using an electrical **capacitance** system that uses electrical currents to measure the amount of water in the stratum corneum layer of the skin.

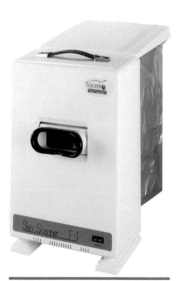

Figure 5-3 Equipro skin scanner.

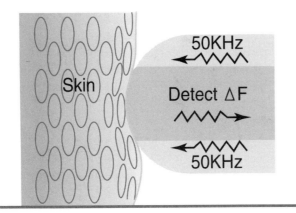

Figure 5-4 Elasticity measurement.

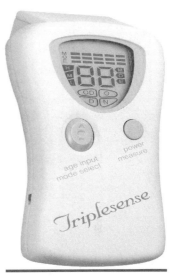

Figure 5-5 Triplesense courtesy of Moritex.

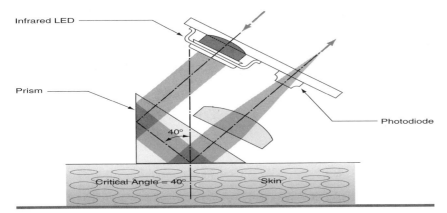

Figure 5-6 Sebum measurement.

The unit has **electrodes** that produce a positive and negative pole. A small electrical charge is sent to the skin and changes as it encounters water. The more moisture the skin has, the higher the reading on the sensor; this is shown as a number value on the face of the sensor. Instructions to interpret the moisture meter are different for each manufacturer.

Why It Works: Advanced Imaging System

Advanced imaging systems use multiple technologies to provide a complete analysis of the skin so the client can see, and so the esthetician can track results. These systems provide a consistent visual image by providing a structured location for the client to place his or her face. The high-resolution camera then takes a picture, which is transferred to a computer. Multiple angles of the face are available as well, and a filtered blacklight can also be used to provide a comprehensive view of the skin.

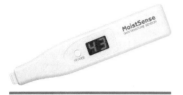

Figure 5-7 Visia complexion analysis system courtesy of Canfield Scientific Inc.

Some systems also use technology called **fluorescence spectroscopy.** Fluorescence spectroscopy measures the chemical properties of tissue by analyzing the intensity and character of light emitted in the form of fluorescence. Photons of light activate certain molecules within the cell, and the calming of the molecule releases fluorescence. The wavelength released is analyzed by the computer system, which then interprets the data and gives a comprehensive analysis.

These advanced analysis systems use computer software based on dermatological scales, comprehensive statistical models, and data on topical skin features. An advanced analysis system gives detailed readings on skin elasticity, moisture level, bacteria, Fitzpatrick skin type, wrinkle count, pigmentation, and skin texture. A client's information is put into the software and a personalized report is produced, but it is still up to the esthetician to be knowledgeable about treatments and products to educate the client. Figure 5-7 shows one analysis system.

HOW TO USE A WOODS LAMP

- Make sure that the client's skin is clean and free of makeup.
- The room must be very dark in order to fully see all the indications.
- Cover your client's eyes.
- Turn on the lamp and note all visual indications.

See Figure 5-8 for a guide to colors and skin type indications for a Woods lamp.

Color	Condition
white fluorescent	thick cornea layer
white spots	random horny layer and dead cells; dandruff
blue-white	normal healthy skin
purple fluorescent	thin skin, lacking moisture
light violet	dehydrated skin
bright fluorescent	hydrated skin
brown	sun damage
yellow	comedones

Figure 5-8 Woods lamp color indications.

How to Use a Skin Scope

- This can be used in many places, as long as the light is filtered out by the tent that covers the client's head.
- Clients do not need to cover their eyes but should be cautioned not to stare directly into the lights.
- Open one end and lock hinges into place.
- Turn on the scope.
- Have clients turn to face the blacklight.

How to Use a Skin Sensor and Moisture Meter

- This is a very manufacturer-dependent machine, which means that you must follow their directions.
- Clean your client's skin, then apply the sensor to the surface of the skin.
- You will need multiple readings throughout the area you are measuring to get an accurate analysis.
- Your manufacturer will have a specific set of instructions for interpreting the analysis.

■ HOW TO BUY

The Woods lamp and skin scope are very solid technical tools. It is always a good idea to buy from a reputable company. Typical price ranges on Woods lamp and skin scopes can be from $150 to $950. Skin sensors can run from $50 for a moisture meter to $500 for the basic elasticity meter. Advanced skin analysis systems can run from $1,500 up to $18,000 for a very sophisticated system with a video camera and computer software.

Make sure your equipment has a safety certification such as a UL listing or a CSA, CE, or ISO certification. UL, CSA, and CE listings indicate that the equipment has been tested for safety. ISO indicates that it has been manufactured per international standards and the manufacturer is tested twice a year.

Buyer's Checklist

- What is the price?
- Do you have an instruction manual, DVD, or on-site training?
- Is the machine UL listed, ISO certified, or CSA tested?
- Does it come with marketing materials?
- Can I buy replacement parts, and what is the price?
- What is the warranty?

TIP **Underwriters Laboratory** is the U.S. organization responsible for testing products for consumer safety. Many international products are not UL certified. Underwriters Laboratory has recently started an international section of certification. The alternative to UL listing is **CSA or CE certification.** The UL mark on a product tells you that the machine has been thoroughly tested and investigated by a team of product safety professionals.

■ SAFETY

- The skin analysis equipment that we have covered is inherently safe.
- Do not allow your client to stare into the blacklight.
- Make sure that any cords or plugs on your equipment are in good working order. No cracks or broken plugs should be evident.

■ MAINTENANCE

Maintenance is one of the most important aspects of owning esthetic machines. Manufacturers will also have their own protocols, so be sure to follow their directions. In general, use these guidelines:

- Use camera lens or eyewear cleaner to remove any dust and debris that have accumulated on the lens.
- Always wipe down the exterior of your skin scope or Woods lamp to remove fingerprints or product residue.
- With more technical equipment, follow your manufacturer's instructions.
- Blacklight bulbs break easily. Use caution transporting and changing bulbs in the Woods lamp and skin scanner.

■ DISINFECTION AND SANITIZATION

- Any part of your skin analysis equipment that the client is in contact with should be sprayed with an EPA-registered high-level disinfectant.
- When using a skin scope, pay attention to the inside of the scope, especially the fabric; spray high-level disinfectant, leave on for ten minutes, and wipe dry.
- Be careful to never spray the blacklight with any wet material.
- The skin sensor will have specific guidelines for you to use.

■ CONTRAINDICATIONS AND CAUTIONS

There are no contraindications for skin analysis equipment. Be aware that some clients have very strong reactions when seeing their skin under a skin scope for the first time.

■ PREPARATION FOR TREATMENT

- Have your client fill out an assessment form.
- Check for contraindications.
- For a normal facial treatment, have your client change into a treatment gown and remove all jewelry.
- When using a skin scope, have your client remain clothed and perform the analysis first.

■ PROTOCOLS

Skin Scope Event

To really educate your clients and sell additional products and services, try a skin scope event.

1. Set up your skin scope in a private area of your space.
2. Have the client cleanse his or her skin, you can offer a makeup application afterward.
3. If the client does not want to remove makeup, you can explain that he or she will not get a true visual of what is happening in the skin, only a good overview.
4. Use your Woods lamp chart and skin analysis sheet to give a detailed account of the photo damage, skin type, and skin condition.
5. Recommend treatments and products to correct the conditions that you can.

Your Protocol:

_____

_____

_____

_____

_____

_____

_____

_____

_____

_____

■ YOUR EQUIPMENT INFORMATION

Manufacturer info:

Name/phone number: _____

Web site: _____

Date purchased: _____   Registration: _____

Warranty info: _____

Replacement part info: _____

TROUBLESHOOTING

I cannot seem to get a good view of the different colors in the skin.

The room has too much light or you have a bulb that has burned out.

My light will not turn on.

Check all cords, and make sure the blacklight bulbs are secured in their sockets. Make sure your GCFI outlet has not been tripped.

All I see is one color (purple or blue) on the client's skin.

Your client has too much makeup on, or you have found the rare normal skin type (blue).

PROS AND CONS

What are the pros and cons of this equipment?

Pros

- Helps give you accurate information about your client's skin.
- Helps you proceed with the correct and safe treatment for your client.
- Can help you identify when a client has a possible fungus or bacteria.
- Woods lamps can be used on surfaces in your treatment room to illuminate areas that need to be cleaned.
- Increase sales of your products and services.
- Advanced analysis systems provide consistent visual information about the client's skin.
- Advanced analysis systems provide a concise written report for the client.
- Advanced analysis systems increase the professional image of the esthetician.

Cons

- Some new technology equipment is very expensive; thoughtfully weigh the impact on your business before purchasing.
- Requires additional training to interpret information.
- Blacklight bulbs are very expensive to replace, so make sure your equipment will be well taken care of.

REFERENCES

1. D'Angelo, J., Dean, P., Dietz, S., Hinds, C., Lees, M., Miller, E., & Zani, A. (2003). *Milady's Standard Comprehensive Training for Estheticians*. New York: Thomson Learning.
2. Lees, M. (2001). *Skin Care: Beyond the Basics*. New York: Thomson Delmar Learning.
3. Nordman, L. (2005). *Professional Beauty Therapy, The Official Guide to Level 3* (2nd ed.). London: Thomson Learning.
4. Simmons, J.V. (1989, 1995). *Science and the Beauty Business: The Beauty Salon and its Equipment* (2nd ed.). United Kingdom: Macmillan Press Ltd.

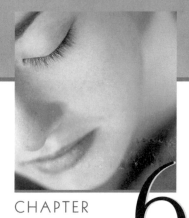

Treatment Bed and Chairs

CHAPTER **6**

A good treatment bed and **ergonomically** correct chair are mandatory for a successful esthetic practice. If you or your clients are uncomfortable during the treatment, it will impact how your business will grow. A client who is uncomfortable is unlikely to come back for further services. See Figure 6-1 for an example.

■ FUNCTIONS

The right treatment bed places your client in a comfortable and safe position during esthetic treatments. The chair provides the esthetician a comfortable and ergonomically correct position to perform the treatment.

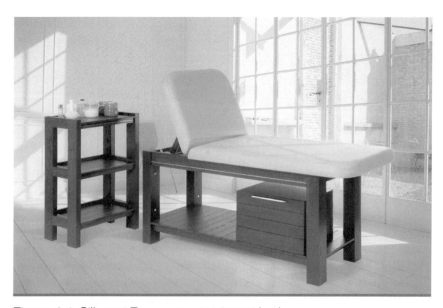

Figure 6-1 Silhouet-Tone soma treatment bed.

■ WHY THEY WORK

Treatment beds come in many shapes and sizes. Primarily, a treatment bed works by creating a soft, comfortable place for the esthetic client to lie on. Most esthetic treatment beds have movable parts for the head and legs. This allows for maximum comfort for the client and helps the esthetician perform various services.

■ HOW TO USE THEM

Use depends on the type of bed that you purchase. There are several options.

Hydraulic Bed

A hydraulic bed is a standard treatment bed placed on a hydraulic base that allows for height adjustment by pressing on the hydraulic lever at the bottom of the bed. The head and legs will generally have a manual adjustment.

When first placing your client on the bed, start at the lowest level with which the client feels comfortable as they lie on the bed, then pump the lever until the bed level is ergonomically correct and comfortable for you. Figure 6-2 shows a hydraulic bed.

Stationary Bed

A stationary bed can be made with a metal or wood frame. All adjustments for the head and legs are manual, and this bed also comes in a portable frame. Removable arms are generally included, but height adjustment is usually not available, unless you are using a bed with a manual adjustment. This system is usually created on a wooden frame.

When using a stationary bed, it is best to adjust the bed to the ergonomically correct height for the esthetician. If needed, a stool may be provided for the client to step up to the bed. If the bed is a standard metal frame esthetic bed, adjust the head and legs before you place your client on the bed. This is a manual adjustment and can be hard to make with the client lying on the bed. Figure 6-3 shows a stationary bed.

Electric Bed

An electric bed allows adjustment of the height, head, and leg position. These beds can come with or without removable arms and have some

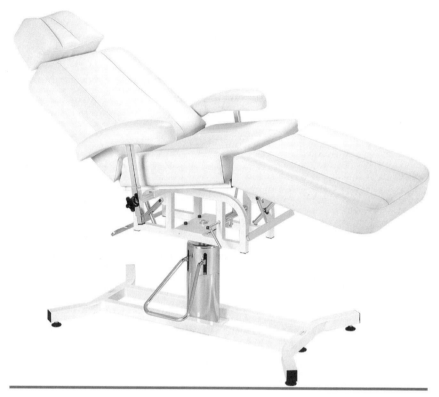

Figure 6-2 Equipro hydraulic bed.

very extensive styles. This bed is either created on a metal frame with wood paneling or made completely of metal. This is the ultimate bed for the esthetician, because it can accommodate any client, including those with disabilities. Figure 6-4 shows an electric bed.

To operate this bed, lower it to a comfortable height for the client, and have the client lie down; then raise the height, and adjust the head and legs by pushing the corresponding button on the control panel at the head of the bed.

Multipurpose Beds

Manufacturers are creating new multipurpose beds that lay flat for massage and body treatments and include a pedicure station and manicure trays. These beds come with many options, including electric adjustment. Figure 6-5 shows a multipurpose bed.

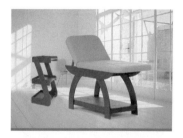

Figure 6-3 Sorisa stationary bed.

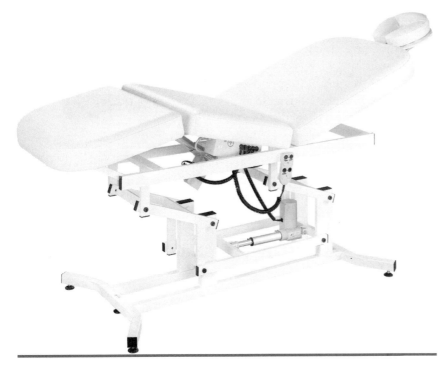

Figure 6-4 Equipro electric bed.

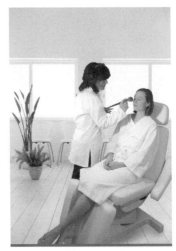

Figure 6-5 Silhouet-Tone Elite Platinum treatment bed.

■ ESTHETIC CHAIRS

The chair that you spend the majority of your time working on should be comfortable and ergonomically correct. A standard office task chair does not always work for long-term use. The size is usually too wide and has less range of motion than a chair made specifically for a treatment bed. You will spend more money for a treatment chair, but it is well worth it when you will spend many hours working on it; Figure 6-6 shows an example.

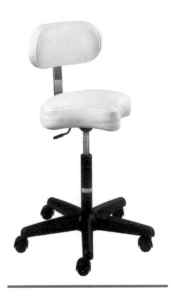

Stools

- Must have a height adjustment
- Must have a well-padded seat
- Must come with at least a two-year warranty
- Must be on movable wheels

See Figure 6-7 for an example of a stool.

Figure 6-6 Equipro technician chair.

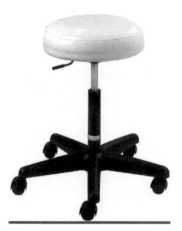

Figure 6-7 Equipro technician stool.

Chairs

- Must have an adjustable backrest or one that fits comfortably for your frame
- Must offer lumbar support
- Height must be adjustable
- Seat must be well-padded
- Should come with at least a two-year warranty

Both stools and chairs can come with a saddle seat, which is shaped like a bicycle seat. Some find it very comfortable, but it is not for everyone. Try to buy your chairs at a show or showroom, where you can sit on them to test them out for comfort, like you might test a mattress. This is definitely a personal comfort issue. If you are an owner buying chairs for staff, make sure you are able to adjust the chair and that it provides adequate back support.

■ HOW TO BUY

A bed is a very important purchase; a quality bed can be expected to last at least seven years. Beds range in price from $350 for a portable bed to $6,000 for an electric multipurpose bed. Comfort and quality are primary concerns, along with ergonomic safety for the technician. Make sure your bed can accommodate any size client, and get the correct weight load. A width of at least 28 inches is preferred for maximum comfort.

If your bed has electrical parts, make sure it has a safety certification, such as an Underwriters Laboratory (UL) listing, a CSA certification, or an International Standards Organization (ISO) certification. UL and CSA listings indicate that the equipment has been tested for safety. ISO certification indicates that it has been manufactured per international standards and that the manufacturer is tested twice a year.

A chair can range in price from $80 to $200, depending on the features with which the chair is equipped. For maximum comfort, look for a chair with a backrest and fully adjustable height. Some manufacturers can give you the option of additional padding in the seat, but all chairs should be on movable castors.

Buyer's Checklist

- What is the price?
- What are the shipping costs?
- Do you have an instruction manual or DVD?
- Is the bed UL listed, ISO certified, or CSA tested?

- Does it come with armrests, or are those sold separately?
- Can the armrests be removed?
- Can extra padding be added to the bed?
- What choices are there for color and covering?
- What is the bed frame made of?
- Is it a multipurpose bed? If so, which services can it accommodate?
- Can I buy replacement parts?
- Can my chair have additional padding placed in the seat?
- What height does the chair adjust to?
- Does the chair backrest adjust?
- Does the chair come in different color coverings?
- What is covered by the warranty, and for how long?

■ SAFETY

Safety concerns deal mainly with the safety of the client getting on and off the bed. Here are some tips:

- If your bed is not adjustable, have a steady stool that a shorter client can step on to get onto the bed.
- Always help your client on and off the bed.
- Make sure you know about any cardiovascular problems that could cause dizziness at the end of the treatment.
- Always check the components of your bed for wear and tear. Manual headrests and leg adjustments can wear over time, and electric beds can have shorts in the wiring.

The safety of an esthetic chair is dependent upon on how the esthetician uses it.

- Always check the castors to make sure they are in working order, and have locks on them if needed.
- Avoid using the chair or stool on a slippery, wet floor.
- Always use ergonomic practices while working to avoid repetitive stress injury. Figure 6-8 provides some simple ergonomic practices.

Back/Body Position	Hands	Arms
Support should be adjusted to fit up to middle of back. Body should be no more than 4 inches away from bed.	Should be at a 90-degree angle with elbows supported on bed.	The client's head should be on the same level as the esthetician's breastbone.

Figure 6-8 Ergonomics chart.

■ MAINTENANCE

Maintenance for a treatment bed is very easy. Manufacturers will also have their own protocols, so be sure to follow their directions. These general guidelines will get you started:

- Clean the covering of the bed daily; make sure the cleaner you use is compatible with the covering and will not discolor it.
- If you have a wood base, use a wood polish or cleaner on a monthly basis.
- Check electric cords and control panels.
- Never use a heating pad uncovered on a vinyl surface. This will cause the vinyl to dry out and crack.
- Essential oils will leave stains that cannot be removed, so be sure to use a cover or padding.

■ DISINFECTION AND SANITIZATION

- Disinfection is primarily applying a spray of EPA-approved high-level disinfectant solution to the surface of the bed or chair after each use.
- Wipe clean after the time specified by the manufacturer, then make the bed.
- Avoid the use of caustic substances such as ammonia, bleach, or scouring scrubs.
- If for some reason you have a blood spill on the surface, follow the OSHA blood spill procedure or one that is mandated by your state licensing board.

■ CONTRAINDICATIONS AND CAUTIONS

Using a treatment bed has no direct **contraindications,** but there are some cautions that relate to the health of your client. This is why the consultation is extremely important to determine contraindications or special needs that your client may have. Do not rely exclusively on the intake form; it is important to verbally get information and clarification from your client. Be aware of special considerations, including the following:

- Pregnancy: Make sure that your client is very comfortable at all times. You may need to purchase a bolster or support to allow the client to be placed safely on the bed.
- Heart problems: Make sure you assist your client on and off the bed; dizziness can occur, which could cause him or her to fall.
- Migraines, severe headaches: Make sure you have the correct neck support for the client. Sometimes tension in the neck and shoulder area can cause headaches.
- High or low blood pressure: Never leave a client with blood pressure issues alone on a treatment bed; help them on and off the bed.

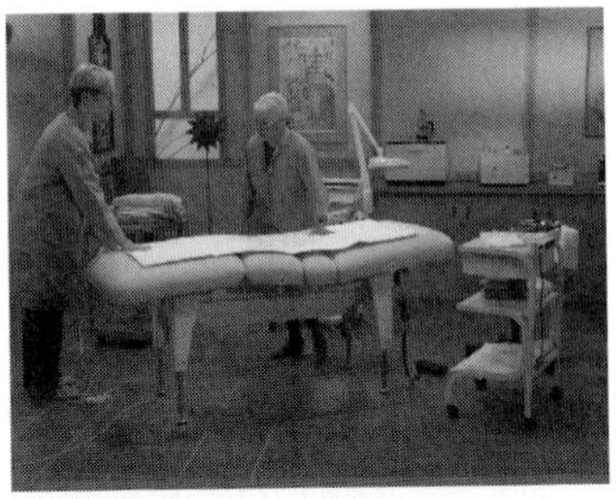

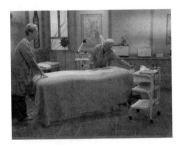

Figure 6-9a Bed warmer. Some look like a fitted sheet and cover the entire bed; others are more like large heating pads. They are found in the linen departments of many stores. In either case, a heat regulator dial sets the temperature from low to high. Purchase one that is made to place under the client. They range in price from moderate to the more elaborate ones made specifically for spa environments that have more water activity.

■ PREPARATION FOR TREATMENT

- Have your client fill out an assessment form.
- Check for contraindications.
- Have your client change into a treatment gown and remove all jewelry.

■ PROTOCOLS

This protocol for the treatment bed is based on setting up your bed for your client. You have two options. Both require that a twin fitted sheet be placed on the bed first.

The Cocoon Wrap

Step 1: Place a heated pad on the bed, then add a twin or double-size blanket. Lay the blanket horizontally if a double-size blanket or vertically if a twin. The head will not be on a twin blanket, so be sure to add a towel underneath the head.

Step 2: Place a flat sheet over the top of the blanket.

Step 3: Place a facial towel flat at head of bed.

Step 4: Place the client on the bed and wrap, starting with one side first then the other. The client should feel very secure but not claustrophobic. If the room is cold, place a comforter or blanket over the client. Figure 6-9a through Figure 6-9k show step-by-step pictures of a cocoon wrap.

Figure 6-9b Fitted sheet (twin size) and light blanket. The fitted sheet is optional, but if used, place it on top of the bed warmer. The light blanket is placed over the sheet and is used to keep the client warm.

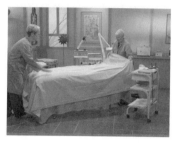

Figure 6-9c Flat sheet (twin size). Drape it over the blanket.

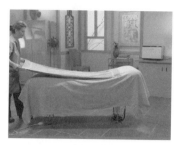

Figure 6-9d Hand towel. Terry or cotton towel. Place it at the top of the bed in the head/shoulder area.

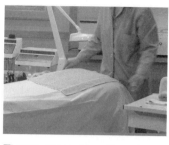

Figure 6-9e Headband. Position it on top of the towel.

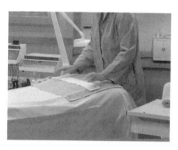

Figure 6-9f Cotton towel. Fold it in half diagonally so that there are two "points" at one side. Position the folded edge even with the bottom edge of the headband (points should be facing you).

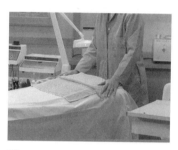

Figure 6-9g Help the client lie down, with the head centered on the wrap and the headband and the body centered on the bed.

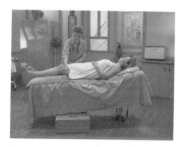

Figure 6-9h Wrap the head, drawing up each side of the towel, one side at a time.

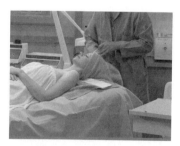

Figure 6-9i Hold the towel with one hand, bring up the headband and close it securely. Check to make sure that the client is comfortable and the head wrap is not too tight.

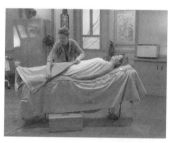

Figure 6-9j Bring up one side of the sheet and blanket, starting at the feet and legs, tapering the covering at the shoulder. Repeat with the other side.

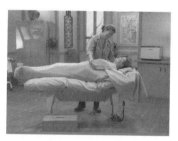

Figure 6-9k Tuck the blanket under the feet, and place a small hand towel at client's décolleté to protect the cocooned covering from spills.

Noncocoon Draping Setup

Step 1: Place a fitted twin-size sheet on the bed.
Step 2: Place a flat twin-size sheet on bed.
Step 3: Place a small facial towel flat at the head of the bed.
Step 4: Place a blanket over top, just like making a twin bed.
Step 5: Pull to one side to help the client get under the sheets.

Your Protocol:

_____

_____

_____

_____

_____

_____

■ YOUR EQUIPMENT INFORMATION

Manufacturer info:

Name/phone number: _____

Web site: _____

Date purchased: _____   Registration: _____

Warranty info: _____

Replacement parts info: _____

TROUBLESHOOTING

My electric bed will not move up and down.

Check all connections to the outlet; check all wires for possible shorts or disconnection. Check to see if you have a circuit breaker on the bed that has been tripped. If the problem is not one of these, contact the manufacturer.

My hydraulic bed is not moving.

Contact the manufacturer; hydraulics require a specialist.

The covering on my bed has been discolored.

Look at the type of surface disinfectant you are using and change it. Some disinfectants with citrus oil can stain lighter-colored beds. If it is dye from an application, like a lash tint, use the lash tint remover or acetone to gently remove it. When in doubt, call your manufacturer for their suggestions.

Q & A

What is the best type of bed to purchase?

That depends on your budget, whether you need a multipurpose bed, and any ergonomic requirements you may have.

The ideal bed is wide and thickly padded with a durable vinyl cover and can have the height, head, and legs adjusted with minimal effort. The rest is décor and depends on how you want the esthetic treatment room to look.

Are heating pads for the treatment beds mandatory?

No; they definitely are very comfortable to the client, but if you have a holistic care philosophy, then the electrical current may go against the healing philosophy due to the disruption of the body's own electrical currents.

REFERENCES

1. D'Angelo, J., Dean, P., Dietz, S., Hinds, C., Lees, M., Miller, E., & Zani, A. (2003). *Milady's Standard Comprehensive Training for Estheticians.* New York: Thomson Delmar Learning.
2. Simmons, J. V. (1989, 1995). *Science and the Beauty Business: The Beauty Salon and its Equipment* (2nd ed.). United Kingdom: Macmillan Press Ltd.
3. Lees, M. (2001). *Skin Care: Beyond the Basics.* New York: Thomson Delmar Learning.
4. Nordman, L. (2005). *Professional Beauty Therapy, The Official Guide to Level 3* (2nd ed.). London: Thomson Learning.

Wax Heaters

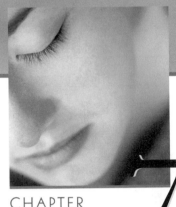

Waxing is one of the most profitable and widely requested esthetic services. It is important to have a high-quality wax heater that will heat the wax to the correct temperature on a consistent basis. It must be able to handle all types of wax, and it must have a temperature control in the 98.6 to 165 degree Fahrenheit range.

CHAPTER 7

■ FUNCTIONS

Heat all types of depilatory wax to correct temperatures. Figure 7-1 shows an example of a wax heater.

■ WHY IT WORKS

Wax heaters come in many shapes and sizes, but all utilize the same general technology. Most have a thermostatically controlled electrical heating

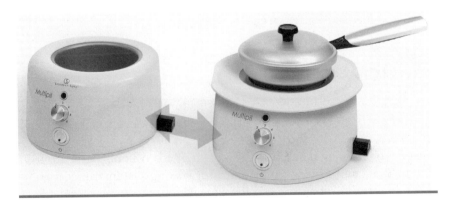

Figure 7-1 Silhouet-Tone wax pot.

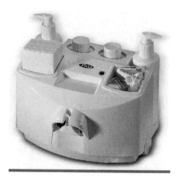

Figure 7-2 PHD waxing system.

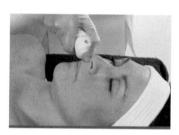

Figure 7-3 PHD lip wax.

element, but the design and use of each pot is generally proprietary to the manufacturer. All wax pots should have a range of temperature from 98.6 to 165 degrees Fahrenheit; the temperature an esthetician must use is based on the type of wax chosen.

Another alternative to warm wax is the disposable cartridge applicator system. Some systems are very advanced, and they have strict temperature controls and disposable applicators for each service; others are a gently warmed wax with a roller head attached. See Figure 7-2 and Figure 7-3 for some examples of waxing systems and products.

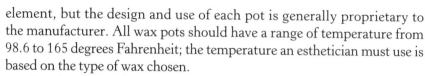

HOW TO USE IT

There are many different techniques to use for waxing, and advanced education in these techniques is always recommended. As far as wax pot use, here are a few suggestions:

- Turn wax on at the lowest temperature at least 15 minutes before your service; this will allow a gentle heating of your wax. Occasionally too much heat too fast can destroy the effectiveness of the wax. Follow the manufacturer's instructions closely.
- Adjust the temperature recommended by the wax manufacturer 2 to 5 minutes before applying.
- If you have a wax pot with an automatic thermostat, you can set the temperature and let it heat to the correct temperature.
- Make sure to remove the lid before heating.
- If you have a disposable applicator waxing system, follow heating directions closely. The heating chamber and holding chamber are separate, so you will heat the cartridge in one chamber, then move the wax applicator to the working chamber.
- Always wipe away any wax dripped from applicators as they happen or immediately after service.

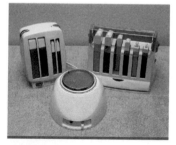

Figure 7-4 Cartridge applicator and wax pot.

HOW TO BUY

Purchase a waxing system from a manufacturer you can trust, and make sure they will be able to replace parts as needed. A wax pot will go through much wear and tear and could be replaced every two years, depending on who is using it and how it is maintained. Wax pots can run from $30 to $250, and a disposable applicator waxing system can cost about $200. Figure 7-4 shows some of the wide variety of wax pots available.

It is important to make sure your waxing equipment has a safety certification, such as an Underwriters Laboratory (UL) listing or a CSA or

International Standards Organization (ISO) certification. UL and CSA listings indicate that the equipment has been tested for safety. ISO certification indicates that the product was manufactured per international standards and that the manufacturer is tested twice a year.

Buyer's Checklist

- What is the price?
- Do you have an instruction manual, DVD, or on-site training?
- Is the machine UL listed, ISO certified, CE marked, or CSA tested?
- Does it come with accessories, or do those have to be purchased separately?
- Can I buy replacement parts?
- What does the warranty cover, and for how long?
- Does the wax pot have a wide temperature range?

■ SAFETY

There is much controversy regarding the safety of wax pots; the primary concerns are with cross-contamination and burns on the skin. For general safety follow these guidelines:

- Do not operate a wax pot with a damaged cord or plug.
- Do not use a wax pot if the thermostat is not working.
- Make sure your unit is properly grounded. Do not overload circuits.
- Keep cord away from heated surfaces.
- Always test the temperature on your wrist before applying wax to the client.
- Do not heat anything but wax in the pot.
- Do not use around an area that has aerosol sprays (for example, in the middle of a hair salon).

■ MAINTENANCE

Maintenance for a wax pot does require consistency and a good system of employing hygienic processes. The waxing area is one of the most overlooked areas of some treatment rooms. Manufacturers have their own protocols, so be sure to follow their directions. In general, follow these guidelines:

- Always clean any wax off of the surface of a wax pot immediately after the service.
- Use the manufacturer's recommended wax remover only.

- Do not allow wax to build up between the heating unit and the removable pot or in between the heating element and the edge of the pot.
- Check your thermostat once a month with an oven thermometer; use your manufacturer's guidelines for the correct range.
- Do not leave unused wax in the pot for a long time.
- Clean pot interior once a month.
- Never use water on your pot.

DISINFECTION AND SANITIZATION

Cross-contamination is a big concern with waxing services. It is very important to work clean when you are performing hair removal services. Here are some general guidelines:

- Always wear gloves when waxing. Blood, lymph, and biological debris will be removed during the service.
- Always clean the skin before applying wax.
- Do not double-dip; that is, do not use an applicator to apply wax over just-waxed skin and then dip that applicator back into the wax pot. This is controversial, although many estheticians feel that the wax pot heats up enough to kill bacteria.
- If using a sanitary wax system, make sure not to reuse the wax applicator on multiple clients.
- Use an EPA-registered high-level disinfectant to clean all surfaces after waxing.
- Put all waxing debris in a separate plastic bag before placing it in the garbage can.

CONTRAINDICATIONS AND CAUTIONS

The consultation is extremely important to determine contraindications or special needs that your client may have. Do not rely exclusively on the intake form; it is also important to verbally get information and clarification from your client. Be aware of the following:

- **Retin A** or **Accutane** use within the last year
- Exfoliation performed within 48 hours before waxing (includes microdermabrasion and chemical peels)

TIP Bacteria growth is influenced by pH, water content, and temperature. Bacteria will grow between 40 and 140 degrees Fahrenheit. Keep that in mind when deciding how to work clean.

- Pregnancy
- Skin inflammation that could be made worse
- Skin disorders or diseases that could be aggravated by treatment
- Very sensitive skin may make treatment uncomfortable for the client
- Nervous client: treatment will be ineffective if the client cannot relax
- Botox: no treatment until 72 hours after injection
- **Epilepsy**
- Cuts and **abrasions**
- Severe bruising
- Recent scar tissue: skin is very sensitive and less resistant
- **HIV**
- **Malignant melanoma:** treatment must be completed and client must be in remission. Obtain physician approval. Do not apply treatment when in doubt about a possible abnormality; instead, refer the client to a dermatologist.

■ PREPARATION FOR TREATMENT

- Have your client fill out an assessment form.
- Check for contraindications.
- Have your client change into a treatment gown and remove all jewelry.
- Clean skin of all dirt and oils.

■ PROTOCOLS

The protocol to use is determined primarily by the wax you use and the type of training you received. Here is an interesting leg-waxing protocol using the disposable applicator waxing system. Figure 7-5 shows an example of a leg wax.

Disposable Applicator Leg Wax

Step 1: Remove the applicator from the heating compartment.
Step 2: Remove the cap from the tube of wax; attach the applicator.

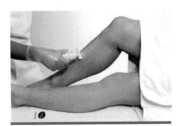

Figure 7-5 PHD leg wax

Step 3: Release the applicator by lifting the lever upwards. Squeeze until a small amount comes out; apply at a 45° angle.

Step 4: Glide slowly down the leg; repeat on the second leg.

Step 5: Press down to close the applicator lid and return it to the heating unit.

Step 6: Using cotton strips, remove wax starting at the ankle; work in small movements.

Step 7: Repeat on the other leg.

Step 8: Finish with soothing lotion.

Step 9: Remove the applicator from the wax tube and discard.

Basic Strip Brow Wax

Figures 7-6a through 7-6m provide a step-by-step illustration of a basic strip brow wax.

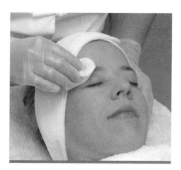

Figure 7-6a STEP 1: Clean area to be waxed.

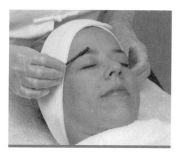

Figure 7-6b STEP 2: Gently comb hair with disposable mascara wand.

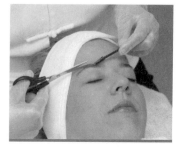

Figure 7-6c STEP 3: Trim hair.

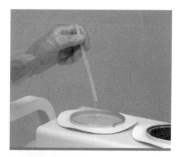

Figure 7-6d STEP 4: Stir wax and test on wrist before applying.

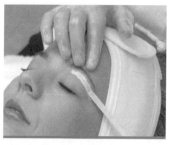

Figure 7-6e STEP 5: Apply wax against hair growth.

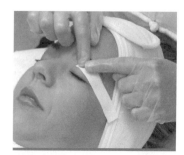

Figure 7-6f STEP 6: Apply strip.

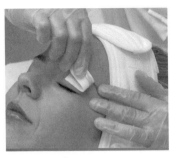

Figure 7-6g STEP 7: Remove strip.

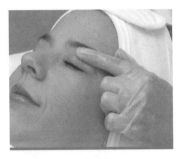

Figure 7-6h STEP 8: Place finger on brow to soothe skin.

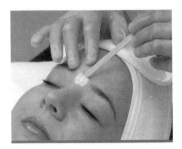

Figure 7-6i STEP 9: Apply wax to area between brows.

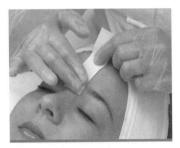

Figure 7-6j STEP 10: Apply strip.

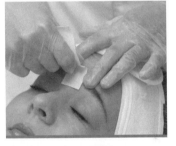

Figure 7-6k STEP 11: Remove strip and apply pressure.

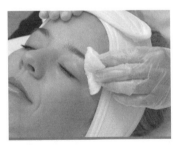

Figure 7-6l STEP 12: Clean area with post-waxing product.

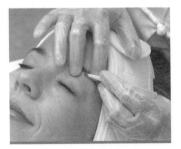

Figure 7-6m STEP 13: Tweeze any remaining hair.

Lip Wax

Hard wax is the best option for gentle hair removal.

Step 1: Clean the area to be waxed with a gentle cleanser.
Step 2: Test the wax on the inside of your wrist.

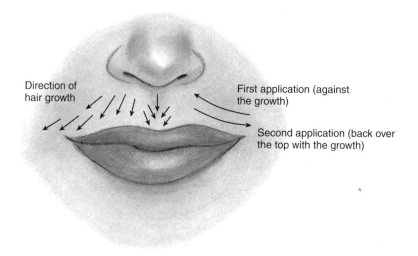

Direction of
hair growth

First application (against
the growth)

Second application (back over
the top with the growth)

Figure 7-7 Direction of application.

Step 3: Apply a thin layer in two directions:

1. Against the direction of hair growth.
2. With the direction of hair growth, as shown in the illustration in Figure 7-7.

Step 4: Pull the edge of the wax and remove against hair growth. Stay close to the skin, and do not lift up.

Step 5: Place your finger on the area to soothe skin.

Step 6: Clean the skin with a post-waxing product.

Your Protocol:

_____

_____

_____

_____

_____

_____

_____

_____

_____

■ YOUR EQUIPMENT INFORMATION

Manufacturer info:

Name/phone number: _____

Web site: _____

Date purchased: _____   Registration: _____

Warranty info: _____

Replacement parts info: _____

TROUBLESHOOTING

Troubleshooting of any waxing systems must be referred to the manufacturer. Risk to the client and esthetician is high when a thermostat is not working or any other electrical malfunction happens.

Q & A

What are the pros and cons of a general wax pot versus a disposable applicator system?

Wax Pot Pros

Effectiveness: A wax pot can be very effective; it has been the standard for many years.
Cost: Wax pots are cost-effective, and waxing is one of the most profitable services.
Ease of use: When personnel are trained, they will find wax pots easy to use.
Safety: Wax pots are safe when procedures are properly followed.

Wax Pot Cons

Training: Use requires minimum training and consistent practice.
Maintenance: Consistent and thorough cleaning is mandatory; cross-contamination can be a huge issue.

Disposable Applicator System Pros

Effectiveness: Systems are effective, but they require a learning curve; application is fast.

Ease of use: Systems are easy to use when personnel are properly trained.

Safety: Systems are safe when procedures are properly followed; no cross-contamination or burns should occur.

Disposable Applicator System Cons

Cost: Disposable applicator systems are more expensive than individual wax pots.

Training: Use does require minimum training and consistent practice.

Maintenance: Consistent and thorough cleaning is mandatory; applicators must be disposed of after each use.

Can I achieve results without a wax?

Only if you are performing hair removal with electrolysis or lasers.

Should I buy or lease a system?

This should be based on your financial situation. In general, a waxing system is such a small expenditure that a leasing company would not finance it unless it is grouped with other equipment.

Is less expensive better?

No. Try to buy from a distributor or manufacturer that is ISO certified or UL listed.

REFERENCES

1. Bickmore, H. (2004). *Milady's Hair Removal Techniques: A Comprehensive Manual.* New York: Thomson Delmar Learning.
2. D'Angelo, J., Dean, P., Dietz, S., Hinds, C., Lees, M., Miller, E., & Zani, A. (2003). *Milady's Standard Comprehensive Training for Estheticians.* New York: Thomson Delmar Learning.
3. Hill, P., & Bickmore, H. (2008). *Milady's Aesthetician Series: Advanced Hair Removal.* New York: Thomson Delmar Learning.
4. Lees, M. (2001). *Skin Care: Beyond the Basics.* New York: Thomson Delmar Learning.
5. Nordman, L. (2005). *Professional Beauty Therapy, The Official Guide to Level 3* (2nd ed.). London: Thomson Learning.

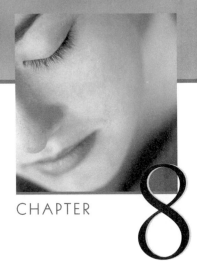

Steamer

The steamer is one of the most important pieces of equipment that the esthetician can own. It is the warmest of the four misting modalities that are used during professional treatments, which are shown in the chart in Figure 8-1. A professional facial is always enhanced by using a steamer, and regardless of your philosophy of skin care, you should incorporate a steamer into your practice.

CHAPTER 8

■ FUNCTIONS

Steaming dilates pores, increases microcirculation in the skin, softens the stratum corneum to facilitate product penetration and extraction of comedones, has an **antiseptic** effect on skin, keeps products moist,

Misting modality	Temperature	Used for
CO_2	Cool	Vasoconstriction, reduction of inflammation, soothing sensitive skin
Vac/spray	Warm–room temperature	Applying toners/fresheners, soothing irritated skin
Lucas spray	Warm–cool	Applying herbal and essential oils, vasodilation, vasoconstriction, calming irritated skin
Steamer	Hot	Vasodilation, facilitating deep cleansing, activating certain products, assisting in extraction

Figure 8-1 The four misting modalities.

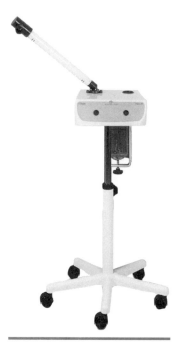

Figure 8-2 Sihouet-Tone steamer.

and is used to provide aromatherapy treatments. Figure 8-2 shows a steamer.

■ WHY IT WORKS

A steamer has a heating element that boils water to create steam, which builds pressure and moves through an arm attached to the unit. The warm mist softens the dead cells on the surface of the skin for easier exfoliation, and increases blood circulation by causing dilation of the blood vessels. This brings nutrients to the area being steamed and increases cell **metabolism**.

Steam penetrates into the hair follicle to soften sebum deposits for easier extraction of comedones and milia; it also activates certain products, such as **proteolytic enzyme peels** and some masks.

Ozone Steam

Most steamers have a switch that will turn on to generate ozone; this happens when steam passes over a UV blue light located within the steamer unit. The ozone generated is slight, but it will produce large, fluffy clouds of steam; this treatment is generally indicated for its antiseptic effects on the skin.

■ HOW TO USE IT

All machines come with manufacturer directions. Basic guidelines to remember are:

- Check that the seal between the water jar and the top of the steamer holder is secure and sealed.
- Pour **distilled water** through the top opening of the steamer.
- Fill to the red line indicated on the glass water jar.
- Turn steamer on; do not turn on the ozone generator until steam is actively moving through the arm. If you would like to add aromatherapy to your steamer, place the product on a coil of cotton and insert it in the opening of the nozzle head. Do not place the coil in the water.
- Place the steamer behind the client or to the side, and point the arm no closer than 16 inches from the client's face.
- Turn on the ozone generator if antiseptic effects are needed.
- Clean steamer at least monthly with vinegar or coffee pot cleaner to prevent blockage in the steamer arm.

TIP Thick, oily skin can tolerate steam application less than 16 inches from the face.

- Do not leave unused water in the steamer.
- Do not overfill.
- Do not use more than 15 minutes on skin; it can cause dehydration.
- Start steam before turning the nozzle toward the client's face.

▪ HOW TO BUY

Steamers can run from a very inexpensive $150 to approximately $1,000. The more expensive models have the option of putting aromatherapy oils directly into the water or offer a cool steam option. Look for models that have glass water holders; plastic can melt and leach chemicals into the water. Make sure that you can easily get replacement parts from your manufacturer or vendor.

Make sure your equipment has a safety certification such as a Underwriters Laboratory (UL) listing, Canadian Standards Association (CSA) or International Standards Organization (ISO) certification, or CE marking. UL and CSA listings indicate that the equipment has been tested for safety. ISO certification indicates that the item was manufactured per international standards and that the manufacturer is tested twice a year. Buying products that have been subjected to testing will help minimize the potential for fire hazards and short circuits in the heating element.

Use due diligence when purchasing an inexpensive steamer. Check with the Better Business Bureau in your area for information on your supplier, and try to see the equipment at a trade show or showroom first.

Buyer's Checklist

- What is the price?
- What are the shipping costs?
- Do you have an instruction manual, DVD, or on-site training?
- Is the machine UL listed, ISO certified, CE marked, or CSA certified?
- Can I buy replacement parts? If so, what are the costs?
- What does the warranty cover, and for how long?
- Can I have the steamer serviced if something happens?
- Where is the machine manufactured?
- Is the base height adjustable?
- Does the steamer allow for the use of essential oils?
- Does it have automatic safety features that shut off the machine if the water runs dry?

> **TIP** **Underwriters Laboratory** (UL) is the U.S. organization responsible for testing products for consumer safety. Many international products are not UL certified, although UL has recently started an international section of certification. The alternatives to UL listing are **CSA certification, CE Marking or International Standards Organization (ISO) certification.** The UL mark on a product tells you that the machine has been thoroughly tested and investigated by a team of product safety professionals.

■ SAFETY

The steamer can cause harm to you and your client if not properly maintained. Here are some guidelines to follow:

- Always check cords before plugging them into outlets.
- Never turn on the steamer without water in the jar.
- Do not let the water fall below the minimum fill line. A good steamer will have an automatic shutoff if the water level falls too low; many inexpensive ones do not have that option.
- Always check to make sure that the seal between the water jar and the steamer unit is in good condition and seals correctly when the jar is screwed in. If it does not, hot steam can boil over and drip out of the sides, which can result in a burn.
- Always make sure your steamer does not have a buildup of minerals, which appears as a white buildup on the heating element. This can mean that the steamer arm is also clogged, which can cause spitting of boiling water when the steamer is turned on.
- Always wait until the steamer has cooled down before filling the water jar. The glass will shatter or the plastic will crack if there is an extreme temperature difference.
- Never put aromatherapy oils directly in the steamer unless your manufacturer specifically allows it. Some oils can be volatile under heat and can lose their effectiveness.

■ MAINTENANCE

Maintenance is one of the most important aspects of owning esthetic machines. Manufacturers will also have their own protocols, so be sure to follow their directions. In general, follow these guidelines:

- Empty your steamer of any water after your last appointment and wipe out the water receptacle.
- Wipe down the arm and main unit with a high-level disinfectant or surface cleaner. It is easy to get a buildup of products on the arm, because you will often rotate the arm after applying products to the face.
- Clean your steamer once a month with vinegar and water; or if you dislike the smell, coffee pot cleaner works as well. Put the mixture into the distilled water and run the steamer until the water reaches the minimum level. Let cool, then wash the water receptacle and dry it.

TIP To clean your steamer with vinegar and water, fill the steamer to the maximum level and put 2 tablespoons of vinegar in the jar. Run the steamer without ozone for 5 minutes, let the steamer cool down, then empty the water jar and refill it with distilled water. Run the steamer until the water is too low to continue. Wait until the unit is cool, clean out water jar, and place the jar back in the steamer.

■ DISINFECTION AND SANITIZATION

Disinfection is very simple with a steamer. It is important to make sure that water is not left in a steamer for long periods of time without changing it. Warm water environments are very hospitable to bacteria.

- Wash down your unit with high-level disinfectant or surface cleaner to remove all product residues. Do not forget the knobs and base of the steamer.
- If you use cotton inside the steamer head for aromatherapy, make sure you dispose of it after use.
- Do not push down too hard when placing the steamer arm head back on; it can crack over time.

■ CONTRAINDICATIONS AND CAUTIONS

The consultation is extremely important to determine contraindications or special needs that your client may have. Do not rely exclusively on the intake form. It is also important to verbally get information and clarification from your client. Pay special attention to the following conditions:

- Pregnancy: Use caution when working with pregnant women. Their skin can be irritated very easily.
- Heart problems: Heat can make someone with a heart problem dizzy. Use caution.
- Skin inflammation: Most heat treatments increase circulation, which makes inflammation worse (e.g., it can cause rosacea to flare up). Use a Lucas spray instead.
- Skin disorders or diseases may be aggravated by treatment.
- Heat treatment on sensitive skin may be uncomfortable for clients.
- Nervous clients: Treatment will be ineffective if the client cannot relax.
- Epilepsy.
- Severe bruising can be uncomfortable for the client.
- High or low blood pressure could be made worse due to the increase in circulation. If it is treated and under control, use caution. Never leave a client with blood pressure issues alone, and always help them on and off the treatment bed.
- Malignant melanoma: Treatment must be completed and the client must be in remission. Obtain physician approval. Do not apply

treatment when in doubt about a possible abnormality; instead, refer the client to a dermatologist.

- Breathing problems, such as uncontrolled asthma and COPD: Check with your client as you apply steam. Never leave clients with breathing problems alone.
- Heat sensitivity.
- **Claustrophobia**.

■ PREPARATION FOR TREATMENT

The steamer is rarely a treatment by itself; it is usually combined with other modalities.

- Have your client fill out an assessment form.
- Check for contraindications.
- Have your client change into a treatment gown and remove all jewelry.
- Make sure the water receptacle is filled with distilled water.
- Turn on the machine a few minutes before use. It can take some time for the heating coil to boil the water.

■ PROTOCOLS

Enzyme Mask Application

Step 1: Perform a first and second cleanse on the skin.
Step 2: Apply enzyme exfoliant or other mask.
Step 3: Place eye pads over the client's eyes.
Step 4: Turn steam on and position the steamer arm over the client's face.
Step 5: Let steam penetrate for the time interval indicated by the skin product manufacturer's instructions. Treatment should last no more than about 15 minutes.
Step 6: Proceed with your product manufacturer's protocol.

See Figure 8-3 for an example of steam application.

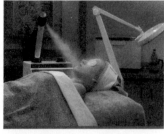

Figure 8-3 The steamer helps to provide stimulation for circulation in the face as well as softens sebum and other debris.

Basic Facial

Step 1: Look at the skin through a magnifying lamp for initial skin analysis.
Step 2: Remove makeup with appropriate makeup remover.
Step 3: Cleanse skin with appropriate cleanser.

Step 4: Remove cleanser with sponges or a warm towel.

Step 5: Apply toner.

Step 6: Perform a skin analysis with a magnifying lamp and Woods lamp. Turn steamer on.

Step 7: Apply exfoliant and steam 10 to 15 minutes, depending on manufacturer instructions.

Optional Step: Use a brush machine under steam for a deep cleanse.

Step 8: Remove exfoliant with sponges or a warm towel.

Step 9: Massage the skin for 15 to 20 minutes.

Step 10: Apply appropriate mask.

Step 11: After 10 minutes, remove the mask with a warm towel or sponges. Follow the manufacturer's directions.

Step 12: Apply toner, appropriate moisturizer, and sunscreen.

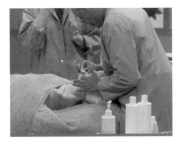

Figure 8-4a Remove makeup.

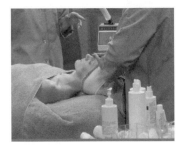

Figure 8-4b Cleanse face.

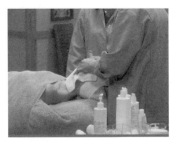

Figure 8-4c Remove cleanser with towel or sponges.

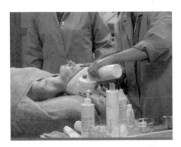

Figure 8-4d Apply toner.

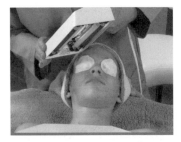

Figure 8-4e Perform skin analysis.

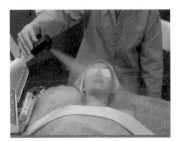

Figure 8-4f Apply steam.

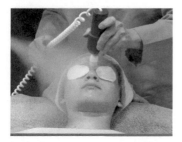

Figure 8-4g Optional step.

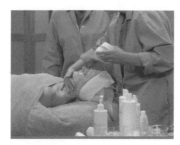

Figure 8-4h Remove exfoliant.

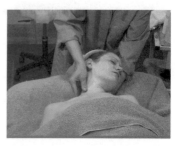

Figure 8-4i Massage.

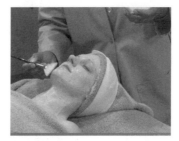

Figure 8-4j Apply mask.

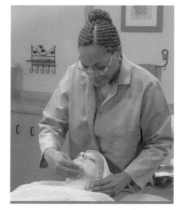

Figure 8-4k Remove mask.

Your Protocol:

_____

_____

_____

_____

■ YOUR EQUIPMENT INFORMATION

Manufacturer info:

Name/phone number: _____

Web site: _____

Date purchased: _____   Registration: _____

Warranty info: _____

Replacement parts info: _____

TROUBLESHOOTING

Steamer will not turn on.

Check to see that the outlet the steamer is plugged into has not been tripped. Usually there is a small button or a fuse located on the underside of the steamer that you can push to reset the electrical circuit if the mechanism has been tripped; this can happen when the automatic safety shutoff is triggered (when the water gets too low).

Hot water is dripping from the bottom of the machine.

Check that the seal between the water receptacle and the unit is completely secure. Check to see if there are any cracks or damage to the seal.

Machine is spitting hot water.

Run a deep clean though the steamer. Check to see that the steamer arm head is not cracked.

Q & A

What are the pros and cons of steamer equipment?

Pros

Effectiveness: Steamers are very effective and are an important part of the professional facial. You cannot perform a thorough and safe extraction without one.
Cost: A steamer is a cost-effective and inexpensive machine.
Ease of use: A steamer is very easy to use.
Safety: Normally, steamers are safe machines, but safety issues can happen with a poorly maintained steamer or a non–UL listed machine.

Cons

Maintenance: A steamer requires consistent and thorough cleaning to avoid any safety issues.
Broad Use: Not all clients can tolerate steam. It is good to have alternate misting systems, such as a Lucas spray or vacuum spray unit.

Can I achieve results without steam equipment?

You can use alternate forms of misting or hot towels, but you will not get the same results as you would with a steamer, especially when trying to perform extractions.

Should I buy or lease?

This decision must be based on your financial situation. In general, a single steamer unit is so inexpensive that a leasing company would not finance it unless it is grouped with other equipment.

Can a steamer make a difference in my practice?

Yes. The steamer is an easy tool to use. If you plan to perform extractions or a removal of comedones, it will make it much easier.

Is less expensive better?

No. Your steamer will go through many hours of use and will wear out quickly if poorly made. If you find a very good bargain steamer, make sure that it is UL or CE listed for electrical safety. It is fine to start with a less expensive model, but realize you will need to replace it sooner.

REFERENCES

1. D'Angelo, J., Dean, P., Dietz, S., Hinds, C., Lees, M., Miller, E., & Zani, A. (2003). *Milady's Standard Comprehensive Training for Estheticians.* New York: Thomson Delmar Learning.
2. Simmons, J. V. (1989, 1995). *Science and the Beauty Business: The Beauty Salon and its Equipment* (2nd ed.). United Kingdom: Macmillan Press Ltd.
3. Lees, M. (2001). *Skin Care: Beyond the Basics.* New York: Thomson Delmar Learning.
4. Nordman, L. (2005). *Professional Beauty Therapy, The Official Guide to Level 3* (2nd ed.). London: Thomson Learning.
5. Nordman, L. (2004). *Beauty Therapy, The Official Guide to Level 2* (3rd ed.). London: Thomson Learning.
6. Gerson, J. (2004). *Milady's Standard Fundamentals for Estheticians.* New York: Thomson Delmar Learning.

Optional Equipment

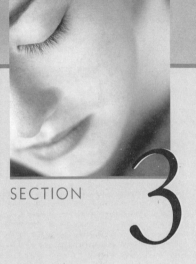

SECTION

3

Hot Cabinet

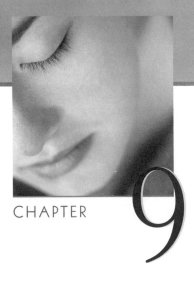

The hot cabinet is commonly called the **hot cabi.** It is used to heat wet towels that remove products from the skin, and also to heat products to apply to the skin. The hot cabinet is an essential piece of esthetic equipment.

CHAPTER 9

■ FUNCTIONS

To heat wet towels to a comfortable temperature to remove masks, cleansers, product residue, and to warm masks and massage creams before application. Figure 9-1 shows an example of a hot cabinet.

■ WHY IT WORKS

The hot cabinet uses an electrical heating element within the unit that can be thermostatically controlled. Electricity flows to the heating element, and the interior of the cabinet heats up by **conduction**. Most hot cabinets have a range of temperature from 135 to 175 degrees Fahrenheit. The units that have a higher temperature, closer to 175°F, have a switch that can be set at 135 degrees or 175 degrees Fahrenheit. A basic hot cabinet has one switch, generally set at 145 degrees, and can hold up to 24 towels. Some hot cabinets have a UV light built in to control bacteria growth, and a double compartment to hold up to 48 towels.

■ HOW TO USE IT

- Turn the unit on. If using a single thermostat control, turn the cabinet on at least 30 minutes prior to service.
- Wet several towels with warm water.

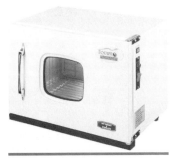

Figure 9-1 Equipro hot cabinet.

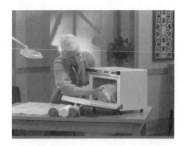

Figure 9-2 Hot cabi use.

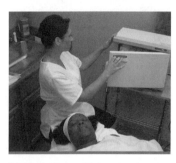

Figure 9-3a Take the hot towel out of the hot cabi.

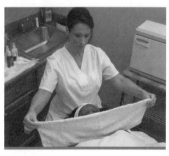

Figure 9-3b Shake out the towel and place it under the chin.

- Roll up the towels and place them in hot cabinet.
- Remove as needed.

Figures 9-2 through 9-3d show an example of step-by-step hot towel use.

HOW TO BUY

Hot cabinets are relatively inexpensive but do not last as long as other pieces of equipment. It is important to make sure your equipment has a safety certification, such as a UL listing or a CSA or ISO certification. UL and CSA listings indicate that the equipment has been tested for safety. ISO indicates that it has been manufactured per international standards and that the manufacturer is tested twice a year.

Buyer's Checklist

- What is the price?
- Do you have an instruction manual or DVD?
- Is the machine UL listed, ISO certified, CE marked, or CSA tested?
- Does the unit come with a UV sanitizer bulb?
- Can I buy replacement parts?
- What does the warranty cover, and for how long?
- Where is the product manufactured?
- Does the unit have a dual temperature switch?

SAFETY

The hot cabinet is a safe machine to use as long as all electrical parts are functioning correctly. Here are some general guidelines:

- Check the cord for any cracks or deterioration.
- Check the plug for missing prongs, unusual wear, or damage.
- Always plug in to a grounded outlet.
- Make sure there are no cracks in the exterior or interior of the cabinet.

MAINTENANCE

Maintenance for a hot cabinet is very easy. Manufacturers will also have their own protocols, so be sure to follow their directions. In general, use these guidelines:

- Always disinfect with an EPA-approved high-level disinfectant at the end of the day.
- Wipe out the cabinet completely. Rust and minerals can build up if not properly cleaned out.
- Empty the moisture overflow tray daily. Mold can grow in the tray.
- Do not leave the cabinet on overnight.
- Wipe down the exterior of the cabinet at the end of the day. Products can be transferred from your hands to the exterior of the cabinet and build up.

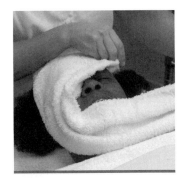

Figure 9-3c Wrap one end of the towel to the forehead.

■ DISINFECTION AND SANITIZATION

- Clean out the interior of your hot cabinet daily.
- Spray with an EPA-approved high-level disinfectant.
- Leave the disinfectant on the surface for 10 minutes or as directed by the manufacturer.
- Wipe dry.
- Change the UV bulb when it burns out. Each bulb has approximately 6,000 hours of use.

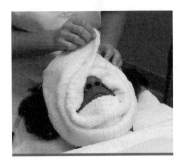

Figure 9-3d Leave the towel on the client, then remove product starting at forehead.

■ CONTRAINDICATIONS AND CAUTIONS

There are no contraindications for the use of the hot cabinet, just general cautions regarding your client's health concerns. The consultation is extremely important to determine contraindications or special needs that your client may have. Do not rely exclusively on the intake form; it is important to verbally get information and clarification from your client. Be on the lookout for these specific conditions:

- Heart problems: Heat can cause dizziness. Use caution.
- Skin inflammation: Most heat treatments increase circulation, which makes inflammation worse.
- Skin disorders or diseases may be aggravated by treatment.
- Sensitive skin may make treatment uncomfortable for the client.
- Claustrophobia: A client can feel smothered by the hot towel.
- Cuts and abrasions: Do not perform facial treatments on open cuts.
- Severe bruising can be uncomfortable for a client.
- High or low blood pressure could be made worse due to the increase in circulation. Even if it is treated and under control, use caution. Never leave a client with blood pressure issues alone, and always help them on and off the treatment bed.

- HIV.
- Malignant melanoma: Treatment must be completed and the client must be in remission. Obtain physician approval. Do not apply treatment when in doubt about a possible abnormality; instead, refer the client to a dermatologist.

■ PREPARATION FOR TREATMENT

- Have your client fill out an assessment form.
- Check for contraindications.
- Have your client change into a treatment gown and remove all jewelry.

■ PROTOCOLS

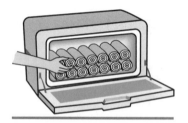

Figure 9-4 Step 1.

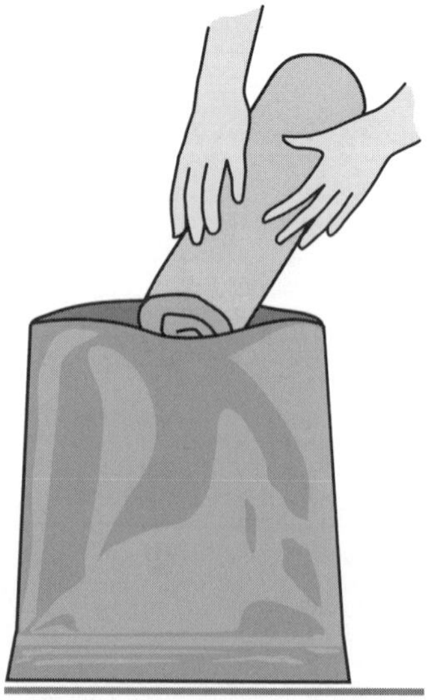

Here is a simple protocol for aromatherapy-infused towels. Clients appreciate the added sensory experience.

Aromatherapy Hot Towels

Step 1: Fill sink with hot water.
Step 2: Place up to six drops of lavender essential oil into the water.
Step 3: Place towels in the sink.
Step 4: Pull the sink plug and let water drain out.
Step 5: Roll towels up and place them in the hot cabinet.

Hot Towel Neck Roll

Figure 9-4 through Figure 9-8 illustrate this protocol step-by-step.

Step 1: Remove towel from the hot cabinet just before applying a facial mask.
Step 2: Place the towel in the plastic bag used for paraffin hand dips.
Step 3: Wrap a dry towel around the plastic bag.
Step 4: Place a towel under the client's neck.
Step 5: Remove the towel from under the client's neck when the mask time is finished.
Step 6: The towel will be cooled down enough to use it to remove the mask.

Figure 9-5 Step 2.

Your Protocol:

_____

_____

_____

_____

_____

_____

_____

_____

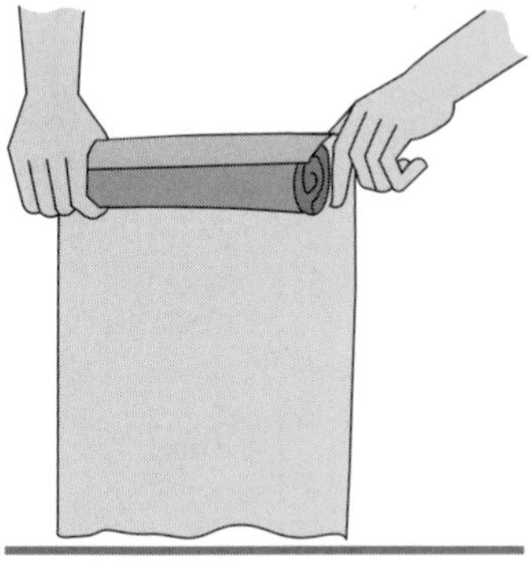

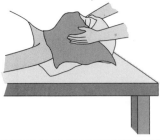

Figure 9-6 Step 3.

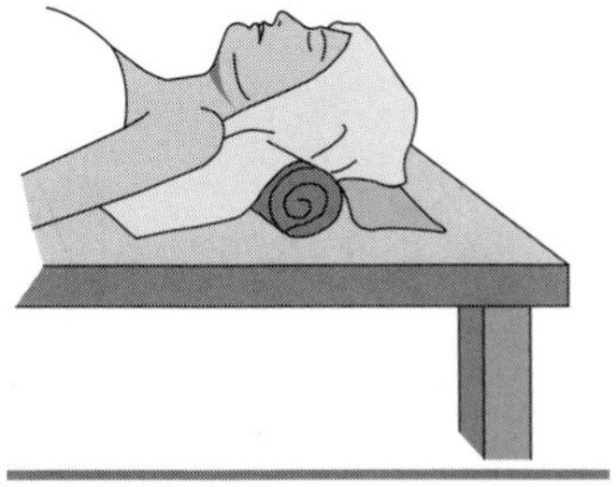

■ YOUR EQUIPMENT INFORMATION

Manufacturer info:

Name/phone number: _____

Web site: _____

Figure 9-7 Step 4.

Date purchased: _____   Registration: _____

Warranty info: _____

Replacement parts info: _____

TROUBLESHOOTING

Troubleshooting a hot cabinet should be referred to your manufacturer due to the sensitive nature of the thermostat. It is very important to maintain the correct temperature within a hot cabinet; incorrect temperatures can lead to a burn or growth of bacteria.

Figure 9-8 Step 5.

Q & A

What are the pros and cons of a hot cabinet?

Pros

Effectiveness: A hot cabinet is very effective for heating towels to a safe temperature.
Ease of use: A hot cabinet is easy to use.
Safety: Hot cabinets are safe when used properly

Cons

Cost: Hot cabinets can be expensive, depending on the model you buy.
Maintenance: A hot cabinet requires consistent and thorough cleaning to prolong the life of unit, and term of use is shorter than many pieces of esthetic equipment.

Can I achieve results without a hot cabinet?

No. Many people have adopted the habit of using a slow cooker to heat towels. This does not provide a controlled, safe temperature; generally, towels get too hot and can burn the technician during removal.

REFERENCES

1. D'Angelo, J., Dean, P., Dietz, S., Hinds, C., Lees, M., Miller, E., & Zani, A. (2003). *Milady's Standard Comprehensive Training for Estheticians.* New York: Thomson Delmar Learning.
2. Lees, M. (2001). *Skin Care: Beyond the Basics.* New York: Thomson Delmar Learning.
3. Nordman, L. (2005). *Professional Beauty Therapy, The Official Guide to Level 3* (2nd ed.). London: Thomson Learning.
4. Simmons, J. V. (1989, 1995). *Science and the Beauty Business: The Beauty Salon and its Equipment* (2nd ed.). United Kingdom: Macmillan Press Ltd.

Brush Machine

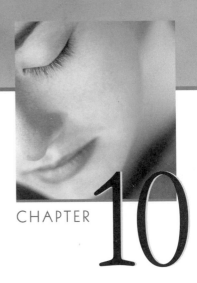

The brush machine is a wonderful way to give a gentle deep cleansing to the skin. It is usually used during the second cleanse and provides a manual exfoliation, which is very important for the health of the skin. It is one of the basic pieces of equipment that can add to the esthetician's professional facial. See Figure 10-1 for an example of a brush machine.

▪ FUNCTIONS

A brush machine provides a manual exfoliation of the stratum corneum, increases microcirculation in the skin, and helps deep cleanse the skin.

▪ WHY IT WORKS

The brush machine works by an electrical circuit attached to a motor, which creates the energy to move the brush attachment in a circular pattern. The speed of the oscillation can be adjusted by a control on the front of the machine.

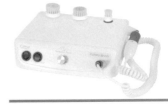

Figure 10-1 Silhouet-Tone brush machine.

Some exciting new technology uses sonic vibration to cleanse the skin: a brush that works on the same principle as the sonic toothbrushes that many of us use. The brush creates a very high oscillation in a back-and-forth movement, which dislodges debris at a deeper level within the skin. This is different than ultrasound, which we will go into later. See Figure 10-2 for a picture of a sonic brush.

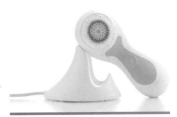

Figure 10-2 Clarisonic brush machine.

▪ HOW TO USE IT

The brush machine is easy to use: the secret is to choose the correct texture of brush for the skin type you are working on. For example, if you

TIP Try to purchase a natural bristle brush for a mechanical brush machine; synthetic can create too much friction on the skin.

are using a stiff bristle brush, it will not be the best choice for sensitive skin. This is the same with the sonic technology.

To use a mechanical brush machine, here are some guidelines:

- Always cleanse the skin first and perform an accurate skin analysis.
- Choose the correct attachment based on skin type and condition. For example, a large, stiff brush would be used for a body treatment, and a small sponge attachment would be fine for sensitive skin.
- Apply a gel cleanser; wet the brush and start at the forehead on the lowest setting. If the skin can tolerate the speed, proceed with one pass over the face.
- Turn up the speed slightly and continue with a second pass. Do not forget the neck and décolleté.
- Do not use longer than 5 minutes.
- You can also perform this with your steam on at the same time.

To Use a Sonic Brush

See Figure 10-3 for a chart of how to use a sonic brush.

- Perform your first cleanse and analysis.
- Choose the correct brush attachment.
- Any cleanser can be used with this technology; it is very gentle.
- You will have specific manufacturer instructions for speed and duration. In general, three ascending beeps indicate a high oscillation, three descending beeps indicate normal, and two beeps indicate normal speed.
- Start with normal speed for the first two minutes, unless the client has very thick, coarse skin. Treatment should last about four minutes.

Step 1	Cleanse skin and perform skin analysis
Step 2	Pick correct attachment: small brush (face), large brush (body treatment), sponge (sensitive skin)
Step 3	Apply cleanser
Step 4	Wet brush; put in handle
Step 5	Place on forehead
Step 6	Turn on low; turn up as skin tolerates
Step 7	Move in circular motion over face and décolleté

Figure 10-3 How to use a sonic brush.

■ HOW TO BUY

The brush machine should be bought from a reputable vendor or manufacturer, and you should have the option of natural bristle brushes. These units can run from $150 to $400 for a digital model.

You should have several attachments that come with the unit:

- A large body brush
- A medium facial brush
- A small facial brush
- One or two sponge attachments

The sonic brush is self-contained and comes with two different brush attachments with normal and sensitive bristles. You can purchase a stronger brush head in addition to these. It does not use the same round oscillations as the mechanical brush, so synthetic brush heads are fine. A sonic system costs around $80, but it is also meant to be sold to your clients at a list price of $195.

Make sure your equipment has a safety certification, such as an Underwriters Laboratory (UL) listing or CSA or ISO certification. UL and CSA listings indicate that the equipment has been tested for safety. ISO certification indicates that a product has been manufactured per international standards and that the manufacturer is tested twice a year. See Figure 10-4 for a chart of features to look for.

Buyer's Checklist

- What is the price?
- Do you have an instruction manual or DVD?
- Is the machine UL listed, ISO certified, CE marked, or CSA tested?
- Does the brush machine have at least three adjustable speeds?
- What brush attachments come with the machine?
- Can I buy replacement parts?
- What are the prices of parts and additional attachments?
- What does the warranty cover, and for how long?
- If the machine breaks, who will service it?

Brush machine	
	Multiple brush heads
	Variable speed
	Comfortable handle
	UL listed

Figure 10-4 Features to look for.

■ SAFETY

Safety for a mechanical brush machine is primarily concerned with electrical safety. Make sure that the electrical cords, plugs, and circuitry are in good working order. Make sure that your brush attachments are fully inserted into the brush handle, and never submerge your brush handle in water when it is plugged in. Do not overload circuits with all of your other equipment, and use a good surge protector.

■ MAINTENANCE

Maintenance is one of the most important aspects of owning esthetic machines. Manufacturers will also have their own protocols, so be sure to follow their directions. In general, follow these guidelines:

- Always unplug your machine when not in use.
- Brush attachments should not be stored in a UV sanitizer or inserted into the brush handle.
- Wipe down the equipment when you are done with each service. Product will leave a dry buildup on the surface, making it sticky and unsightly.
- Do not store your brushes with the bristles down.
- Follow the manufacturer's instructions for recharging if you are using a sonic brush.
- Never leave your brush heads in wet disinfectant overnight.
- Do not use a manual exfoliant with a brush attachment; you can only use a manual exfoliant with a sponge attachment.

■ DISINFECTION AND SANITIZATION

See Figure 10-5 for a chart of disinfection and maintenance. Here are some general guidelines:

- Always wash your brush attachments in soap and water.
- Remove them from the soapy water, rinse well, and pat dry.
- Store in a closed container with the bristles up.
- UV sanitizer can be used to help dry brush attachments, but do not leave them in liquids for more than 30 minutes. Over time, the bristles will yellow.

Disinfection	Maintenance
Wash & rinse attachments	Do not store in UV sanitizer
Soak in EPA-approved high-level disinfectant 15 minutes (per manufacturer's directions)	Wipe down equipment when done
Dry and place in closed container; store upright if possible	Do not store with brush bristles down or leave in high-level disinfectant overnight

Figure 10-5 Disinfection and maintenance steps.

CONTRAINDICATIONS AND CAUTIONS

The consultation is extremely important to determine contraindications or special needs that your client may have. Do not rely exclusively on the intake form. It is also important to verbally get information and clarification from your client. Pay special attention to clients with the following conditions:

- Pregnancy.
- Skin inflammation: Most mechanical exfoliation treatments increase circulation, which can make inflammation worse.
- Skin disorders or diseases may be aggravated by treatment.
- Treatments on sensitive skin may be uncomfortable for a client.
- Nervous clients: Treatment will be ineffective if the client cannot relax.
- Botox: No treatment until 72 hours after injection.
- Cuts and abrasions: Electrical current will concentrate in the area, because bodily fluids act as a conductor.
- Severe bruising will most likely be uncomfortable for the client.
- Recent scar tissue: Recently scarred skin is very sensitive and less resistant, so use caution when using electrotherapy. High frequency is okay when used six weeks after injury or surgery, if there is no pulling of the skin.
- HIV.
- Malignant melanoma: Treatment must be completed and the client must be in remission. Obtain physician approval. Do not apply treatment when in doubt about a possible abnormality; instead, refer the client to a dermatologist.

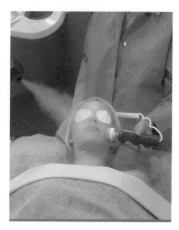

Figure 10-6 Mechanical brush application.

▪ PREPARATION FOR TREATMENT

- Have your client fill out an assessment form.
- Check for contraindications.
- Have your client change into a treatment gown and remove all jewelry.
- Cleanse skin and perform an accurate skin analysis.

▪ PROTOCOLS

Listed below is a basic manual exfoliation with steam that can be used with most brush machines.

Manual Exfoliation with Brush Machine and Steam

Step 1: Cleanse skin and remove cleanser.

Step 2: Choose appropriate brush attachment; turn on steamer.

Step 3: Apply gel cleanser.

Step 4: Wet brush attachment, and start at the forehead with a gentle speed while steam starts on the skin.

Step 5: Continue throughout the face, working towards the neck and décolleté.

Step 6: Repeat again if needed.

Step 7: Remove cleanser and proceed with balance of treatment.

Your Protocol:

_____

_____

_____

_____

_____

_____

_____

_____

_____

_____

■ YOUR EQUIPMENT INFORMATION

Manufacturer info:

Name/phone number: _____

Web site: _____

Date purchased: _____ Registration: _____

Warranty info: _____

Replacement parts info: _____

TROUBLESHOOTING

My brush attachments have gotten yellow and matted in the center.

The brush attachments have been stored bristle-side down or in a UV sanitizer for too long. They need to be replaced.

My brush attachment will not stay in the brush handle.

The attachment connector may be worn down, or you may not be pushing the attachment into the handle with enough force. Make sure you feel a click when you push it in. Run it before it touches the client's face. Sonic brushes have a specific way that the head must be placed on, so you will have to refer to the manufacturer for their directions.

Q & A

What are the pros and cons of brush machines?

Pros

Effective results: These machines provide safe and effective manual exfoliation.
Cost: Brush machines are inexpensive to purchase.
Ease of use: They are easy to use.

Cons

High-maintenance: The machine must be wiped down after every service, and brush attachments must be maintained well.
Client discomfort: Some clients with sensitivity find the brush attachments too rough. Sonic may be a good alternative to them, except for clients with a tactile sensitivity.

Client contraindications: Brushes are not for use on all clients. A thorough client intake form must be completed and reviewed prior to treatment.

REFERENCES

1. D'Angelo, J., Dean, P., Dietz, S., Hinds, C., Lees, M., Miller, E., & Zani, A. (2003). *Milady's Standard Comprehensive Training for Estheticians.* New York: Thomson Delmar Learning.
2. Lees, M. (2001). *Skin Care: Beyond the Basics.* New York: Thomson Delmar Learning.
3. Nordman, L. (2005). *Professional Beauty Therapy, The Official Guide to Level 3* (2nd ed.). London: Thomson Learning.
4. Simmons, J. V. (1989, 1995). *Science and the Beauty Business; The Beauty Salon and Its Equipment* (2nd ed.). United Kingdom: Macmillan Press Ltd.

Disinfection and Sanitization Machines

Disinfection is a mandatory step required by every state board. It protects clients, as well as the esthetician, from disease. Disinfection is a very important part of keeping everyone in the spa, salon, or medi-spa healthy and protected. In this chapter we will look at the autoclave, bead sterilizer, UV sanitizer, and ultrasonic cleaner, and we will cover the basic principles of disinfection and sanitization.

CHAPTER 11

■ FUNCTIONS

Disinfect or sanitize any implements that come in contact with a client and are not discarded after each service.

■ WHY SANITIZE?

Estheticians' close contact with clients creates a situation that requires decontamination to prevent the spread of bacteria and viruses between client and esthetician. By not following aseptic procedures, not cleaning up correctly after a treatment, or not using the correct chemical and mechanical cleaning items, the esthetician can foster an environment that puts themselves and others at risk. Estheticians routinely come into contact with bodily fluids such as blood, pus, and saliva. Even if they are not visible to the esthetician, bacteria are still present.

Bacteria

Bacteria are always present on skin and other surfaces. They are considered **microorganisms,** and they have three phases: growth, active, and inactive. Bacteria in the inactive stage form spores, which can live through many unfavorable conditions. It is impossible to kill inactive bacteria

111

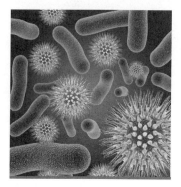

Figure 11-1 Bacteria.

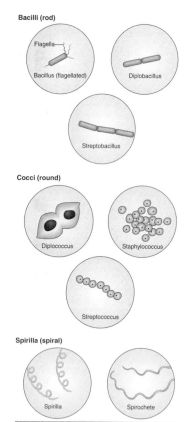

Figure 11-2 Bacterial shapes.

without sterilization. Bacteria can be classified as either good or bad. Nonpathogenic bacteria are helpful, but pathogenic bacteria are harmful and cause disease. There are different classifications of **pathogenic bacteria,** and these are shown in Figure 11-1.

Cocci

Cocci are round and come in three types: staphylococci, streptococci, and diplococci.

Diplococci are paired, and they cause bacterial pneumonia, sinusitis, and inflammation in the lungs. **Streptococci** are bacteria that resemble a string of beads, and they are pus forming. Strep throat is caused by this kind of bacteria. **Staphylococci** are also pus forming, but they grow in clusters. Commonly called "staph," this kind of bacteria can cause infection and may be resistant to treatment. MRSA (methicillin-resistant staphylococcus aureus bacterium) is included in this group.

Bacilli

Bacilli are the most common bacteria; they are rod-shaped. **Spirilla** are spiraled and long. **Lyme disease** and **syphilis** are caused by these bacteria.

See Figure 11-2 for a chart of the different types of bacteria.

Parasites are also included in the pathogenic bacteria group, and they are classified as either vegetable or animal parasites. Parasites need a host in order to survive, much like a virus; without a viable host, they will die. Mold is one of the most common parasites, and it poses a problem for most people. See Figure 11-3 for an example of pathogenic bacteria.

- Vegetable parasites are called **fungi;** these include molds, yeasts, and mildew. Ringworm and favus are vegetable parasites.
- Animal parasites are very contagious and include **scabies, lice,** and itch mites.

Viruses

A **virus** is not a microorganism that can live on its own; it must have a host. It does not have a cellular structure; it consists of a single type of nucleic acid. Viruses penetrate cell walls and become part of them, as shown in Figure 11-4.

A virus can infest most plants, animals, and bacteria. Viruses are responsible for **smallpox, chickenpox, AIDS, hepatitis,** and many more diseases. In esthetics, the main viruses that cause concern are the **herpes** group, **papovirus,** and **retrovirus.**

The herpes group includes:

- **Fever blisters** and cold sores, caused by herpes simplex 1
- **Genital herpes,** caused by herpes simplex 2
- Chickenpox, caused by the varicella virus
- **Mononucleosis,** caused by the Epstein-Barr virus

The papovirus group includes:

- Common warts, or *verruca vulgaris*
- Flat warts, or *verucca plana*

The retrovirus group includes:

- AIDS, caused by Human Immunodeficiency Virus (**HIV**)
- Cancer
- Hepatitis

See Figure 11-5 for a general illustration of a virus.

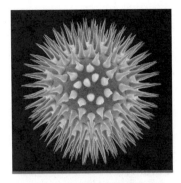

Figure 11-3 Pathogenic bacteria.

■ ASEPTIC PROCEDURE

Aseptic procedure refers to the process of handling disinfected and sanitized implements to avoid recontamination. The equipment discussed in this chapter will aid you in your disinfection process, but there are some basic procedures that must be followed.

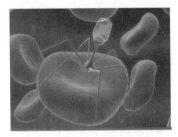

Figure 11-4 Virus entering cell.

Hand Washing

This is the simplest and most important step, so simple that it is often overlooked by both technicians and clients. It is the first step in any aseptic procedure, and it must be done before applying gloves. Hand washing should include scrubbing nails; see Figures 11-6 and 11-7.

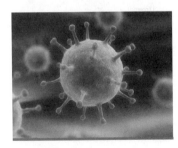

Figure 11-5 Virus.

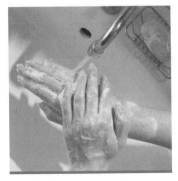

Figure 11-6 Washing hands is a mandatory step.

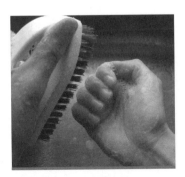

Figure 11-7 Scrubbing nails.

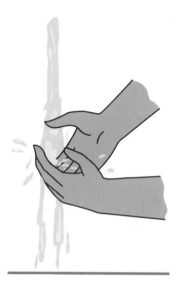

Figure 11-8a Step 1.

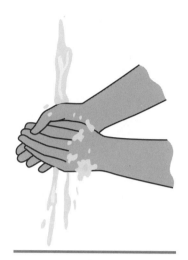

Figure 11-8b Steps 2 and 3.

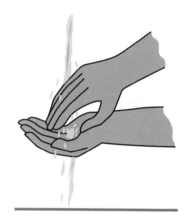

Figure 11-8c Step 4.

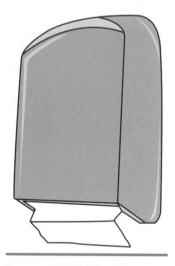

Figure 11-8d Step 5.

If you simply apply soap and immediately rinse it off, it will not be effective. Here is a simple but thorough process that is followed by health care practitioners.

Step 1: Wet hands with warm water, as shown in Figure 11-8a.

Step 2: Dispense soap.

Step 3: Work soap into a lather, and be sure to wash above the wrists. Use a fingernail brush if available for under fingernails. Rub hands together for a minimum of 15 seconds, as shown in Figure 11-8b. Tip: sing the Happy Birthday song as you wash to be sure you are washing long enough.

Step 4: Rinse thoroughly (see Figure 11-8c), grab a towel, and turn off the faucet with the towel. Do not touch the faucet with your clean hands.

Step 5: Dry hands with a towel (see Figure 11-8d).

Apply Gloves

Gloves, as shown in Figure 11-9, are essential when working with the public. There is much controversy among estheticians about using gloves throughout a facial, but there are specific times that gloves should always be used, preferably throughout the entire treatment. Keep in mind that allergic reactions to latex gloves are common. It is better to use nonlatex gloves. Check with your medical supply distributor to see what is available.

Effective Cleaning

All of the equipment in this chapter requires debris to be removed from the implements before use. Some of the equipment requires an EPA-registered disinfectant process first. See Figure 11-10 for a chart of commonly used disinfectants.

Effective cleaning also applies to procedures used during treatment and after the treatment is done. During treatment, it is important to not cross-contaminate surfaces that come into contact with the client. For example, if you touch your client's face and then reach for a bottle, the bottle has been contaminated and will need to be disinfected. All implements that have been disinfected should be kept covered prior to use. This can be done by laying a towel over the implements. After the service, all linens, surfaces, and implements should be cleaned (see Figure 11-11). Linens and implements should be stored in a clean, dry place. Do not place dirty implements or linens close to clean ones, and be aware of airborne contaminants. It is important for the esthetician to always be aware of the proper disinfection procedures. Be sure to review the many

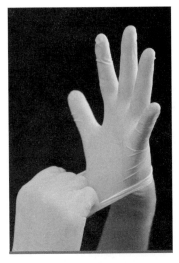

Figure 11-9 Put gloves on.

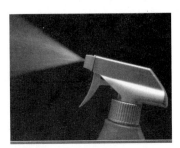

Figure 11-11 Spray all surfaces after treatment.

Name	Form	Strength	How to Use
Quaternary Ammonium Compounds (Quats)	Liquid or tablet	1:1000 solution	Immerse implements in solution for 20 or more minutes.
Formalin	Liquid	25% solution	Immerse implements in solution for 10 or more minutes.
Formalin	Liquid	10% solution	Immerse implements in solution for 20 or more minutes.
Alcohol	Liquid	70% solution	Immerse implements or sanitize electrodes and sharp cutting edges for 10 or more minutes.

Figure 11-10 Commonly used disinfectants.

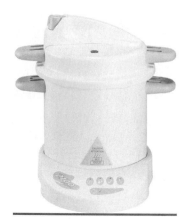

Figure 11-12 Autoclave.

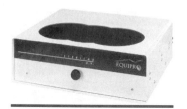

Figure 11-13 UV sterilizer.

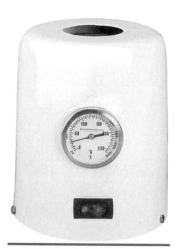

Figure 11-14 Glass bead sterilizer.

textbooks that are available for more details on disinfection, sanitation, and microbiology.

HOW IT WORKS

Listed below are the most common types of machines used for disinfection.

Autoclave

The only true means of sterilization is an **autoclave,** shown in Figure 11-12. **Sterilization** is the total destruction of all microorganisms, and the autoclave accomplishes this with a combination of heat, steam, and pressure. Not all **implements** can be autoclaved; glass, for example, will crack under the pressure. An autoclave has a metal chamber into which metal implements, sponges, and other materials can be enclosed with an air-sealed door. The chamber heats up to above the boiling point, usually to a final temperature of 260 degrees Fahrenheit. With sufficient pressure, the autoclave will sterilize materials for 20 minutes. After the steam is vented, the materials are placed in clear sterilization pouches and sealed. There are very specific guidelines for using an autoclave that are required by both state and federal agencies.

UV Sterilizer

The UV sterilizer does not offer a true sterilization. It is used after a wet disinfection process to store and dry implements. The **UV-C** short-range light destroys microorganisms, but it cannot be relied on for the full disinfection that is required for esthetic procedures. The UV-C light is used in a closed cabinet that protects the esthetician from exposure. It usually has a timer or a switch that is activated when the door is opened to turn on the UV-C bulb. The effectiveness of the equipment depends on having a closed environment, correct wavelength output from the bulb, and no debris on the surface of the object being irradiated. The cabinet must be made of aluminum to prevent rust. A UV sterilizer, such as the one shown in Figure 11-13, can store glass without the risk of the glass breaking.

Glass Bead Sterilizer

A glass bead sterilizer, like the one shown in Figure 11-14, is a small container filled with glass beads that are electrically heated. Some have heated air that is also circulated within the unit, and some units can reach 446 degrees Fahrenheit, but these cannot be relied upon for full sterilization. The glass bead sterilizer is not an FDA-approved sterilizer, but it can be used in the esthetic industry for an additional level of disinfection. It is especially useful for small metal implements, such as small scissors and tweezers.

Ultrasonic Cleaner

An ultrasonic cleaner, like the one shown in Figure 11-15, uses sound waves in the range of 15 to 400 **kilohertz.** This creates a process called **cavitation,** which you will learn more about in the ultrasound chapter. Cavitation causes the cleaning solution in the ultrasonic cleaning tank to vibrate at a high rate of speed, which causes air bubbles to explode with force, sending the solution into the smallest cavities of the implements being cleaned. The force of the mini explosions is enough to remove biological debris; this type of cleaning is indicated for metal implements, jewelry, and even microdermabrasion diamond-tip heads. An ultrasonic cleaner can be used as a primary disinfectant if the solution used in the ultrasonic cleaner is approved by your state board.

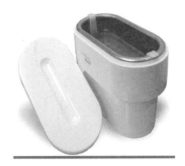

Figure 11-15 Ultronics Ultrasonic.

▪ HOW TO USE IT

All of the equipment listed in this chapter has very specific manufacturer directions that must be followed. We provide some general guidelines here, but it is best to check the manufacturer's recommendations prior to using any equipment.

Autoclave

- Clean all implements with soap and water or 70% solution of alcohol.
- Make sure all debris is removed.
- Place item in an autoclave envelope, seal it, and insert the envelope into the autoclave.
- Follow directions for your equipment settings; usually, 30 minutes is adequate.

TIP Autoclaves are required by state agencies and the CDC to be tested at least monthly for biological spore growth. Make sure you know your state requirements.

UV Sterilizer

- Clean all implements with soap and water.
- Pat dry.
- Soak in EPA- and state-approved high-level disinfectant for the recommended time, usually 15 to 20 minutes.
- Rinse.
- Pat items dry and place them in the UV sterilizer.
- Set the timer for 30 minutes.

Glass Bead Sterilizer

- Clean all implements with soap and water.
- Pat dry.
- Soak in EPA- and state-approved high-level disinfectant solution for the recommended time, usually 15 to 20 minutes.
- Rinse.
- Pat items dry and place them in the glass bead sterilizer; only place small, metal implements in a bead sterilizer.
- Set timer for 30 minutes.

Ultrasonic Cleaner

- Clean all implements with soap and water.
- Pat dry; make sure all soap residue has been removed.
- Place implements in the ultrasonic cleaner's soaking tank.
- Close the lid and turn the unit on for no more than 10 minutes.
- Remove implements and rinse off any remaining solution.
- Pat dry and place in a UV sterilizer.
- Set timer for 30 minutes.

TIP Always use the correct disinfectant for your ultrasonic cleaner. Some other solutions will cause a film to build up on the interior that is very hard to clean.

With all of your disinfection and sanitizing equipment, remember to make sure that your equipment has a safety certification, such as a UL listing or a CSA or ISO certification. UL and CSA listings indicate that the equipment has been tested for safety. ISO certification indicates that the item was manufactured per international standards and that the manufacturer is tested twice a year.

■ HOW TO BUY

Here are some helpful questions to ask when looking to buy.

Buyer's Checklist

- What is the price?
- Is this a state-approved disinfection process?
- Do you have an instruction manual or DVD?
- Is the machine UL listed, ISO certified, or CE or CSA tested?
- Does it come with cleaning solution, or does that have to be purchased separately?
- Can I buy replacement parts?

- What is covered under the warranty, and for how long?
- Where was the equipment manufactured?

■ SAFETY

Manufacturer's directions for safe use are very important with each of these machines. The general rules for safety are as follows:

- Always check electrical cords and plugs to make sure they are in good working order.
- If using a liquid disinfectant, make sure it is changed on a regular basis and per the manufacturer's directions for effectiveness.
- Do not plug equipment in near a sink if you can avoid it.
- Always use an outlet equipped with a **ground fault circuit interrupter (GFCI).**
- Do not look directly at a UV light.

■ MAINTENANCE

Autoclave

- The autoclave must be spore tested on a monthly basis or per your state's regulatory requirements. The test strips are supplied by various companies, and these can be sent in for immediate testing. Once testing is complete, you will be provided with a printed report stating your current level of compliance. Some states allow in-house testing, and the manufacturer can direct you to an appropriate testing facility.
- Always wipe out your autoclave after each use to avoid moisture buildup.
- Make sure the seal on the lid or door is in good working order; there should be no cracks or lifting.
- Clean the autoclave's exterior often.

UV Sterilizer

- Wipe out your UV sterilizer after each use; do not leave moisture in the chamber.
- Do not put soaking wet implements in a sterilizer; always pat them dry first.
- Change bulbs after 6,000 hours of use.
- Make sure bulbs do not have any residue buildup on them.
- Clean the exterior of your UV sterilizer often.

Glass Bead Sterilizer

- Glass bead sterilizers have a cleaning solution that the beads must be soaked in as soon as they appear to have a film buildup. Follow the manufacturer's directions.
- Clean the sterilizer's exterior often.
- Check all cords and plugs.

Ultrasonic Cleaner

- Change the liquid disinfectant on a regular basis. As soon as debris is seen in the liquid, change it.
- Scrub the chamber with soap and water to remove any residue.
- Do not submerge the ultrasonic cleaner in water; use a clean sponge to wipe it down.
- Clean the exterior and lid often; the disinfectant solution can cause a filmy buildup, like soap scum, if not used correctly.
- Check all cords and plugs.

TIP Do not use your ultrasonic cleaner on dirty implements; always remove debris first. This will make cleanup much easier and less expensive.

■ YOUR EQUIPMENT INFORMATION

Manufacturer info:

Name/phone number: _____

Web site: _____

Date purchased: _____ Registration: _____

Warranty info: _____

Replacement parts info: _____

TROUBLESHOOTING

Because disinfecting and sterilization equipment is regulated by state and federal agencies, any problem you encounter with your equipment must be referred to your manufacturer immediately. This is because it could affect you or your client's health and safety.

Q & A

What are the pros and cons of the different disinfection and sanitization equipment?

Autoclave pros

Effectiveness: The most effective form of sanitization is an autoclave. It provides hospital-level sanitization that is very safe. Some states are starting to require the use of this equipment in esthetic practices.
Ease of use: An autoclave is easy to use with minimal training.
Safety: Autoclaves are very safe to use. Operator misuse can cause spores to grow, but mandatory testing will alert you to any problems.

Autoclave cons

Cost: An autoclave is an expensive piece of equipment. The least expensive ones start at $1,000, but the cost may go as high as $6,000.
Maintenance: Autoclaves require consistent and thorough cleaning and mandatory testing.

Glass bead sterilizer pros

Effectiveness: Glass bead sterilizers provide an effective form of high-heat disinfection.
Ease of use: Bead sterilizers are easy to use with minimal training.
Safety: This type of sterilizer is very safe.

Glass bead sterilizer cons

Cost: Glass bead sterilizers are expensive, and most states do not recognize them as an adequate primary form of disinfection. A wet disinfection solution will still need to be used.
Maintenance: Consistent and thorough maintenance is required.

UV sterilizer pros

Ease of use: UV sterilizers are easy to use with minimal training.
Safety: UV sterilizers are very safe. Be aware that if the machine malfunctions, the UV-C bulb will stay on after the door is opened; you should never look directly at a UV-C bulb, so this can be dangerous.
Cost: A UV sterilizer is an inexpensive piece of equipment.

UV sterilizer cons

Effectiveness: At the esthetic level, UV sterilization is not considered an effective level of disinfection. States require a wet disinfection solution. UV sterilizers are mainly used for sanitary storage.
Maintenance: UV sterilizers require consistent and thorough cleaning.

Ultrasonic cleaner pros

Ease of use: Ultrasonic cleaners are easy to use with minimal training.
Safety: These machines are very safe and can be used as a primary disinfectant if the wet solution you use is approved by your state.
Cost: Ultrasonic cleaners are inexpensive.
Effectiveness: These are considered an effective form of disinfection when a state-approved disinfectant solution is used.

Ultrasonic cleaner cons

Maintenance: These machines require consistent and thorough cleaning.

Can I achieve results without disinfection and sanitization equipment?

Yes, if you are using a state-approved wet disinfectant system. Manufacturer directions must be followed closely, and staff must be properly trained on all aspects of disinfection.

REFERENCES

1. D'Angelo, J., Dean, P., Dietz, S., Hinds, C., Lees, M., Miller, E., & Zani, A. (2003). *Milady's Standard Comprehensive Training for Estheticians*. New York: Thomson Delmar Learning.
2. Simmons, J. V. (1989, 1995). *Science and the Beauty Business, The Beauty Salon and its Equipment* (2nd ed.). United Kingdom: Macmillan Press Ltd.
3. Lees, M. (2001). *Skin Care: Beyond the Basics*. New York: Thomson Delmar Learning.
4. Nordman, L. (2005). *Professional Beauty Therapy, The Official Guide to Level 3* (2nd ed.). London: Thomson Learning.
5. Pugliese, P. (2005). *Advanced Professional Skin Care Medical Edition*. Bernville, PA: The Topical Agent.
6. Gerson, J. (2004). *Milady's Standard Fundamentals for Estheticians*. New York: Thomson Delmar Learning.

Vacuum Spray Machine

The vacuum spray machine is usually combined with other pieces of esthetic equipment and is commonly known as an *eight-in-one* or a *six-in-one*. This machine is often underutilized by estheticians. The vacuum spray machine, like the one shown in Figure 12-1, is actually two machines in one; it provides vacuum suction and a vapor spray.

▪ FUNCTIONS

Vacuum suction improves blood and **lymphatic flow**, reduces swelling and puffiness, and provides gentle exfoliation. Sprays are used to calm and hydrate the skin and to apply toner.

▪ HOW IT WORKS

A vacuum supplies negative air pressure, which is created by an electric motor attached to a pump. The vacuum pump reduces atmospheric pressure; this creates negative airflow from the cup attachments, which are connected to the hose at the end of the unit. The spray is generated by positive air pressure created by the electric motor, and it flows through a tube connected to a spray bottle. The entire unit is regulated by a control valve that you can adjust for various levels of pressure.

The Vacuum

The vacuum feature used in esthetic treatments is aimed at improving lymph flow and circulation. Increased lymph flow is beneficial for removing **toxins** from the body, increasing cellular respiration, and

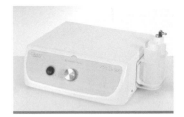

Figure 12-1 Silhouet-Tone Cirrus Vacuum Spray Machine.

improving the overall health of the skin. The vacuum may be used to loosen impacted comedones, but it will not "vacuum" them out of the skin.

Lymph System

Vacuum treatments are designed to move lymph through the lymph nodes. There are some machines that are designed to provide a very precise lymph drainage massage. To understand how this works, it is important to understand the lymph system; this is a defensive system with several important functions, including the following:

- Removal of bacteria and foreign material
- Drainage of excess fluids for elimination
- Movement of immune cells to areas where they are needed
- Transportation of digested fats to blood vessels
- Repair of injured tissues
- Removal of excess protein from tissues for deposit in the bloodstream, which reduces inflammatory response

The lymph system consists of lymph nodes, lymph vessels, and lymph fluid. It is not affected by the heart, like blood circulation; lymph is moved by muscular contraction. **Edema** is a symptom of a poorly functioning lymph system, and it can be assisted by lymphatic drainage massage as well as vacuum massage.

Lymph vessels collect lymph fluid from the lymph capillaries and move it through the lymph nodes in afferent vessels; after it has been filtered, it then moves out via efferent vessels into the blood. Figure 12-2 shows an illustration of the lymph system.

The immune response triggers the macrophages and lymphocytes within the lymph nodes. The macrophages attack foreign particles and debris carried in lymph fluids, and lymphocytes create antibodies to fight bacteria. All of this material is deposited into the bloodstream with the lymph fluid. Figure 12-3 shows an illustration of a lymph node.

It is important for the esthetician to understand the significance of the lymph nodes of the head and neck, which are shown in Figure 12-4. Advanced training in lymphatic drainage is mandatory when specialized massage aimed at moving the lymph is needed. Using a vacuum will not provide the same effects as a lymphatic drainage massage, but it will move lymph fluid. It is important to always work in the same direction the flow of blood takes toward the heart. This is a simplified explanation of the lymph system; the esthetician is urged to study further on this subject.

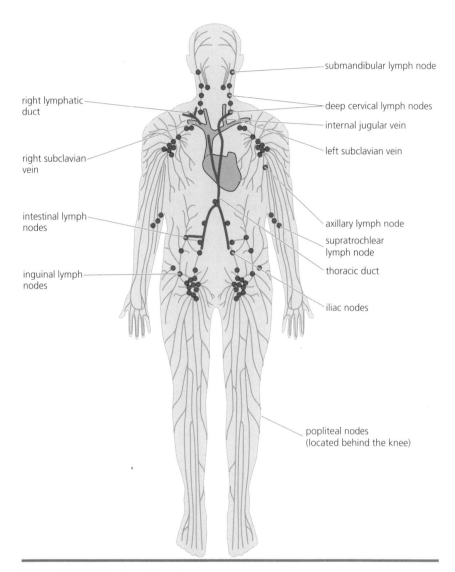

Figure 12-2 The lymph system.

Spray

The spray portion of the machine is used to hydrate the stratum corneum with toners, fresheners, or herb-infused water. This is one of the four misting modalities referred to in the steamer chapter. The mist is usually applied at room temperature or cooler, which also helps reduce irritation.

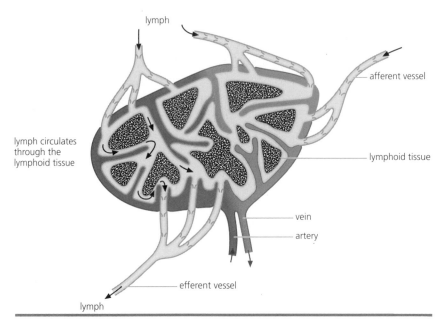

Figure 12-3 The lymph node.

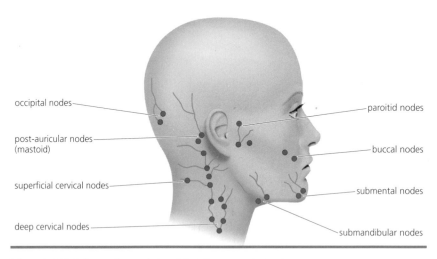

Figure 12-4 Lymph nodes of the face and neck.

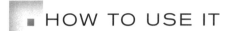 ## HOW TO USE IT

To perform a correct vacuum suction treatment, training is needed on the use of the correct vacuum cup, sometimes called a **ventouse.** These cups come in many sizes, from a 10–inch for bodywork to a small comedone ventouse. Figure 12-5 shows a chart of the different sizes.

Glass cup	Picture	Use and effect
Body cup: various diameters available from 2-10 cm	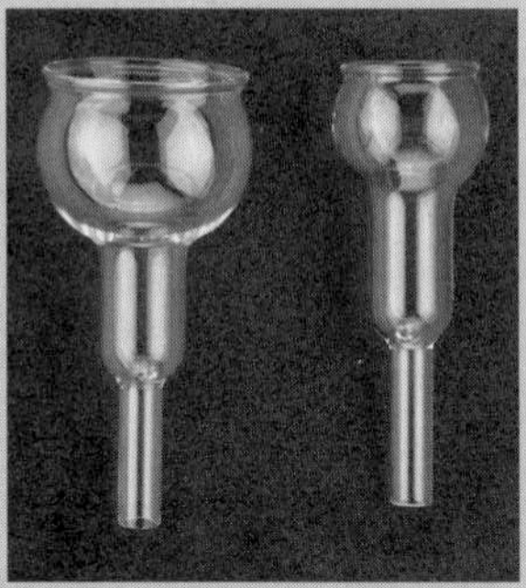	All areas of the body including the back where muscular tension may also be relieved
Facial cup: various diameters available from small to medium	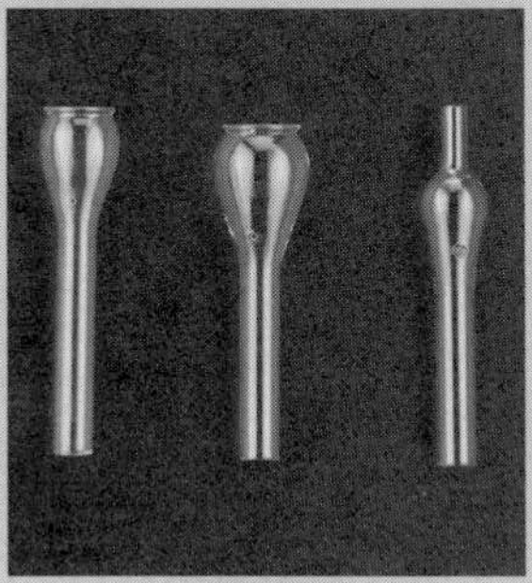	General skin cleansing; lymphatic drainage of the face and neck; treatment of fatty deposits (double chin condition)
Comedone ventouse	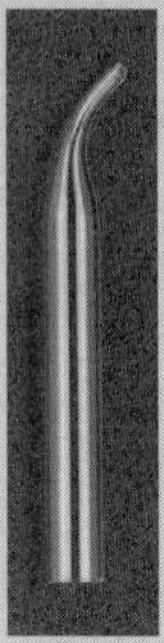	Mechanical comedone extraction; congested areas around the chin and nose
Flat ventouse	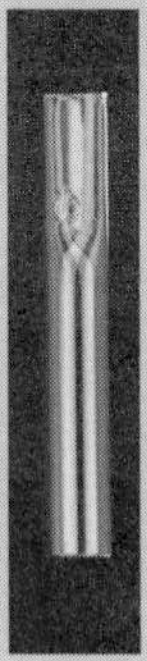	Treatment of expression lines; can also be used for general skin cleansing

Figure 12-5 Chart of ventouse (vacuum cup) sizes.

Vacuum spray machine	Multiple ventouse (vacuum) attachments
	Variable speed
	Two empty spray bottles
	UL listed

Figure 12-6 Features to look for.

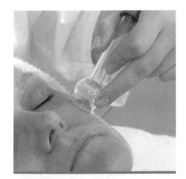

Figure 12-7 Vacuum application.

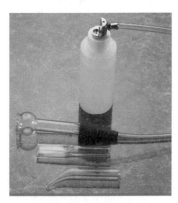

Figure 12-8 Vacuum spray accessories.

After choosing the correct size vacuum cup for the application, apply a lubricant to the skin and perform gliding movements towards the lymph nodes while placing your finger over the hole in the ventouse. This process is the same for a body application, such as the one shown in Figure 12-7.

For a spray application, fill the spray bottle with the appropriate toner, adjust the spray level, and put your finger over the hole in the top of the bottle. A fine mist will be released over the skin. Be sure to apply eye pads and fully mist the skin for maximum benefit. See Figure 12-8 for an example of accessories to use in treatment.

Make sure your equipment has a safety certification such as a UL listing or a CSA or ISO certification. UL and CSA listings indicate that the equipment has been tested for safety; with any electrical equipment, this is very important. ISO certification indicates that the equipment has been manufactured per international standards and that the manufacturer is tested twice a year.

■ HOW TO BUY

Listed below are some helpful questions to ask before you buy.

Buyer's Checklist

- What is the price?
- Does the item come with an instruction manual or DVD?
- Is the machine UL listed, ISO certified, or CSA or CE tested?
- Does it come with multiple ventouses, or do these have to be purchased separately?
- What do the ventouses cost?
- Can I buy replacement parts?

- What is covered under the warranty, and for how long?
- Where was the machine manufactured?

Figure 12-6 provides a chart that shows some features to look for.

SAFETY

Vacuum suction treatment can cause bruising, so it is important to perform the treatment properly. Always follow manufacturer recommendations in addition to these general guidelines:

- Never pull the vacuum cup away from the skin without turning off the suction.
- Do not apply too much vacuum suction to the skin.
- Do not overtreat an area.
- Do not apply treatment to breast tissue.
- Do not use a vacuum cup that is too small for a treatment area.
- Do not increase vacuum pressure while the cup is stationary on the skin; only increase it while gliding across the skin.
- Always check cords and attachments before turning the machine on.

Safety measures concerning the spray portion of the unit are minimal. Here are the general guidelines:

- Do not spray while the client's eyes or mouth are open.
- Do not put heated liquid in the spray bottle.

MAINTENANCE

Maintenance is important with every esthetic machine, and these standard guidelines should be followed, along with any recommendations from the manufacturer:

- Always wipe down every surface with an EPA-registered high-level disinfectant.
- Remove debris and lubricant with soap and water after each treatment.
- Do not store tubes in a UV sterilizer; they will yellow.
- Replace tubes as soon as they start to change color or appear to have debris buildup.

- Do not allow spray bottle tips to become clogged with excess product.
- Do not pull the plug out of the outlet by pulling on the cord.

■ DISINFECTION AND SANITIZATION

It is very important to disinfect ventouses after each use. Use this easy-to-follow system:

- Wash the vacuum cups with soap and water.
- Take a small, flexible brush or pipe cleaner and insert it into the cup to remove any debris.
- Soak in an EPA-registered high-level disinfectant solution according to the manufacturer's instructions.
- Remove after the recommended time; rinse and pat dry.
- Place in a UV sanitizer to finish drying.
- Wipe down the tube. If you see debris in the tube, try to clean it or replace the tube.

To disinfect the spray bottle:

- Wash with soap and water.
- Soak in an EPA-registered high-level disinfectant solution for the recommended time.
- Rinse with clean water.
- Place upside down to dry.

See Figure 12-9 for a chart of disinfection and maintenance steps.

TIP Place a thin piece of gauze at the connection between the ventouse (vacuum cup) and the hose. This will catch any debris that may come loose.

Disinfection	Maintenance
Wash and rinse attachments	Can store vacuum attachment but not spray bottles in UV sanitizer
Soak in EPA–approved high level disinfectant 15 min (per manufacturer's directions)	Wipe down equipment when done
Dry and place in closed container	Do not leave in EPA–approved wet disinfectant overnight

Figure 12-9 Disinfection and maintenance steps.

CONTRAINDICATIONS AND CAUTIONS

The consultation is extremely important to determine contraindications or special needs that your client may have. Do not rely exclusively on the intake form. It is also important to verbally get information and clarification from your client. A vacuum spray treatment has the following contraindications:

- Pregnancy: Use caution when working with pregnant clients; they can be very sensitive.
- Heart Problems: A heart in a compromised condition is unable to cope with an increased constriction or dilation of blood vessels; this can lead to fainting or a heart attack.
- Blood vessel disorders: **Arteriosclerosis,** or hardening of the arteries, affects the arteries' ability to handle increased blood flow. Fainting can occur when treatments cause increased dilation of the blood vessels.
- Skin inflammation: Most vacuum treatments increase circulation, which can make inflammation worse.
- Skin disorders or diseases: These may be aggravated by treatment.
- Very sensitive skin: Treatment may be uncomfortable for clients with this skin type.
- Lack of tactile sensation (e.g., numbness due to stroke): A client will not be able to gauge the intensity of the vacuum flow; this can damage skin.
- Reduced skin elasticity: Skin can be further damaged by the suction.
- Stretch marks and scar tissue: Skin can be damaged further by the stretching motions that occur during treatment.
- Broken and **varicose veins:** Suction can cause more damage.
- Botox: Treatment should be avoided for 72 hours after injection.
- Severe bruising: This condition will make treatment uncomfortable for the client.
- High or low blood pressure: Blood pressure conditions can be made worse due to the increase in circulation. Even if blood pressure issues are being treated and are under control, you must still use caution. Never leave a client with blood pressure conditions alone, and help them on and off the treatment bed.
- HIV or history of cancer: Vacuum treatment moves lymph through the lymph system, which can aggravate immune system problems. Always ask for medical guidance before treating clients with these diseases.

- History of blood clots (**thrombosis**) or **embolism**: Treatment could aggravate these conditions and could cause a heart attack or stroke.
- Malignant melanoma: Medical treatment must be completed and the client must be in remission. Obtain physician approval. Do not apply treatment when in doubt about a possible abnormality; instead, refer the client to a dermatologist.

PREPARATION FOR TREATMENT

TIP It is important that the skin be warm and hydrated before using the vacuum treatment. Make sure to apply steam first.

- Have your client fill out an assessment form.
- Check for contraindications.
- Have your client change into a treatment gown and remove all jewelry and contact lenses.
- Analyze the skin using a magnifying lamp.
- Explain the procedure.
- Make sure to test all equipment before applying treatment.
- Inspect all wires and electrodes.
- Follow manufacturer's instructions to set up your vacuum spray machine.

PROTOCOLS

TIP Avoid vacuum treatment around the delicate eye area.

The vacuum spray machine can be used on the face and body. Here is a standard protocol for the face:

- After cleansing and steaming, spray the appropriate toner with the machine's sprayer, as shown in Figure 12-10.
- Apply the appropriate lubricant evenly to the skin.
- Pick the correct ventouse for the area being treated (refer to Figure 12-5).
- Turn the machine on, and test the equipment on the back of your hand.
- Start at the lowest vacuum setting.
- Place your finger over the hole on the side of the vacuum cup. Start at the upper chest, and move upward toward the lymph node. Refer to Figure 12-11a.
- Release your finger from the hole in the vacuum cup at the end of each stroke.
- Move the vacuum upward, starting at the base of the neck and ending at the side. See Figure 12-11b. Repeat four times.

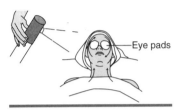

Figure 12-10 Turn on the machine, place one finger on top of the spray bottle, and apply spray in upward circular movements about 12 inches from the face.

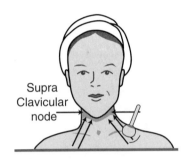

Figure 12-11a Move vacuum cup in an upward motion toward the supra-clavicular node.

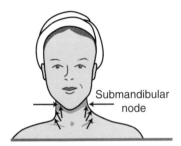

Figure 12-11b Move vacuum cup in an upward motion toward the sub-mandibular node.

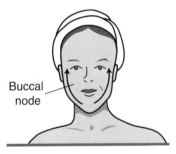

Figure 12-11c Move vacuum cup in an upward motion toward the side of the ear.

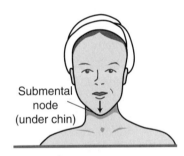

Figure 12-11d Move vacuum cup in a downward motion toward the submental node.

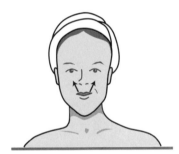

Figure 12-11e Move vacuum cup in an upward motion toward the parotid node.

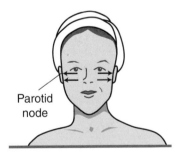

Figure 12-11f Move vacuum cup horizontally toward the parotid node.

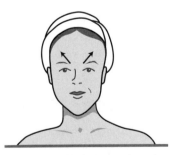

Figure 12-11g Move vacuum cup in an upward motion toward the hairline.

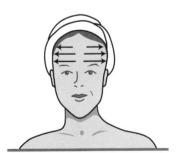

Figure 12-11h Move vacuum cup horizontally toward the side of the forehead.

- Move the vacuum upward, from the center of the chin to just below the ear. See Figure 12-11c.
- Move the vacuum downward, from under the lower lip to the top of the chin, as shown in Figure 12-11d.
- Move the vacuum upward, from the side of the mouth up toward the nose, as shown in Figure 12-11e.
- Move the vacuum from the side of the nose horizontally toward the ear, as shown in Figure 12-11f.
- Move the vacuum upward, from the center of the eyebrows to the hairline. See Figure 12-11g.
- Move the vacuum horizontally, from the center of the forehead to the hairline. Repeat three times. See Figure 12-11h.
- Continue with the rest of the facial treatment.

Comedone Treatment

- Perform the basic facial steps, up to the steaming and exfoliating stage.
- Spray astringent on the skin.
- Place the comedone ventouse on the area to be extracted, but *do not* let the ventouse glide on the skin.
- Use your finger over the hole in the ventouse to hold the vacuum still; release it in a pulsing movement.
- Follow with manual extraction or another treatment.

YOUR EQUIPMENT INFORMATION

Manufacturer info:

Name/phone number: _____

Web site: _____

Date purchased: _____ Registration: _____

Warranty info: _____

Replacement parts info: _____

TROUBLESHOOTING

My spray will not come out in an even, light mist.

Your spray head may be clogged. Perform a thorough cleaning and try again. If it still will not spray, replace the spray head.

I am not getting any suction when I turn on my machine.

Check all electrical attachments and the outlet to make sure nothing has been tripped. Call your manufacturer if it is still not working; the motor could have problems.

Q & A

What are the pros and cons of the vacuum spray machine?

Pros

Effectiveness: The vacuum works very well to move lymph fluid, and it creates a rosy glow in the skin.
Cost: The machine is cost-effective and inexpensive.
Safety: The spray machine is very safe, but the vacuum treatment can cause bruising if misused.

Cons

Ease of use: Before performing treatment, estheticians must not only be trained in the correct use of the vacuum machine but also in the correct movements.
Training: Training and practice are required to perform a safe and effective vacuum treatment. The spray portion is very easy to learn.
Maintenance: Consistent and thorough cleaning is required to avoid clogging.

Can I achieve results without the vacuum spray machine?

Yes. Lymph can be moved by manual lymphatic drainage massage, and you can use a spray bottle, Lucas spray, or carbon dioxide spray.

Should I buy or lease my machine?

Usually this machine is included in multiple modality machines, which can be leased. When buying separately, it probably would be better to purchase your vacuum sprayer, unless you are combining it with a large equipment order.

REFERENCES

1. D'Angelo, J., Dean, P., Dietz, S., Hinds, C., Lees, M., Miller, E., & Zani, A. (2003). *Milady's Standard Comprehensive Training for Estheticians*. New York: Thomson Delmar Learning.

2. Gerson, J. (2004). *Milady's Standard Fundamentals for Estheticians.* New York: Thomson Delmar Learning.

3. Hill, P., & Todd, L. (2008). *Milady's Aesthetician Series: Advanced Face and Body Treatments for the Spa.* New York: Thomson Delmar Learning.

4. Nordman, L. (2005). *Professional Beauty Therapy, The Official Guide to Level 3* (2nd ed.). London: Thomson Learning.

Lucas Spray Pulverizer

The Lucas spray pulverizer is also known as a *Lucas Championniere*. It is unique among atomizers and is used widely in Europe by most estheticians. It was originally used to spray **carbolic acid** (phenol) in operating rooms as an antiseptic during surgery, a practice introduced in 1860 by Dr. Joseph Lister. The modern version was adapted from Dr. Lister's invention by Lucas Championniere. Not only is the Lucas spray extremely effective in cleansing the skin, the spray can also be used to carry essential oils, skin fresheners, and astringents to the skin in a very fine mist without altering the molecular structure of the product. Figure 13-1 shows a photo of a Lucas spray pulverizer.

■ FUNCTIONS

The Lucas spray pulverizer sprays a fine mist to hydrate and cleanse the skin; it may also be used to apply astringents to oily skin and to calm sensitive skin.

■ HOW IT WORKS

The Lucas spray uses a metal chamber that is filled with distilled water. This chamber is heated with an electrical coil, which creates steam that expands and creates pressure; this in turn forces the steam out of a small opening in the front of the sprayer. There are two glass jars on the front: one holds the active ingredient to be pulverized, and the other catches the condensation. Both have clear plastic tubes attached to the bottom of the nozzle. As the steam is forced through the nozzle, it creates a vacuum that pulls up the active ingredients and sprays them out with the mist. The temperature of the mist is controlled by altering the temperature of the active ingredients in the glass jar.

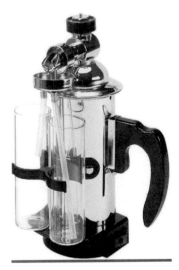

Figure 13-1 Equipro Lucas spray.

137

■ WHAT IT DOES TO THE SKIN

The Lucas spray creates a very fine mist of water and active ingredients that allows the hydrating solution to penetrate the stratum corneum. True absorption depends on the molecular structure of the active ingredients in the pulverizer. This is an excellent modality for applying essential oils to the skin, because the fine mist does not heat up the essential oils, which can alter the molecular structure of the product. This is one of the four misting modalities used in esthetic treatments, and can range from warm temperatures to very cool.

■ HOW TO USE IT

Here are the guidelines for using a Lucas spray:

- Always use distilled water.
- Remove the knob at the top of the unit.
- Place a funnel in the opening, and pour distilled water in until you see the level reach the red water-level line on the back of the unit.
- Fill the appropriate jar with active ingredients; these may be essential oils, fresheners, astringents, and or herbal tinctures.
- Turn the unit on.
- The unit will heat up quickly, and a fine mist will begin to flow, pulling up the active ingredients.
- Apply mist to the skin in a consistent pattern over the treatment area.
- Turn off the unit when you are finished spraying the mist. Figure 13-2 shows a step-by-step use chart.

Step 1	Unscrew knob at top of Lucas spray.
Step 2	Fill unit with distilled water. Do not go above red line.
Step 3	Fill right side jar with active ingredients.
Step 4	Plug in and turn on unit.
Step 5	When mist starts, apply to skin in an even smooth pattern.
Step 6	Remove and turn off when skin is saturated.

Figure 13-2 Step-by-step use chart.

■ HOW TO BUY

The Lucas spray has a long history, but the technology has remained essentially the same. Prices range from about $375 to $395, depending on the supplier. Look for a supplier that can guarantee a two-year warranty and supply the accessories you will need.

The sprayer is a sensitive electrical machine, so make sure your equipment has a safety certification, such as a UL listing or a CSA or ISO certification. UL and CSA listings indicate that the equipment has been tested for safety. ISO certification indicates that the equipment was manufactured per international standards and that the manufacturer is tested twice a year. Using safety-tested machines will prevent the potential for fire hazards and short circuits in the heating element.

Buyer's Checklist

- What is the price?
- What are the shipping costs?
- Do you provide an instruction manual, DVD, or on-site training?
- Is the machine UL listed, ISO certified, or CE or CSA listed?
- Can I buy replacement parts? If so, what are the costs?
- What is covered under the warranty, and for how long?
- Can you service the Lucas spray?
- Where was the machine manufactured?
- Does the machine have any automatic safety features that shut it off if the water runs dry?

Figure 13-3 shows a chart of features to look for when you buy.

Lucas spray	Metal casing, well-made
	Small cleaning tool included
	Replacement glass available
	UL listed

Figure 13-3 Features to look for.

■ SAFETY

The Lucas spray is a safe machine, but there are some guidelines to follow to avoid burn injuries and damage to the machine:

- Never touch the metal part of the unit when the machine is on.
- Never open the top of the unit when the machine is on.
- Never run all of the water out of the machine.
- Always check the cord to make sure it is in good condition.
- Plug the unit into a GFCI-grounded outlet.

■ MAINTENANCE

The Lucas spray is a high-maintenance esthetics machine. It is very important to follow these general guidelines for cleaning and maintenance. Keep in mind that many suppliers also have guidelines to follow.

- Never use anything other than distilled water in the Lucas spray. It is impossible to clean out the interior of unit once minerals build up.
- Do not use any oil-based products such as grapeseed oil, jojoba oil or any other massage oil in the sprayer.
- Use the small wire brush that comes with your unit to clean the sprayer nozzle after each use.
- Wipe down exterior surfaces to keep them free from residue after the unit is turned off and cool.
- Wash out both glass jars after each use.

Figure 13-4 shows a maintenance chart for Lucas sprays.

Disinfection	Maintenance
Wash and rinse attachments	Do not run all water out of sprayer
Soak glass cups in EPA-approved high-level disinfectant for 15 minutes (per manufacturers directions)	Wipe down exterior of equipment when done; clean sprayer nozzle with small wire brush
	Clean and rinse glass cups after each use

Figure 13-4 Disinfection and maintenance.

■ DISINFECTION AND SANITIZATION

Only the esthetician makes contact with a Lucas spray; therefore, general cleaning and maintenance guidelines are sufficient to disinfect it.

■ CONTRAINDICATIONS AND CAUTIONS

The Lucas spray is a wonderful machine for many conditions, and it has no contraindications regarding its use. The only caution to keep in mind is that some clients may have a general sensitivity to some of the active ingredients used in the unit. There is no substantial heat generated by the machine that would warrant any vascular contraindications.

■ PREPARATION FOR TREATMENT

- Have your client fill out an assessment form.
- Check for contraindications.
- Have your client change into a treatment gown and remove all jewelry and contact lenses.
- Analyze the skin using a magnifying lamp.
- Explain the procedure.
- Make sure to test the equipment before applying treatment.
- Fill Lucas sprayers with distilled water and active ingredients.
- Follow the manufacturer's instructions to set up your Lucas spray.

■ PROTOCOLS

Listed below are protocols for treatment room use.

Aromatherapy Lucas Spray

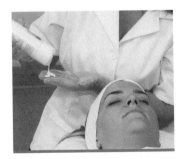

Figure 13-5a Perform first and second cleansing.

Step 1: Perform the first and second cleansing on the skin. See Figure 13-5a.

Step 2: Apply a manual scrub exfoliant, and use it per the manufacturer's instructions. See Figure 13-5b.

Step 3: Use a warm towel to remove product, as shown in Figure 13-5c.

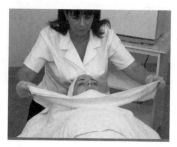

Figure 13-5b Apply manual exfoliant.

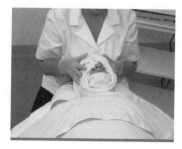

Figure 13-5c Use warm towel to remove product.

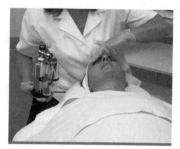

Figure 13-5d Spray in an even pattern.

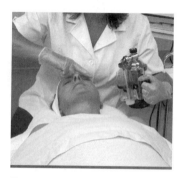

Figure 13-5e Spray in an even pattern.

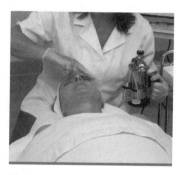

Figure 13-5f Spray in an even pattern.

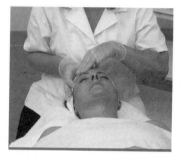

Figure 13-5g Gently massage product into skin.

Step 4: Place eye pads on the client, turn on the Lucas spray, and fill the appropriate jar with distilled water or premade hydrosol with the appropriate essential oils for the client's skin type.

Step 5: Place a bath towel across the client's chest, cover the hair, and place a towel behind the neck and shoulders.

Step 6: Spray until the skin is saturated, approximately 1 to 2 minutes. See Figures 13-5d, 13-5e, and 13-5f.

Step 7: Gently massage excess product into the skin, as shown in Figure 13-5g.

Step 8: Remove residue from the skin with a tissue.

Step 9: Proceed with the rest of the facial treatment.

Your Protocol:

_____

_____

_____

_____

■ YOUR EQUIPMENT INFORMATION

Manufacturer info:

Name/phone number: _____

Web site: _____

Date purchased: _____   Registration: _____

Warranty info: _____

Replacement parts info: _____

TROUBLESHOOTING

The Lucas spray is a machine that must be serviced by the supplier.

The spray will not turn on.

Check to make sure the outlet the steamer is plugged into has not been tripped, and check the cord for cracks or deterioration. If this does not correct the problem, contact your supplier.

Hot water is dripping from the bottom of the machine.

There is a crack in the base of the unit. Unplug the machine immediately and contact your supplier.

The machine is spitting hot water.

There is a mineral buildup inside the machine from not using distilled water. Call your supplier to see how to get the unit serviced, and *do not* try to run vinegar or any other product through the unit to remove mineral buildup.

Q & A

What are the pros and cons of a Lucas spray pulverizer?

Pros

Effectiveness: This machine is very effective and has a long history of use.
Ease of use: The sprayer is easy to use with minimal training.
Broad use: The sprayer can be used on all clients.

Cons

Safety: The sprayer is a very safe machine, but safety issues can occur with a poorly maintained unit or through operator misuse.
Cost: This is an expensive machine.
Maintenance: Consistent and thorough cleaning will prevent any safety issues. Use only distilled water to avoid issues with mineral buildup.

Can I achieve results without a Lucas sprayer?

You can use alternate forms of misting, or hot towels, but you will not get the same results that you would from using a Lucas spray.

REFERENCES

1. D'Angelo, J., Dean, P., Dietz, S., Hinds, C., Lees, M., Miller, E., & Zani, A. (2003). *Milady's Standard Comprehensive Training for Estheticians.* New York: Thomson Delmar Learning.
2. Lees, M. (2001). *Skin Care: Beyond the Basics.* New York: Thomson Delmar Learning.
3. Nordman, L. (2005). *Professional Beauty Therapy, The Official Guide to Level 3* (2nd ed.). London: Thomson Learning.
4. Simmons, J. V. (1989, 1995). *Science and the Beauty Business: The Beauty Salon and its Equipment* (2nd ed.). United Kingdom: Macmillan Press Ltd.

Infrared Heat Lamp

This piece of equipment is one of the radiant heat modalities frequently used in body treatments. It can also be used for facial treatments and is a safe modality with proven results. An infrared heat lamp uses both radiant heat and infrared rays to provide many beneficial results.

CHAPTER 14

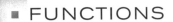 FUNCTIONS

Infrared heat causes dilation of the blood vessels, increased circulation, increased metabolism, reduced muscle stiffness, increased secretion of sweat and sebum, gentle pain reduction, warming within the skin, and it increases the effectiveness of some esthetic treatments.

HOW IT WORKS

Most of the lamps that are available for esthetic use are incandescent with a built-in reflector and red-tinted glass. These lamps are usually fitted with dimmers to give more of an infrared output. The lamp is positioned over the face or body, about 17 to 23 inches from the skin.

The infrared light from the lamp penetrates the skin, and the radiant heat warms the skin; however, the lamp is used primarily to heat the skin. Heat lamps come in a one- or three-head model.

WHAT IT DOES TO THE SKIN

Radiant heat causes dilation of the blood and lymph vessels within the skin; this in turn creates more blood and lymph flow, helping with the nutrition of the cells and the elimination of toxins. The sweat glands are also activated by the internal heat created and will secrete at a higher rate, which also helps the organs eliminate toxins. When heat rays penetrate, the nerves convey a tingling sensation that interrupts the pain signal, thus gently relieving the body's interpretation of pain.

Infrared rays create little if no direct heating of the skin. Instead, they cause a reaction within the skin that causes the blood vessels to dilate; this brings the body's natural warmth to that area of the skin, causing the feeling of deep heat. Infrared rays are especially soothing because there is little stimulation of the nerve endings.

Higher temperatures applied to the skin increase the rate of metabolism in the body. This acts much like a fever does when a virus or bacteria invades the body; this action increases the removal of toxins, and repairs to damaged tissues are speeded up. Edema, or swelling of the tissues, is reduced by the increased blood and lymph flow, which eases pain. Sweat and sebum secretions are increased, which creates a deep cleansing effect in the skin.

All of these effects also help products applied to the skin absorb at a faster rate. Warm, hydrated skin has a better absorption rate, which leads to improved results for your esthetic treatments.

■ HOW TO USE IT

The heat lamp is very easy to use. Figure 14-1 demonstrates an infrared heat lamp application.

- Turn lamp on 10 minutes prior to use to get the full heating effects.
- When treating the face, place a mask and eye pads on your client before positioning the lamp over your client's face. If you are using the lamp for a body treatment, apply the body mask first.
- Place the lamp about 17 to 23 inches from the area you are going to heat.
- The treatment should take 10 minutes for the face and up to 30 minutes for the body.

Figure 14-2 shows a chart with guidelines for heat lamp use.

■ HOW TO BUY

The heat lamp you purchase must be UL or CE or CSA listed. Use the same cautions you would for choosing electrotherapy equipment. Prices vary widely with this equipment; they can range from $250 for a one-bulb lamp to $500 for a three-bulb lamp (refer to Figure 14-1 for an example).

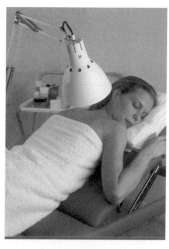

Figure 14-1 Infrared heat lamp application.

Step 1	Turn on lamp 10 minutes prior to application
Step 2	Apply product to skin (body, face mask or both)
Step 3	Apply eye pads
Step 4	Position lamp 17 to 23 inches from skin
Step 5	Leave on for 10 minutes (face) or 30 minutes (body)
Step 6	Turn on low; turn up as skin tolerates
Step 7	Move in circular motion over face and décolleté

Figure 14-2 How to use a heat lamp.

Look for even distribution of heat from the bulbs. To test this, shine the light on a white wall or white paper; you should have an even distribution of red light. Figure 14-3 shows what features to look for when you buy.

Buyer's Checklist

- What is the price?
- Do you have an instruction manual or DVD?
- Is the machine UL listed, ISO certified, or CSA or CE tested?
- Does it come with a stand, or does that have to be purchased separately?
- Where can I buy replacement parts?
- Can I purchase replacement bulbs? If so, what do they cost?
- What does the warranty cover, and for how long?

Heat lamp	Infrared output
	Multiple arms
	Even distribution of light
	UL listed or CE mark
	Metal guard on lamp casing
	Replacement bulbs available
	Warranty

Figure 14-3 Features to look for.

TIP Overexposure to an infrared heat lamp can result in burns, headaches, and fainting. Use caution and follow directions.

■ SAFETY

There are definite safety considerations when using a heat lamp. Some general guidelines are as follows:

- Check for electrical safety. Always inspect plugs, cords, and the lamp head for cracks or damage.
- Make sure the angle joints on the lamp remain tight. A loose joint could cause the arm to fall on a client.
- The lamp should be properly guarded so that the technician or client cannot get burned by touching the bulb accidentally.
- The lamp should be very stable on its base.
- Lamps must be plugged into three-prong grounded wall outlets. Make sure that you do not overload the outlet. A ground fault circuit interrupter, or GFCI, is required on all outlets within six feet of a water source. For the purposes of a facial room, it is a good idea to have GFCIs for all the equipment you will be working with.

■ MAINTENANCE

Maintenance is very easy. Here are some general guidelines:

- Always clean your lamp after each use by wiping it down with a gentle cleaner or soap and water.
- Check bulbs on a weekly basis. If they do not heat up within 10 minutes, change them.
- Make sure the safety guard on your lamp is secure.

■ DISINFECTION AND SANITIZATION

The only disinfection that needs to take place is to wipe off the lamp wherever you touch it. For tips on maintenance, see the chart in Figure 14-4.

■ CONTRAINDICATIONS AND CAUTIONS

The consultation is extremely important to determine contraindications or special needs that your clients may have. Do not rely exclusively on the intake form; it is important to verbally get information and clarification from your client. A heat lamp has an overall impact on the body, so you must be very thorough in your client intake process.

Disinfection	Maintenance
Any area in contact with client or technician requires disinfection	Wipe down outer part of lamp after each use
	Check bulbs weekly
	Check safety guard daily; make sure it is tight

Figure 14-4 Disinfection and maintenance.

- Pregnancy: Use caution when working on pregnant clients; they can be very sensitive.
- Heart problems: A heart in a compromised condition is unable to cope with increased constriction or dilation of blood vessels. This can lead to fainting or a heart attack.
- Blood vessel disorders: Arteriosclerosis, or hardening of the arteries, affects the arteries' ability to handle increased blood flow. Fainting can occur during heat treatments due to increased dilation of the blood vessels.
- Skin inflammation: Most heat treatments increase circulation, which can make inflammation worse.
- Very sensitive skin or loss of skin sensation: Clients with sensitive skin will be uncomfortable, and those with loss of sensation will not be able to tell when they are heating up too much.
- Cuts and abrasions: Do not perform treatments on any area that is in the process of healing.
- Severe bruising: This condition will make treatment uncomfortable for the client.
- High or low blood pressure: Either condition could be made worse due to the increase in circulation that occurs during heat treatments. Even if the condition is being treated and is under control, use caution. Never leave a client with blood pressure issues alone, and help them on and off the treatment bed.
- HIV: Always use the OHSA bloodborne pathogen guidelines to protect both client and technician.
- History of blood clots (thrombosis) or embolism: Treatment can aggravate these conditions and may cause a heart attack or stroke.
- Malignant melanoma: Treatment must be completed, and the client must be in remission; obtain physician approval before proceeding. Do not apply treatment when in doubt about a possible abnormality; instead, refer the client to a dermatologist.

■ PREPARATION FOR TREATMENT

- Have your client fill out an assessment form.
- Check for contraindications.
- Have your client change into a treatment gown and remove all jewelry and contact lenses.
- Analyze the skin with a magnifying lamp.
- Explain the procedure.
- Make sure to turn the lamp on 10 minutes before applying treatment.
- Inspect the lamp; make sure there are no electrical problems.
- Follow the manufacturer's instructions for the setup of your lamp.

■ PROTOCOLS

Heat lamps are used primarily in body treatments, and they can be used to provide a heating effect over a facial mask if needed. Here we discuss the basic protocol, but the products and procedures that work best should be based on the equipment manufacturer's recommendations and the skin care products that will be used.

Body Use

- Prepare the bed for a body treatment.
- Turn on the heat lamp.
- Have the client lie down and drape according to state requirements. This treatment works best on exposed skin.
- Use skin care products as directed by the manufacturer.
- Place the lamp 17 to 23 inches from the area being treated.

Leave on no less than 10 minutes. Rotate between areas if you have a one-bulb lamp. Treatment should not exceed 30 minutes.

Facial Use

- Prepare treatment bed for facial treatment.
- Turn on lamp.
- Remove makeup or perform the initial skin cleansing.
- Perform a second cleansing; you can use your steamer and brush machine to do this.
- Exfoliate skin.
- Massage the skin using the heat lamp to warm the skin during the massage. Keep the lamp away from the client's face.

- Apply serum.
- Apply mask. The heat lamp is used mainly at this phase to help with penetration and relaxation; place it at least 17 inches from the face, and cover the client's eyes.
- Use the heat lamp for no more than 10 minutes.
- Apply finishing cream.

Your Protocol:

_____

_____

_____

_____

_____

_____

_____

_____

YOUR EQUIPMENT INFORMATION

Manufacturer info:

Name/phone number: _____

Web site: _____

Date purchased: _____ Registration: _____

Warranty info: _____

Replacement parts info: _____

TROUBLESHOOTING

My lamp will not turn on.

Check all cords and check your outlet. The circuit may have been tripped.

I turn my lamp on, but the light is slow to light up or does not light up at all.

Make sure the bulb is firmly screwed in but not too tight. If that does not work, change the bulb, making sure that the bulb attachment is not loose.

Q & A

What are the pros and cons of the infrared heat lamp?

Pros

Effectiveness: A heat lamp is very effective for heating up tissues and providing some pain relief. It is wonderful to use when performing body treatments, because it warms the client without overwarming the room.

Ease of use: Infrared lamps are an easy modality to use with minimal training.

Safety: These lamps are very safe.

Training: No in-depth training is required prior to use.

Cons

Cost: A safe, quality lamp can be expensive. The ideal lamp has three heads and can run up to $600.

Frequency of use: Infrared heat lamps are used infrequently by estheticians.

What are the same results without using an infrared lamp?

Yes. There are other options for getting the same results in facial and body treatments, such as galvanic current, heated body wrap blankets, and steam.

Should I buy or lease my infrared lamp?

This decision should be based on your financial situation. In general, a infrared heat lamp represents such a small dollar amount that a leasing company would not finance it unless you grouped it with other equipment.

REFERENCES

1. D'Angelo, J., Dean, P., Dietz, S., Hinds, C., Lees, M., Miller, E., & Zani, A. (2003). *Milady's Standard Comprehensive Training for Estheticians*. New York: Thomson Delmar Learning.
2. Nordman, L. (2005). *Professional Beauty Therapy, The Official Guide to Level 3* (2nd ed.). London: Thomson Learning.
3. Simmons, J. V. (1989, 1995). *Science and the Beauty Business: The Beauty Salon and its Equipment* (2nd ed.). United Kingdom: Macmillan Press Ltd.

Electric Masks, Mitts, and Booties

Electric masks, mitts, and booties are used as heat therapy treatments that can be added to an existing treatment. Such treatments are cost-effective, easy, and therapeutic. Figure 15-1 shows some of these items.

■ FUNCTIONS

Electric warming accessories increase skin temperature with an occlusive mask or covering. This helps products penetrate and provides an increase in the microcirculation of the skin.

■ HOW IT WORKS

All masks, mitts, and booties essentially work in the same way. A heating coil is encased within a plastic covering; as the coil heats up, the heat radiates through the insulated plastic covering and increases the temperature of the enclosed skin.

Temperatures range from 100 to 120 degrees Fahrenheit and are adjusted using a controller much like you might find in a heating pad, with low, medium, and high settings.

■ WHAT IT DOES TO THE SKIN

The occlusive heat creates an ideal environment for products to be absorbed into the skin. This aids with hydration and also increases microcirculation, which leads to better cell respiration, enhanced removal of waste products, and a soothing of sensory nerve endings. Heat also creates a stress-reducing effect by relaxing muscles. In addition, heat can reduce joint stiffness for clients with **arthritis**.

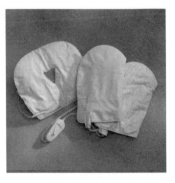

Figure 15-1 Heat mask and gloves.

153

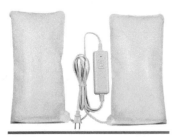

Figure 15-2 Equipro mitts.

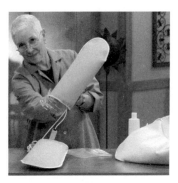

Figure 15-3 Electric mitts on hands.

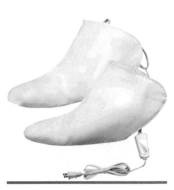

Figure 15-4 Equipro booties.

■ HOW TO USE IT

Here are some general guidelines to follow when using electrical warming devices:

Electric Mask

- Plug the mask into a grounded outlet.
- Turn it to the highest setting for five minutes before application.
- Place skin care product on skin.
- Place eye pads over client's eyes.
- Place moistened gauze or other occlusive mask over the skin care product.
- Adjust the mask to the lowest heat setting and place it on the client's face.
- Secure the mask with the band attached to it.
- Leave the mask on for no more than seven minutes.

Electric Mitts

Figure 15-2 shows one kind of electric mitt, and Figure 15-3 shows some mitts in use.

- Plug the mitts into a grounded outlet.
- Turn them to the highest setting five minutes before application.
- Place skin care product on the client's hands.
- Place the client's hands in a plastic covering.
- Turn the mitts to a low or medium heat setting, depending on the client's preference.
- Place the client's hands in mitts.
- Leave them on for no more than 15 minutes.

Booties

Figure 15-4 shows an example of electric booties.

- Plug the booties into a grounded outlet.
- Turn them to the highest heat setting five minutes before application.
- Disinfect feet with instant sanitizer or wipe with them a **benzalkonium chloride towelette.**
- Apply products to the feet; for example, apply an aromatherapy massage blend or an algae mask.
- Place the client's feet in a plastic covering.

- Adjust heat to a medium or high setting, depending on the client's preference.
- Place the client's feet in booties.
- Leave them on for no more than 15 minutes.

Figures 15-5, 15-6, and 15-7 show charts of how to use masks, mitts, and booties.

Step 1	Turn on mask 5 minutes prior to application
Step 2	Apply product to hands
Step 3	Put hands in plastic covering
Step 4	Turn heat to low or medium (depending on client)
Step 5	Put hands in mitts
Step 6	Leave on 10-15 minutes
Step 7	Remove mitts and massage product into hands

Figure 15-5 How to use the electric mask.

Step 1	Turn on mitts (high) 5 minutes prior to application, then turn on low
Step 2	Apply product to skin
Step 3	Apply eye pads
Step 4	Apply gauze mask
Step 5	Apply mask to face
Step 6	Leave on 15 minutes
Step 7	Remove and continue with facial steps

Figure 15-6 How to use the electric mitts.

Step 1	Turn on booties 5 minutes prior to application
Step 2	Disinfect feet with instant sanitizer or towelette
Step 3	Apply products to feet
Step 4	Place feet in plastic covering
Step 5	Turn temperature to level desired by client
Step 6	Leave on 15 minutes
Step 7	Remove and follow with foot massage

Figure 15-7 How to use the electric booties.

TIP **Underwriters Laboratory** (UL) is the U.S. organization responsible for testing products for consumer safety. Many international products are not UL certified, but Underwriters Laboratory has recently started an international section of certification. The alternative to UL listing is CSA certification. The UL mark on a product tells you that the machine has been thoroughly tested and investigated by a team of product safety professionals.

HOW TO BUY

It is very important that the masks, mitts, and booties you use have a safety certification, such as a UL listing or CSA or ISO certification. UL and CSA listings indicate that the equipment has been tested for safety. An ISO certification indicates that it has been manufactured per international standards and that the manufacturer is tested twice a year.

Buyer's Checklist

- What is the price?
- Does the item come with an instruction manual?
- Is the equipment UL listed, ISO certified, or CSA or CE tested?
- What is covered under the warranty, and for how long?
- Where was the equipment manufactured?

Figure 15-8 shows a chart of features to look for when you buy.

SAFETY

It is important for any electrical equipment you buy to have the proper safety listing and clear directions for use. Here are some general guidelines to follow:

- Always check the cord and plug to make sure there are no cracks or other deterioration.
- Heat up the equipment before applying it to your client's skin; always test the heat on yourself before applying it to your client.
- Do not submerge any electrical equipment in water.
- Do not place wet towels on top of electrical equipment.
- Always unplug electric masks, mitts, and booties after use.

Electric mask	Multiple temperature settings
Mitts	Easy clean surface
Booties	Even distribution of heat
	UL listed/ CE mark
	Warranty

Figure 15-8 Features to look for.

■ MAINTENANCE

Maintenance is very easy, but it must be completed after each use to prolong the effectiveness of the equipment.

- Always wipe out the interior of the mask, mitts, or booties after each use with an EPA-approved high-level disinfectant.
- Do not wrap the power cord around the mask, mitts, or booties; this can cause cracking of the electrical wire.
- Never place hands or feet in the mitts or booties without covering them in plastic first.
- Wipe down the exterior of masks, mitts, or booties after each use.
- Store in a clean, dry, enclosed space to avoid any debris buildup.

■ DISINFECTION AND SANITIZATION

When using electric masks, mitts, or booties, it is always important to make sure any product residue from the previous treatment has been removed. Here are some general guidelines you should follow:

- Always use a plastic covering for the client's hands and feet.
- Always use a gauze, cotton, or plastic occlusive mask before applying the electric mask to the client's face.
- Follow your state's disinfection procedures after each use; make sure you do not submerge any electrical devices in any wet material.
- Always dry out the interior of mitts and booties after each use.
- Wipe the back of the electric mask to dry it.

Figure 15-9 shows a chart that provides tips on disinfection and maintenance.

Disinfection	Maintenance
Disinfect interior after each use with EPA–registered disinfectant	Wipe down inside and outside after each use
Do not submerge in water to disinfect	Always use plastic around hands and feet before placing inside
Store in clean dry place	Dry interior and exterior before storing

Figure 15-9 Disinfection and maintenance.

■ CONTRAINDICATIONS AND CAUTIONS

The consultation is extremely important to determine contraindications or special needs that your client may have. Do not rely exclusively on the intake form; it is also important to verbally get information and clarification from your client. There are some contraindications for heat treatments.

- Pregnancy.
- Heart problems: A heart in a compromised condition is unable to cope with an increased constriction or dilation of blood vessels. Such stresses can lead to fainting or a heart attack.
- Blood vessel disorders: Arteriosclerosis, or hardening of the arteries, affects the arteries' ability to handle increased blood flow. Fainting can result due to the increased dilation of the blood vessels during heat treatments.
- Skin inflammation: Most heat treatments increase circulation, which can make inflammation worse.
- Skin disorders or diseases may be aggravated by treatment.
- Very sensitive skin may make treatment uncomfortable for the client.
- Lack of tactile sensation, such as numbness due to stroke, may not allow the client to gauge the intensity of the heat applied, which could cause damage to the skin if the temperature gets too high.
- Botox: No treatment can be applied until 72 hours after any Botox injection. Botox treatment paralyzes muscles, so any treatment to stimulate muscle would be ineffective.
- Cuts and abrasions: Do not apply any treatment to an area with open cuts and abrasions.
- High or low blood pressure could be made worse due to the increase in circulation. Even if these conditions are being treated and are under control, use caution. Never leave a client with blood pressure issues alone, and help them on and off the treatment bed.
- HIV.
- Malignant melanoma: Treatment must be completed, and client must be in remission; obtain physician approval before proceeding. Do not apply treatment when in doubt about a possible abnormality; instead, refer the client to a dermatologist.

■ PREPARATION FOR TREATMENT

- Have your client fill out an assessment form.
- Check for contraindications.

- Have your client change into a treatment gown and remove all jewelry and contact lenses.
- Analyze the skin using a magnifying lamp.
- Explain the procedure.
- Make sure to test all equipment before applying treatment.
- Inspect all wires and plugs.
- Follow the manufacturer's instructions.

■ PROTOCOLS

Listed below are useful protocols for correct use.

Multilayer Mask for Combination Skin

Step 1: Perform first and second cleansing.

Step 2: Perform gentle exfoliation, such as a manual scrub with a brush machine or an enzyme mask with steam.

Step 3: Apply hydrating serum.

Step 4: Gently massage serum into skin.

Step 5: Apply light, gel-based mask.

Step 6: Apply gauze mask.

Step 7: Apply clay-based mask in eighth-inch thickness.

Step 8: Apply plastic occlusive mask.

Step 9: Apply electric mask on a low heat setting for 10 minutes.

Step 10: Remove product with a warm or cool towel, and proceed with the rest of the treatment.

Algae Hand and Foot Treatment

Step 1: Cleanse hands and feet with a gentle sanitizer.

Step 2: Perform a gentle salt or sugar scrub, and remove excess with warm towels.

Step 3: Apply hydrating algae serum.

Step 4: Gently massage product into skin.

Step 5: Apply algae mud mask.

Step 6: Apply plastic covering to hands and feet.

Step 7: Apply electric mitts and booties on a medium heat setting for 10 to 15 minutes.

Step 8: Remove mitts or booties and remove excess product with a warm or cool towel.

Step 9: Massage hydrating lotion into the client's skin.

Your Protocol:

_____

_____

_____

_____

_____

_____

_____

_____

_____

_____

_____

_____

_____

■ YOUR EQUIPMENT INFORMATION

Manufacturer info:

Name/phone number: _____

Web site: _____

Date purchased: _____   Registration: _____

Warranty info: _____

Replacement parts info: _____

TROUBLESHOOTING

Troubleshooting electric masks, mitts or booties should be referred to your manufacturer or vendor due to the sensitive nature of the thermostats contained in these units. It is very important to maintain the correct temperature with this equipment, because incorrect temperatures can lead to burns or growth of bacteria.

Q & A

What are the pros and cons of using electric masks, mitts, or booties?

Pros

Effectiveness: These units are very effective for providing heat treatments, and they have a long and safe track record with visible benefits.
Cost: These items are cost-effective and inexpensive.
Ease of use: They are all very easy to use.
Safety: This equipment is safe, unless operator instructions are not followed or heat is increased too much for the client's safety.

Cons

Maintenance: Consistent and thorough cleaning provides a safe and effective treatment.

Can I achieve the same results without this equipment?

Yes. There are nonelectric mitts and booties that can be heated in a hot cabinet or microwave. The heat does not last as long, but it is effective. Hot towels are another alternative, but these also cool quickly.

REFERENCES

1. D'Angelo, J., Dean, P., Dietz, S., Hinds, C., Lees, M., Miller, E., & Zani, A. (2003). *Milady's Standard Comprehensive Training for Estheticians.* New York: Thomson Delmar Learning.
2. Gerson, J. (2004). *Milady's Standard Fundamentals for Estheticians.* New York: Thomson Delmar Learning.
3. Lees, M. (2001). *Skin Care: Beyond the Basics.* New York: Thomson Delmar Learning.
4. Nordman, L. (2005). *Professional Beauty Therapy, The Official Guide to Level 3* (2nd ed.). London: Thomson Learning.
5. Nordman, L. (2004). *Professional Beauty Therapy, The Official Guide to Level 2* (3rd ed.). London: Thomson Learning.
6. Simmons, J. V. (1989, 1995). *Science and the Beauty Business: The Beauty Salon and its Equipment* (2nd ed.). United Kingdom: Macmillan Press Ltd.

CHAPTER 16

Paraffin Heaters

Paraffin heaters are used to heat paraffin wax and keep it at a consistent, safe temperature for facial and body applications. It is used in other applications, such as in physical therapy; it has many benefits for the skin, as well as creating a very soothing therapeutic treatment. Figures 16-1 and 16-2 show examples of a paraffin spa and facial paraffin heater.

■ FUNCTIONS

Paraffin increases microcirculation within the skin, hydrates the skin, and creates an occlusive mask for better penetration of products. Heated wax can also be used to relieve muscle aches and pains.

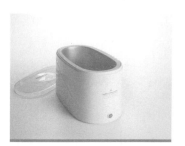

Figure 16-1 Amber paraffin spa.

■ HOW IT WORKS

Paraffin is heated to an average temperature of 126 to 134 degrees Fahrenheit in a metal pot by an electrical heating element enclosed in a plastic housing. It takes 8 to 10 hours for a large-capacity heater to melt a block of paraffin, but a smaller facial unit takes less time. All professional paraffin heaters have a temperature-control thermostat.

Recently available to the esthetics market is a single-use heater, which employs a proprietary heating system to heat paraffin dispensed into individual packets. Packet sizes are available for both hands and feet, but a facial application is not available at this time.

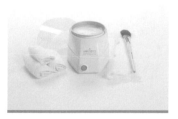

Figure 16-2 Amber facial paraffin spa.

■ WHAT IT DOES TO THE SKIN

The heat from the paraffin increases the blood supply to the skin, which increases microcirculation. When the warm paraffin is applied, moisture is drawn from the underlying layers of the skin; the moisture surfaces and mixes with the applied treatment product. This occlusive mask creates an ideal environment for the absorption of the treatment product applied under the paraffin mask, which results in optimally hydrated skin. Figure 16-3 shows an example of a facial paraffin spa.

Another alternative available to estheticians is **parafango.** This is **fango** (mud) mixed with paraffin. The results are the same as with paraffin, but with the additional benefit of minerals that help revitalize the skin and increase circulation. Figures 16-4 and 16-5 show the application and removal of a parafango treatment.

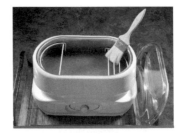

Figure 16-3 Parafango pot.

■ HOW TO USE IT

A paraffin heater is quite easy to use. The grade of paraffin and the quality of the paraffin heater are important for a safe and effective application. Here are a few guidelines for paraffin use:

- A large paraffin-heating unit should be kept on during operating hours due to the length of time it takes to melt the paraffin, usually 8 to 10 hours. A smaller unit can be heated in less time.
- Place a paraffin block or paraffin beads in the unit.
- Turn the unit on. Most professional units have an internal thermostat that regulates operating temperature, as well as a secondary safety thermostat.
- See the Protocols section on page 165 for specific applications.

Make sure your equipment has a safety certification, such as a UL listing or a CSA, CE, or ISO certification. UL, CSA, and CE listings indicate that the equipment has been tested for safety. ISO certification indicates that the unit was manufactured per international standards and that the manufacturer is tested twice a year.

■ HOW TO BUY

Buyer's Checklist

- What is the price?
- Does the unit come with an instruction manual or DVD?
- Is the machine UL listed, ISO certified, or CSA or CE tested?
- Does it come with paraffin and accessories, or do those have to be purchased separately?
- Can I buy replacement parts?
- What is covered under the warranty, and for how long?

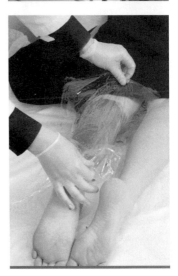

Figure 16-4 Application of parafango.

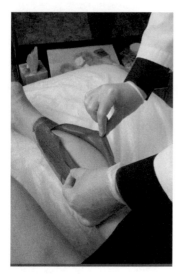

Figure 16-5 Removal of parafango.

Paraffin Heater	Automatic temperature control
	Non-flammable plastic on outside
	Even distribution of heat
	Large oval interior to maximize dripping comfort
	UL listed / CE mark
	Warranty
	Grounded cord

Figure 16-6 Features to look for when you buy a paraffin heater.

Figure 16-6 shows a chart of features to look for when you buy.

■ SAFETY

Paraffin heaters are very safe. The only concern would be a malfunctioning thermostat that could cause the paraffin to become too hot, so it is a good idea to test the unit once a month.

Testing Guidelines:

Step 1: Place a piece of cardboard large enough to cover the top of the paraffin heater over the unit.

Step 2: Make sure the heater is full of wax.

Step 3: Puncture a hole in the center of the cardboard.

Step 4: Place a meat thermometer in the center of cardboard. The thermometer must have a range between 80 and 180 degrees Fahrenheit.

Step 5: Turn the unit on and wait for it to heat up to operating temperature. The thermometer should register a temperature between 124 and 139 degrees Fahrenheit.

- Never put used paraffin back in the heater; this will cause cross-contamination.
- Always clean hands and feet before dipping them in wax.

TIP You can use gauze to dip into the paraffin to wrap around hands and feet, or you can use a gauze mask dipped in paraffin to layer on the face.

■ MAINTENANCE

- Clean your paraffin tank unit once a month.
- Always wipe down the exterior of the tub after each use.
- Check for cracking or paraffin buildup on the exterior.

How to Clean a Paraffin Tank

- Place a long piece of gauze in the melted paraffin. Make sure it touches the bottom and sides of the tub with the ends hanging over the edge for easy grasping.
- Turn off the unit.
- As soon as unit has cooled and the paraffin is solid, lift out the gauze.
- Clean the interior of the tub with an EPA-approved high-level disinfectant.
- Replace the paraffin and turn the unit back on.

DISINFECTION AND SANITIZATION

This is a modality that requires care and diligence to keep the growth of bacteria and fungi under control. In a study done by the University of Oregon in 1996, it was found that if proper disinfection protocols are followed, bacteria and fungi will not live in paraffin. Based on this information, we can assume the following:

- Most bacteria and fungi cannot survive without oxygen, water, or a food source. Neither can survive in temperatures above 120 degrees Fahrenheit. Properly functioning paraffin heaters operate at temperatures of 128 degrees or above.
- Paraffin is not a food source for fungi, and the molecular structure of paraffin is too heavy to house bacteria.
- Paraffin does not contain any oxygen or water. If some solid does get into the paraffin, the paraffin will encapsulate the foreign matter and keep it from contaminating its surroundings.
- Dipping a hand, foot, or other extremity into the paraffin does not contaminate it. For example, when the hand is dipped, the paraffin encapsulates the hand so that it does not even come in contact with the paraffin left in the heater.
- Proper disinfection procedures must always be followed.
- Always clean the area to be dipped with an effective antimicrobial soap or waterless gel.
- Never put used paraffin back into the pot.
- Always keep a lid on the pot.
- Clean the pot at least once a month, or as soon as you see debris of any kind.
- Never dip any body part with any skin abrasion or open cut. This includes cuticles that have been picked open.

Disinfection	Maintenance
Never place used paraffin wax back into pot	Clean paraffin pot once a month or as soon as any debris is found in wax
Use an EPA-approved disinfectant once a month to clean pot	Always keep lid on when not in use
Spray EPA-approved disinfectant on exterior after each use	Check temperature once a month; should be 124-139 degrees
Always disinfect client's hands and feet before dipping	Check exterior for cracking daily
	Wipe down exterior after each use

Figure 16-7 Disinfection and maintenance steps.

Figure 16-7 gives maintenance and disinfection steps for paraffin heaters.

■ CONTRAINDICATIONS AND CAUTIONS

There are very few contraindications for using paraffin. The consultation is still important to determine contraindications or special needs that your client may have. Do not rely exclusively on the intake form; it is also important to verbally get information and clarification from your client.

- Pregnancy: Use caution when working with pregnant clients. They can be very sensitive.
- Blood vessel disorders: Arteriosclerosis, or hardening of the arteries, affects the arteries' ability to handle increased blood flow. Fainting can occur when increased dilation of the blood vessels occurs during heat treatments.
- Skin inflammation: Heat treatments increase circulation, which could make inflammation worse.
- Skin disorders or diseases: These may be aggravated by treatment.
- Very sensitive skin: Clients with this skin type may be very uncomfortable during treatment.
- Botox: No treatment should be performed until 72 hours after injection.
- Cuts and abrasions: Do not perform services on clients with any open abrasions.

- Severe bruising: Bruising will make treatment uncomfortable for your client.
- High or low blood pressure: Either of these could be made worse due to the increase in circulation. Even if such conditions are treated and under control, use caution. Never leave a client with blood pressure issues alone, and help them on and off the treatment bed.
- HIV: Use OSHA guidelines for bloodborne pathogens when working on HIV-infected clients. This will ensure safety for the client and technician.
- Malignant melanoma: Treatment must be completed, and client must be in remission. Obtain physician approval before proceeding. Do not apply treatment when in doubt about a possible abnormality; instead, refer the client to a dermatologist.

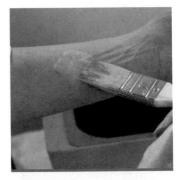

Figure 16-8 Test paraffin on wrist or forearm.

■ PREPARATION FOR TREATMENT

- Have your client fill out an assessment form.
- Check for contraindications.
- Have your client change into a treatment gown and remove all jewelry and contact lenses.
- Analyze the skin using a magnifying lamp.
- Explain the procedure.
- Make sure your paraffin heater has been on a sufficient amount of time and that it is working properly.

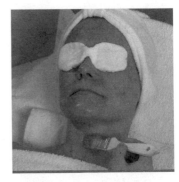

Figure 16-9 Apply first layer of paraffin.

■ PROTOCOLS

Here are some helpful protocols for treatment room use.

Basic Application of Paraffin Mask

Modified from *Milady's Standard Fundamentals for Estheticians*.

Step 1: Test the temperature of the paraffin on your wrist or on the inside of your forearm, as shown in Figure 16-8.

Step 2: Apply the first layer of paraffin to the face with a brush, as shown in Figure 16-9. As an alternative, you can dip a gauze mask first, then apply the mask to the face, but make sure your client has eye pads on first.

Step 3: Apply gauze mask with the nose area cut out. If the client feels uncomfortable, cut a hole for the mouth as well, as shown in Figure 16-10.

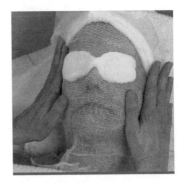

Figure 16-10 Apply gauze mask.

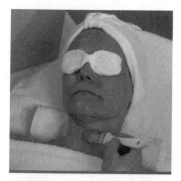

Figure 16-11 Add layers of paraffin.

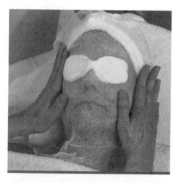

Figure 16-12 Loosen mask.

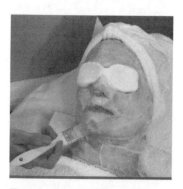

Figure 16-13 Carefully lift off mask in one piece.

Step 4: Begin adding layers of paraffin to the gauze. The mask should be approximately a quarter of an inch thick. See Figure 16-11.

Step 5: Leave the mask on for 15 minutes.

Step 6: Use a wooden spatula to loosen the mask at the hairline and remove it. Refer to Figures 16-12 and 16-13.

Step 7: Proceed with the balance of the facial treatment.

Paraffin Facial for Dry Skin

Step 1: Cleanse skin with a gentle cleanser for dry or dehydrated skin.

Step 2: Remove the cleanser with soft gauze or a warm towel.

Step 3: Apply a gentle enzyme mask to the skin; use products per the manufacturer's instructions.

Step 4: Steam for 7 to 10 minutes.

Step 5: Remove the mask with a warm towel.

Step 6: Spray a toner that is appropriate for dry or dehydrated skin.

Step 7: Blot the toner with tissue.

Step 8: Apply a massage cream or oil for dry or dehydrated skin.

Step 9: Perform a stimulating massage treatment for 8 to 10 minutes. (Refer to Chapter 19 for an indirect massage protocol).

Step 10: Dip the gauze mask in melted paraffin, or apply paraffin to the skin with a mask brush.

Step 11: Leave the mask on for up to 15 minutes, according to manufacturer's directions.

Step 12: Remove the mask and apply a hydrating serum, using light effleurage movements.

Step 13: Apply a finishing cream with an SPF of 15 or higher.

Your Protocol:

_____

_____

_____

_____

_____

_____

_____

■ YOUR EQUIPMENT INFORMATION

Manufacturer info:

Name/phone number: _____

Web site: _____

Date purchased: _____ Registration: _____

Warranty info: _____

Replacement part info: _____

TROUBLESHOOTING

Troubleshooting a paraffin heater should be referred to your manufacturer due to the sensitive nature of the thermostat. It is very important to maintain the correct temperature of a paraffin heater, because incorrect temperatures can lead to a burn or to the growth of bacteria.

Q & A

What are the pros and cons of a paraffin heater?

Pros

Effectiveness: Paraffin provides a very effective hydrating treatment, and it is truly relaxing for the client.
Cost: Paraffin heaters are very cost-effective and inexpensive.
Ease of use: These units are very easy to use.
Safety: Paraffin heaters are very safe.

Cons

Maintenance: These units require consistent and thorough cleaning to ensure a long life.

Can I achieve the same results without a paraffin heater?

No. You need a paraffin heater to provide a warm paraffin treatment. As far as stimulating the circulation of the skin is concerned, there are other electrotherapy modalities that work. Warm paraffin provides a truly relaxing spa experience when applied correctly.

REFERENCES

1. D'Angelo, J., Dean, P., Dietz, S., Hinds, C., Lees, M., Miller, E., & Zani, A. (2003). *Milady's Standard Comprehensive Training for Estheticians.* New York: Thomson Delmar Learning.
2. Simmons, J. V. (1989, 1995). *Science and the Beauty Business, The Beauty Salon and its Equipment* (2nd ed.). United Kingdom: Macmillan Press Ltd.
3. Lees, M. (2001). *Skin Care: Beyond the Basics.* New York: Thomson Delmar Learning.
4. Nordman, L. (2005). *Professional Beauty Therapy, The Official Guide to Level 3* (2nd ed.). London: Thomson Learning.
5. Burke, M. Topping, C., Rodia, R. M., Spencer C., & Henigan, C. (1996). "Are You Getting More Than Soft Hands from a Paraffin (Wax) Bath?" Oregon State University, Eugene, OR. Available online at http://www.therabathpro.com.
6. Gerson, J. (2004). *Milady's Standard Fundamentals for Estheticians.* New York: Thomson Delmar Learning.

Electrotherapy Equipment

SECTION

4

Electrical Theory and Priniciples

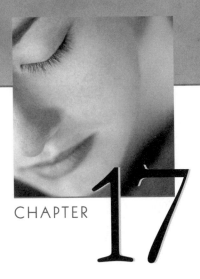

CHAPTER 17

▪ ELECTROTHERAPY AND ESTHETICS

The science of electricity is important for the esthetician to understand. You do not need to be a scientist to understand how electricity will affect the body, but you must understand basic theories to make an educated decision. Most esthetic equipment uses electricity, even the most advanced antiaging modalities. To start to understand the **electrotherapy** machines used in skin care, it is helpful to understand the three types of electric currents, how electricity works, and the terms used to measure electrical current. In addition to the basics of electricity, it is important to understand how electrical energy affects the body, especially the skin.

▪ WHAT IS ELECTRICITY?

Electricity is the flow of negative **electrons** along a **conductor,** which creates a chemical, thermal, or mechanical action. It is a form of energy that is around us at all times. Our bodies even produce electrical charges. To understand electricity, we must understand the atom, which is the building block of all matter. Figure 17-1 shows an illustration of an atom.

An atom has at its center a nucleus, which is made up of positively charged protons and neutrons, which have no charge. The orbit around the nucleus is filled with electrons, and these orbiting electrons travel in bands, or shells, around the nucleus. Electrons are negatively charged. The most important orbit to consider for a discussion of electricity is the outer ring, or **axis;** this band is also called the **valence shell,** and it is easier to displace an electron on this outer ring. These electrons may be shared with other atoms, so they are known as **free electrons.** When an atom gains or

173

Carbon Atom

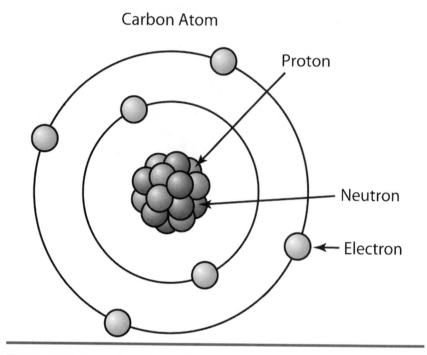

Figure 17-1 Illustration of a carbon atom.

loses electrons, an electrical charge is created. When the outer ring gains an electron, the atom has a negative charge; if it loses an electron, it has a positive charge. So, surrounding each atom is an electrical charge, which either attracts or repels other electrons in other atoms. When these electrons flow along a conductor, electricity is created. Examples of conductors are copper, steel, water, body fluids, and **carbon.**

For electricity to work, such as in our esthetic machines, it must form a circuit. A **circuit** is a conductor connected to components to form a consistent pathway through which electricity can move. See Figure 17-2 for an example.

There are four types of circuits. A **closed circuit** is an electrical current that follows a continuous path between positive and negative poles. A **complete circuit** is the entire path an electrical current follows: from its source, through a conductor, and back to the source again. An **open circuit** is when the flow of electricity is interrupted by a switch or device that breaks the connection. A **short circuit** happens when there is a break in the insulator. To keep the electricity flowing through the center of the conductor, the circuit must use an insulator. An **insulator** is a substance that does not allow electricity to flow through it. For example, plastic and rubber are used as insulation on common electrical wires.

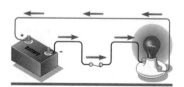

Figure 17-2 A complete circuit.

■ TYPES OF CURRENTS

Electricity comes in three forms: *static, direct current (DC),* and *alternating current (AC).* **Static electricity** is created when a large number of atoms gain or lose electrons, giving an object an electrical charge. In a very arid environment, friction between your body and an object, such as a rug, will cause you to lose electrons to the rug. When you touch a conductor, such as a doorknob, you may see a spark and feel a little shock.

Direct current occurs when electrons move in one direction only. This current is even and uninterrupted. For skin care purposes, DC creates a chemical reaction in the skin; this is called **electrolysis.** This term is also used to mean the permanent removal of hair, but it is actually the chemical reaction that takes place within the skin. Galvanic current is an example of direct current. Figure 17-3 shows a diagram of a DC current.

Alternating current is the flow of electrons in a back-and-forth movement. The most common AC waveform is a sine wave. In electrotherapy it is referred to as a **sinusoidal current.** It is important to note that alternating current does *not* create a chemical reaction within the skin, only a mechanical reaction. **Faradic current** is another waveform that uses an interrupted AC current to create mechanical effects in the body. Alternating current is the current that all of our electrical appliances and outlets use. **Hertz** is the speed at which an AC current reverses direction. Another term for Hertz is **frequency.** Figure 17-4 shows a diagram of an AC current, and Figure 17-5 shows a table of different currents.

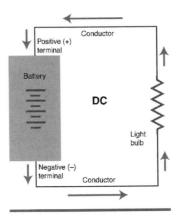

Figure 17-3 Direct current.

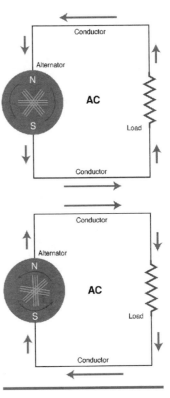

Figure 17-4 Alternating current.

Current	Description
Alternating current (AC)	High frequency; no chemical reaction in skin; another term is sine or sinusoidal current
Sinusoidal	Another term for AC; higher voltage machine used in body therapy; not used by estheticians
Faradic	Interrupted AC current; stimulates muscles; no chemical reaction; used in muscle regeneration
Direct current (DC)	Galvanic current and microcurrent; creates chemical reaction in skin based on polarity
Microcurrent	DC with AC measured in microamps; refers to a modality, not a current; used for skin rejuvenation and other healing techniques

Figure 17-5 Currents and their uses.

■ MEASURING ELECTRICITY

There are three aspects to measuring electric current: *force, flow,* and *resistance.* **Voltage** is the measured push rate, or the force with which the electrical current is being delivered along a conductor. For example, a standard household circuit is 120 volts; larger appliances use 220 volts. Most esthetic machines use the standard 120-volt outlet. **Mains** is the term used for the alternating current that flows from your outlet. Figure 17-6 shows an example of a voltage diagram.

An **ampere** is the measurement used for current flowing along the path of a circuit. This unit of measurement is named after the French physicist **André-Marie Ampère.** A higher rate of electrical current flowing through a circuit will result in a higher amperage. Esthetic machines use microamperes and milliamperes. These strengths are well below the level of danger of electric shock. See Figure 17-7 for a diagram of amperage.

An **ohm** is a measurement of the resistance an electrical current faces as it moves through the circuit. Ohms cannot be measured; they have to be calculated using **Ohm's law.** This is an equation that measures the relationship between volts and amps. See Figure 17-8 for a chart of common electricity measurement.

Electrical power used by a machine is measured in **watts** and **kilowatts.** This is determined by another equation: watts = volts × amps. Esthetic machines will have the voltage and the power rating in watts listed on the machine. This means that you will not have to calculate electrical power use.

TIP Ohm's Law:

ohms = volts ÷ amps

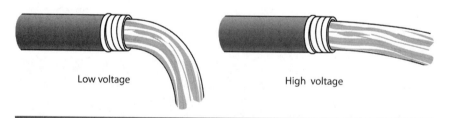

Low voltage   High voltage

Figure 17-6 Voltage diagram.

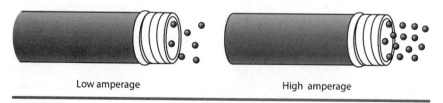

Low amperage   High amperage

Figure 17-7 Amperage diagram.

Measurement	Description
A	Ampere: a measure of the electron flow (current). Too strong for esthetic treatments
mA	Milliampere: 1/1000 of an ampere used w/ galvanic current; no stronger than 3 mA for the face and 8 mA for the body
uA	Microampere: 1/1,000,000 of an ampere; used in microcurrent Nanoampere: 1/1,000,000,000 of an ampere; *new in microcurrent application*

Figure 17-8 Electricity measurement chart.

■ ELECTRICITY AND THE BODY

To understand how electrotherapy machines work, it is important to understand the direct effect that electricity has on the body. Our spinal column is the communication pathway for chemical electrical signals coming from the brain. These electrical signals travel through our nerves to impact all of the major physiological processes in the body. See Figure 17-9 for an illustration.

Our bodies are electrical organisms; they even generate their own electricity. Let us look at how our body is affected by electricity.

- Heart: Without internal electrical pulses, our heart would stop. **Pacemakers** were developed to help a heart that is damaged and unable to produce these pulses.
- Nervous system: Electrical signals drive all sensing and motor actions through the nerve cells.
- Brain: Electrical impulses can be measured in the brain using an **electroencephalogram (EEG).** Scientists are still researching how electricity works in the brain.
- Wound healing: The cell is charged by storing electrically charged particles of **adenosine triphosphate (ATP).** For a damaged cell to heal, electricity of the right current and strength can be applied to the body and transported via the **ion channels,** thus facilitating the natural healing process.
- Muscular movement: Muscles must be stimulated by the electrical charges of the nervous system to function.

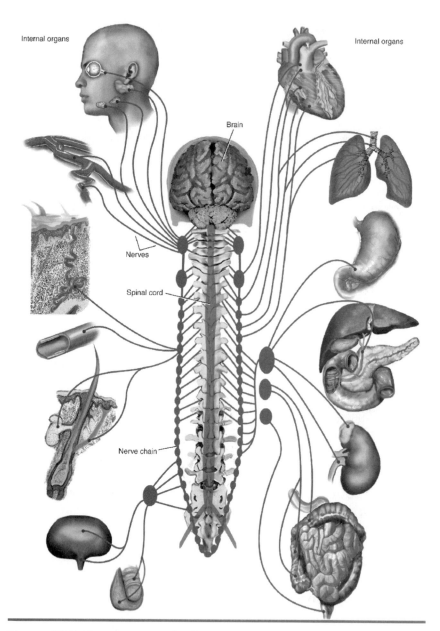

Internal organs

Internal organs

Brain

Nerves

Spinal cord

Nerve chain

Figure 17-9 Nerve communication.

Many other systems of the body are affected by electricity. Many theories regarding how electricity functions in the body are not accepted by Western medicine, but they are widely used throughout the world nevertheless. Research is ongoing and has produced some interesting results.

■ THE HEALING THEORY

In the case of injury or cell degeneration, electrical signals are impaired. Electricity follows the path of least resistance, which means that the electrical current will move around the area of trauma. This is called the **Arndt/Schultz law.**

Every cell in the body is like an electrical generator and can be seen as a self-healing organism. If there is damage to any area of the body, the flow of electricity is impaired, and self-healing cannot occur. The technology of using external electrical currents for healing is called **electrophysiology.** In esthetics, many of these principles are used for repairing damaged skin, fighting aging, and improving the overall appearance. The theory of healing with electricity is interesting and warrants more research by estheticians.

■ ELECTRICITY CAN HARM

As well as being beneficial to the body, electricity can be very harmful. Electrical current passing through the body at high voltage—a current greater than 500 volts—will cause deep burns and destroy tissue. High voltages passing through the body can also short-circuit the nerve impulses, causing biological processes to stop or become abnormal. Sometimes this results in death or permanent injury. See Figure 17-10 for a chart of potential damage that electricity can cause.

Many scientists believe that **electromagnetic pollution** creates unhealthy frequencies of electricity that also harm the body. These frequencies are thought to create stress reactions within the body that can cause fatigue, mental illness, weakening of the immune system, and other diseases. Electromagnetic pollution can come from any of our

1 mA	Barely perceptible
16 mA	Painful shock, no loss of muscle control
20 to 50 mA	Painful shock, local muscle control is lost
100 to 200 mA	Normal heartbeat effected, person is attached to circuit. Death may result
> 200 mA	Severe burns, muscular contraction, heart will stop for as long as current running through body. Duration of shock will determine if heart can be restarted. Death likely

Figure 17-10 Effects of electrical current on the body.

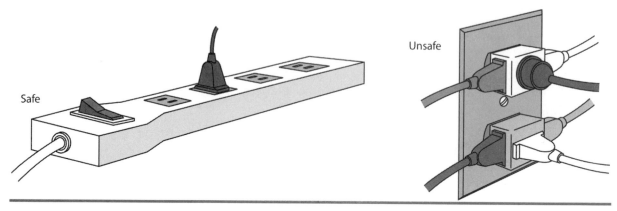

Figure 17-11 Safe and unsafe outlets.

frequently used appliances, computers, and power lines. This is a controversial subject, and many research studies are ongoing regarding this controversial topic.

Electrical Safety

Working with electrical equipment requires due diligence to make sure that both the client and technician are safe. Here are some general guidelines:

- Always check equipment before use for cracks in electrical cords.
- Use only UL, CE or CSA listed equipment.
- Do not overload outlets. See Figure 17-11 for an example.
- Never handle electrical equipment with wet hands.
- Always use a power strip with multiple electrical cords. See Figure 17-12 for an example.
- Never clean equipment that is plugged into an outlet.
- Do not allow cords to become twisted or bent.
- Remove the electrical plug by pulling on the plug, not the cord.
- Do not try to fix electrical wiring unless you are qualified.
- Do not touch two metal objects together if electrical current is moving through either of them. See Figure 17-13 for an example.

You will see in the following chapters that each type of current has a different effect on the body. We will be focusing on the effects of electrotherapy on the skin, but with the knowledge that more than just the surface of the skin will be impacted.

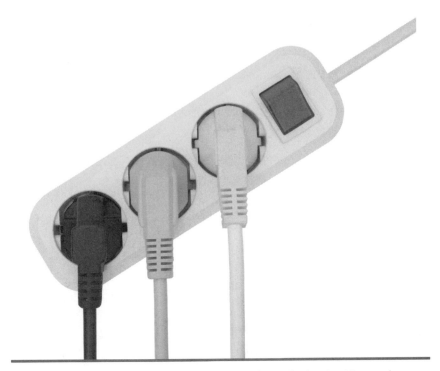

Figure 17-12 Always use a power strip with multiple electric cords.

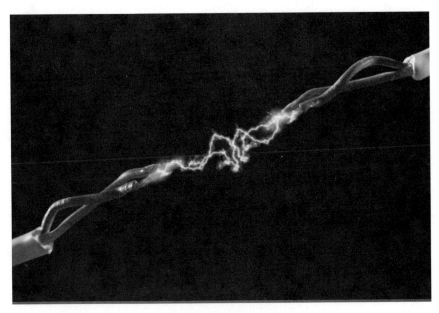

Figure 17-13 Never touch open wires together.

REFERENCES

1. Dean, P., Dietz, S., Hinds, C., Lees, M., Miller, E., & Zani, A. (2003). *Milady's Standard Comprehensive Training for Estheticians.* New York: Thomson Delmar Learning.

2. Simmons, J. V. (1989, 1995). *Science and the Beauty Business: The Beauty Salon and its Equipment* (2nd ed.). United Kingdom: Macmillan Press Ltd.

3. Lees, M. (2001). *Skin Care: Beyond the Basics.* New York: Thomson Delmar Learning.

4. Nordman, L. (2005). *Professional Beauty Therapy, The Official Guide to Level 3* (2nd ed.). London: Thomson Learning.

5. Cooper, M. A. (2003). *Merck Manual of Medical Information: Electrical Injuries.* New Jersey: Merck Research Laboratories.

6. Becker, R. O., & Selden, G. (1985). *The Body Electric.* New York: William Morrow.

7. Starwynn, D. (2002). *Microcurrent Electro-Acupuncture.* Arizona: Desert Heart Press.

8. Gerson, J. (2004). *Milady's Standard Fundamentals for Estheticians.* New York: Thomson Delmar Learning.

High-Frequency Machine

The high-frequency (HF) machine is one of the technologies most commonly used by estheticians. It is a safe, effective, and versatile tool that is affordable and easy to use. In this chapter we will explore the basics of how electricity is used in the HF machine, how to use the machine, why it works, and protocols for use and safety. See Figure 18-1 for an example of a high-frequency machine.

CHAPTER 18

■ FUNCTIONS

The HF machine is used after extraction to kill bacteria and **coagulate** open lesions. It is also used for indirect massage to stimulate the skin and to aid absorption of products by warming the skin.

The HF machine uses an alternating electrical current or sinusoidal current at 100,000 hertz or more. Estheticians use low frequency and high frequency, which are voltages in the range of 100,000 to 250,000 hertz.

Using AC current was pioneered by the scientist **Nikola Tesla** in the late 1800s. Higher frequency, low-voltage current is used for **epilation**, or hair removal.

The major components of an HF machine are the **capacitor** and the **inductance coil.** A capacitor is responsible for smoothing out the "bumps" in the electrical current, much in the same way that shocks function on an automobile. The capacitor holds electrical charges and produces an alternating current. The inductance coil acts like a transformer; it is also called an **Oudin coil.** High-frequency energy is not easy to control via a wire, so the Oudin coil is used in the electrode holder to help control the charge. The electrode holder is an attachment that is plugged into the HF machine, and which is held by the esthetician. An electrode is inserted within it to apply the HF energy.

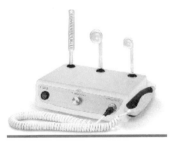

Figure 18-1 Silhouet-Tone equipment.

TIP Nikola Tesla is the inventor that convinced U.S. power companies to use AC current to transport electricity long distances. It is what we use today when we plug our appliances into a wall outlet.

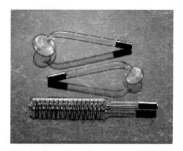

Figure 18-2 High-frequency electrodes.

ELECTRODES

Electrodes have different shapes and sizes, which affect the skin in different ways. The electrode has a metal cap that conducts electricity from the holder. Inside the glass, air has been removed, which creates a vacuum; this vacuum contains a small amount of gas. Usually, neon gas is used, but some electrodes contain argon gas, which gives off a violet or blue glow. Electrodes that contain argon are called **Macintyre violet ray tubes.** Neon gas creates a pink or orange glow. The current that passes through the electrode creates a small amount of ozone, as does the oxygen on the surface of the skin.

There are various sizes of glass electrodes. An **intensifier electrode** is also known as a **mushroom electrode.** Estheticians usually work with two sizes of electrodes: small and large. The small electrode has a more stimulating effect on the skin, because the HF machine works on the point of contact. A small point of contact with the skin will deliver more energy to that area, which works for coagulating open papules and pustules in a technique known as **sparking.** Most HF machines come with a specific sparking electrode that looks like a small cylinder. Also included with most machines is a **saturator electrode** with an **intensifier coil** that is used for indirect high frequency; this looks like a long tube with a metal coil running through the middle, and this is the electrode the client holds as you perform a manual massage with the unit turned on. Figure 18-2 shows a picture of different electrodes.

The gas sealed in the glass electrode creates a small amount of UV light. Because it is sealed, the gas cannot escape. The colors created by the different gases do not affect the treatment outcome; rather, it is the size of the electrode, the intensity of the current, and the method of application that determine results. See Figure 18-3 for a list of common electrodes and their applications.

HOW TO BUY

HF machines are available in two basic varieties: as individual units or in a **combination machine** that has other equipment built in with it. The approximate price for an individual machine is around $200 to $450, but combination machines start at $1,000 and can go as high as $3,500. All machines have the same technology; differences in price relate to the quality of materials and range of support the company you choose has to offer. Make sure your equipment has a safety certification such as a UL listing or a CSA, CE, or ISO certification. UL, CSA, and CE listings

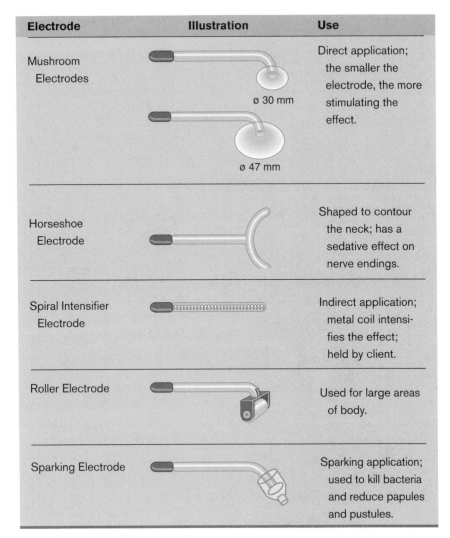

Electrode	Illustration	Use
Mushroom Electrodes	ø 30 mm ø 47 mm	Direct application; the smaller the electrode, the more stimulating the effect.
Horseshoe Electrode		Shaped to contour the neck; has a sedative effect on nerve endings.
Spiral Intensifier Electrode		Indirect application; metal coil intensifies the effect; held by client.
Roller Electrode		Used for large areas of body.
Sparking Electrode		Sparking application; used to kill bacteria and reduce papules and pustules.

Figure 18-3 High-frequency electrodes and their uses.

indicate that the equipment has been tested for safety. ISO indicates that it has been manufactured per international standards and that the manufacturer is tested twice a year.

Buyer's Checklist

- What is the price?
- Do you have an instruction manual, DVD, on-site training, or technical support?
- Is the machine UL, CSA, or CE listed? Is it ISO certified?

TIP **Underwriters Laboratory** (UL) is the U.S. organization responsible for testing products for consumer safety. Many international products are not UL certified, but UL has recently started an international section of certification. The alternative to UL listing is CE or CSA certification. These marks on a product tells you that the machine has been thoroughly tested and investigated by a team of product safety professionals.

- Does the machine come with electrodes, or do those have to be purchased separately?
- Can I buy replacement parts? If so, how much are they and what parts are available?
- What is covered under the warranty, and for how long?
- Do you have a loaner program if my machine breaks?
- Where was this equipment manufactured?

■ WHY IT WORKS

High-frequency energy is absorbed by water molecules, which are vibrated and made warm. This leads to heat production, which increases circulation in the skin and dilates blood vessels, thus increasing lymph flow and blood flow to spread out the heat. Increased circulation is beneficial to the skin and increases cell metabolism to speed healing in damaged tissues. Increased circulation also increases sebum and perspiration secretion; this helps deep-clean the skin and increases hydration.

A single electrode is used to transmit superficial AC current around the point of contact; this means that it affects the specific area only. For example, if you are trying to warm the skin to facilitate absorption, you will have to move the electrode around the face in a consistent pattern.

HF sparking works by stimulating the skin, producing an antiseptic effect as well as tightening and toning. The antiseptic action comes from the heat, which kills bacteria, and from the low level of ions that creates ozone.

HF has no polarity; therefore, it cannot create a chemical change. This means that it *does not create a chemical change within the product* which increases epidermal penetration.

> **TIP** HF is the one treatment that really reduces inflamed pustules and papules. Try the sparking technique several times over the inflamed area.

■ PRODUCT ABSORPTION AND THE SKIN

To better understand how HF treatments affect the skin, you need to understand the process of absorption. **Dermal absorption** is a controversial subject, but here are some basic scientific facts:

- The rate of absorption is directly affected by the concentration of the substance and the area over which it is applied. For example, lidocaine applied in small areas is safe; applied to large areas such as the legs (especially with occlusion) can lead to overdose.
- The thickness of the stratum corneum determines the degree of absorption. Areas where this skin layer is thinner, such as the

genitals, are much more receptive to absorption than, say, the soles of the feet.

- A damaged skin barrier will facilitate absorption at a faster rate. This is why estheticians should always exfoliate before applying serums, and massage and remove the lipid barrier before doing a chemical peel.
- **Occlusion** of the skin will enhance penetration of a product. Occlusion entails applying a substance to the skin that air cannot penetrate. You can purchase plastic masks that will create an occlusive environment in the skin.
- The composition of the product affects its penetration. It is not one certain ingredient that makes the difference; it is molecular weight and how the ingredient is carried in the product. If the ingredient carrier damages the lipid barrier, then absorption will happen at a faster rate.
- **Lipid-soluble** products will absorb better than others. Any product that is similar to the intercellular "cement" (a substance that contains lipids and amino acids that make up the skin's moisture barrier) will be readily accepted by the skin. Below the stratum corneum, the epidermis is hydrophilic, or "water loving"; this means it absorbs water easily. The challenge is to find a carrier that will benefit the lipophilic stratum corneum and the hydrophilic epidermis.
- Increasing the temperature of the skin aids absorption. This why high frequency can indirectly affect how a product is absorbed. Generally speaking, warmer skin facilitates absorption at a higher rate.

■ WHAT IT DOES TO THE SKIN

- Direct high frequency is warming, stimulating, and antiseptic.
- Indirect high frequency is warming and soothing.
- Increases oxygenation of the skin.
- Increases coagulation and will help heal any open lesions after extraction. UV light and ozone have antiseptic properties, but be sure to follow with the appropriate antibacterial lotion on extracted areas, because the ozone created by high frequency is minute.

■ HOW TO USE IT

There are several types of high-frequency applications that you can perform: direct, indirect, and sparking.

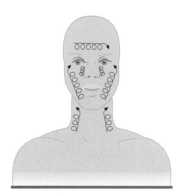

Figure 18-4 Application of direct high frequency.

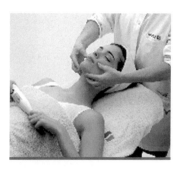

Figure 18-5 Application of indirect high frequency.

For **direct application,** you can apply cream under a gauze mask or use gauze alone. Make sure the equipment is turned off, choose an electrode, and firmly place it in a holder. Turn the machine on. Place your finger on the electrode before placing it against the client's skin to avoid an electrical shock.

Release your finger, adjust the power level based on the client's comfort level with the treatment, and move the electrode in a smooth pattern over the skin without lifting the electrode off the skin. Apply for 8 to 10 minutes for oily skin and 5 minutes for dry skin. Figure 18-4 shows the pattern of application.

Indirect application works by having the client hold the long electrode and holder while the esthetician performs a soothing effleurage massage on the skin. This will produce a warming and soothing effect that is especially effective with aging, sensitive, and rosacea clients. Massage up to 10 minutes maximum.

Indirect application is also known as **Viennese massage.** This technique is indicated for increasing cell metabolism, which will help with aging, dull, and stressed skin. See Figure 18-5 for an example of indirect application.

Sparking is beneficial on papules and pustules. Use the electrode to create minute sparks directly on the lesion. Apply a finger to the electrode, place the electrode over the lesion, gently lift the finger, and spark the area. Place your finger back on the electrode and turn the unit off.

Another term used for sparking is **fulguration.** According to Webster's Dictionary, fulguration is "the act or process of flashing, like lightning." In the medical profession, fulguration is a term used for the removal or destruction of diseased tissue with a controlled electric current. It is important to note that HF treatment will not destroy diseased tissue; if it could, it would be considered a Class III medical device by the FDA, in which case the FDA would not allow the use of high frequency by estheticians.

■ SAFETY

The potential for small electrical shocks is a possibility when using the HF machine, but in general, HF machines are very safe to use. The situations that increase the potential for such shocks include lack of proper machine upkeep, a poorly grounded plug, broken wires, damaged electrodes or electrode holders, and poorly made equipment.

All electrical work performed in the United States must meet the National Electrical Code. In addition, equipment should be UL listed.

TIP Always clean electrodes and the electrode holder to avoid electric shock; product residue will act as a conduit for the high frequency.

TIP Do not allow your client to hold the glass electrode too close to the handle; this can cause small electric shocks.

UL listing is important due to the fact that an independent agency has certified that the equipment has been tested as safe. CSA is another independent testing agency that many North American manufacturers use, and CE testing is used in the European Union. These are good certifications to have and can be an alternative to a UL listing. Unfortunately, there is no governing body that inspects esthetic machines unless they are classified by the FDA. See Chapter 1 for more information on FDA regulations and UL listing.

Wall outlets should be the three-prong grounded type. Make sure that you do not overload the outlet. A ground fault circuit interrupter (GCFI) is required on all outlets within six feet of a water source. For the purposes of a facial room, it is a good idea to have them.

It is a myth that any products containing sulfur or alcohol will burn the skin during a high-frequency treatment. The current is so small that it would be impossible. The problem with sulfur and alcohol and HF applications is the irritation to the skin and the texture of some products when exposed to high frequency. The most that can happen with an HF application is that small shocks may be delivered to the client and esthetician if the machine is not in good working condition. This can be uncomfortable but is not fatal.

TIP Never place an electrode in the holder by pushing with the palm of your hand. The glass could break and cause injury.

■ MAINTENANCE

Maintenance is one of the most important aspects of owning esthetic machines. Maintenance for an HF machine is very easy. Manufacturers will also have their own protocols, so be sure to follow their directions. In general, use these guidelines:

- Clean electrodes and electrode holders after each use.
- Use isopropyl alcohol on a saturated cotton tip to clean out the electrode holder once or twice a month.
- Do not store electrodes in a UV sterilizer.
- Check all wires before use. Do not use the equipment if cracked or loose wires are visible.

■ DISINFECTION AND SANITIZATION

- Disinfect electrodes by saturating the glass portion in contact with the skin with a state-approved high-level disinfectant.
- Do not submerge metal ends in the disinfectant solution.

- Place electrodes in a UV sanitizer for 20 minutes for additional disinfection, but do not store electrodes in the sanitizer.
- Store electrodes in the container that came with your machine or in surgical envelopes. These are available from medical and esthetic suppliers.

■ CONTRAINDICATIONS AND CAUTIONS

The consultation is extremely important to determine contraindications or special needs that your client may have. Do not rely exclusively on the intake form; it is also important to verbally get information and clarification from your client.

- Metal implements in the body and pacemakers: Electricity will concentrate in areas where a conductor is present, and pacemakers will be interrupted.
- Pregnancy: Do not use electricity on pregnant clients.
- Heart problems.
- Skin inflammation: Most electrical treatments increase circulation, which can make inflammation worse.
- Skin disorders or diseases: These may be aggravated by treatment.
- Very sensitive skin: Clients with this skin type may be very uncomfortable during HF treatments.
- Migraines or severe headaches: Treatment may cause worsening of an existing headache, but it has not been known to cause them.
- Lack of tactile sensation (e.g., numbness due to stroke): Clients suffering from sensation loss will not be able to gauge the intensity of the current, which could result in injury.
- Nervous clients: Treatment will be ineffective if the client cannot relax.
- Excessive metal dental work: Treatment will concentrate the current around the metal, but porcelain veneers will not. Clients with braces will be very uncomfortable.
- Metal piercings in the body, including tongue piercings: Current will concentrate around the metal.
- Botox: Treatment is not recommended until 48 hours after injection. The treatment paralyzes muscle, so any treatment to stimulate muscle would be ineffective.
- Epilepsy: Can possibly trigger a seizure.
- Cuts and abrasions: Electrical current will concentrate in the area, because bodily fluids act as a conductor.
- Severe bruising: Bruising makes treatment uncomfortable.
- High or low blood pressure: Such conditions could be made worse due to the increase in circulation. Even if these conditions are be-

ing treated and are under control, use caution. Never leave the client alone, and help them on and off the treatment bed.

- Recent scar tissue: Scarred skin is very sensitive and less resistant. Use caution when using electrotherapy. High frequency is okay six weeks after injury or surgery, if no pulling of the skin occurs.
- HIV: Follow OSHA guidelines to ensure safety for the client and technician.
- History of blood clots (thrombosis) or embolism: Treatment could aggravate the condition and cause a heart attack or stroke.
- Malignant melanoma: Treatment for the malignancy must be complete, and the client must be in remission. Obtain physician approval. Do not apply HF treatment when in doubt about a possible abnormality; instead, refer the client to a dermatologist.

■ PREPARATION FOR TREATMENT

- Have your client fill out an assessment form.
- Check for contraindications.
- Have your client change into a treatment gown and remove all jewelry.
- Analyze the skin using a magnifying lamp.
- Explain the procedure. Your clients may become uncomfortable if they do not understand that the buzzing noise or slight ozone smell are normal.
- Make sure to test all equipment before applying treatment to your clients. After testing your electrode, disinfect the surface before applying it to a client's skin.
- Inspect all wires and electrodes.
- Follow the manufacturer's instructions for setting up and priming your HF machine.

■ PROTOCOLS

Direct Application

Step 1: Pick the correct electrode for the application. Refer back to Figure 18-3 for a description of the different electrodes. See Figure 18-6 for an example of HF direct application.

Step 2: Place gauze and/or cream on the client's face, as shown in Figure 18-7.

TIP What do you do when you discover the client has some contraindication to treatment? Explain that you would not want to make any existing condition worse, and explain how the treatment may do that. Offer a different service if possible, or advise the client that treatment may be possible with some modification; for example, staying away from the area of a severe bruise, or asking your to client remove her piercings.

TIP When in doubt, refer the client to a physician. For insurance purposes, the client should provide you with a doctor's note or a signed waiver of liability.

TIP Always remember to check for contraindications with any electrotherapy treatment. Client comfort and safety are top priorities.

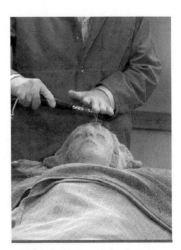

Figure 18-6 Direct HF with gauze mask.

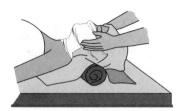

Figure 18-7 Putting gauze on the face.

Step 3: Turn power on.

Step 4: Place your finger on the electrode to break the current. See Figure 18-8.

Step 5: Place the electrode on the client's face, take your finger off the electrode, and increase the current intensity to the desired level; current should feel strong but not irritating. See Figure 18-9.

Step 6: Move the electrode in a circular motion over the skin's surface. See Figure 18-10 for the appropriate pattern.

Treatment should last approximately 8 and 10 minutes for oily or combination skin and 5 minutes for dry skin.

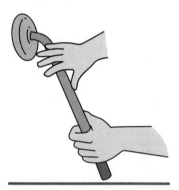

Figure 18-8 Place finger on HF before placing on the face.

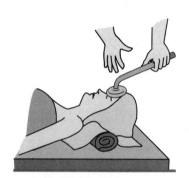

Figure 18-9 Remove finger after the HF electrode is on the face.

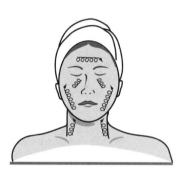

Figure 18-10 Pattern of HF application.

Indirect Application

Step 1: Place the spiral electrode into the handle, and have the client hold the handle with one hand and the electrode with other. See Figure 18-11.

Step 2: Apply massage cream.

Step 3: While touching the client's skin with one hand, turn on the machine. See Figure 18-12.

Step 4: Increase the current until the client feels a warm tingling sensation.

Step 5: Place both hands on the client's face and perform a gentle face, neck, and shoulder massage. Do not use tapotement movements. When massaging over bony areas, reduce the intensity of the current. See Figure 18-13.

Step 6: Perform massage for 8 to 10 minutes.

TIP Remember to check your client's comfort level and skin reaction frequently. Increased redness indicates good circulation; bright flushing redness means that the current is too strong.

Step 7: When finished, maintain contact with the client's skin with one hand, and turn off the machine with the other. See Figure 18-14.

Step 8: Remove the electrode from the client's hand.

Step 9: Continue light massage for 5 to 8 minutes longer without electrical current.

Step 10: Follow with the rest of the facial protocol (e.g., toner, mask, and moisturizer).

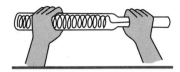

Figure 18-11 Have client hold the electrode for indirect HP application.

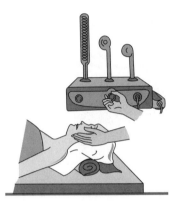

Figure 18-12 Touch client's face while turning on the HF.

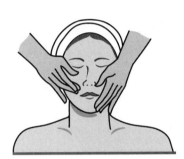

Figure 18-13 Indirect massage pattern.

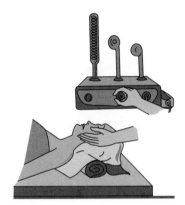

Figure 18-14 Keep hand on client's face when turning off.

Fast and Easy Extraction with High Frequency

Step 1: Clean skin with appropriate cleanser. See Figure 18-15.

Step 2: Tone with astringent. See Figure 18-16.

Step 3: Steam skin with proteolytic enzyme mask for up to 10 minutes.

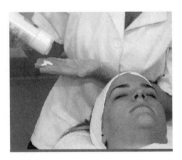

Figure 18-15 Apply cleanser.

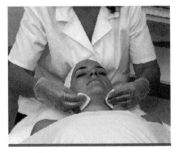

Figure 18-16 Apply astringent with cotton or gauze.

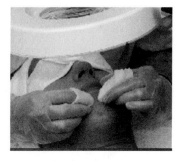

Figure 18-17 Perform extraction.

Step 4: Cover client's eyes, put on gloves, and proceed with extraction. See Figure 18-17.

Step 5: Apply non–alcohol-based acne product to help kill bacteria. Do not use essential oils; they can be volatile under heat.

Step 6: Apply gauze to face. See Figure 18-18.

Step 7: Proceed with the high-frequency application with the electrode. Use for up to 8 to 10 minutes for the direct method or 6 to 8 minutes if using the sparking method. See Figure 18-19.

Step 8: Massage in finishing cream appropriate for oily, acne-prone skin with light effleurage movements. See Figure 18-20.

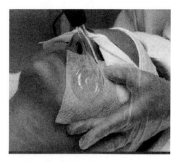

Figure 18-18 Place gauze on face then use HF sparking. Can be done without gauze.

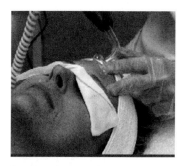

Figure 18-19 Apply HF.

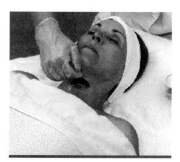

Figure 18-20 Apply appropriate moisturizer.

High-Frequency Facial Treatment for Dry or Dehydrated Skin

Step 1: Cleanse skin with a gentle cleanser made for dry or dehydrated skin.

Step 2: Remove cleanser with soft gauze or a warm towel.

Step 3: Spray appropriate toner.

Step 4: Apply a gentle enzyme mask to the skin according to manufacturer's instructions.

Step 5: Steam for 7 to 10 minutes.

Step 6: Remove the mask with a warm towel.

Step 7: Spray a toner appropriate for dry or dehydrated skin.

Step 8: Blot with tissue.

Step 9: Apply a massage cream or oil for dry or dehydrated skin. Hazelnut and jojoba oil work well.

Step 10: Perform an indirect massage treatment for 8 to 10 minutes; refer to the protocol above.

Step 11: Apply the appropriate mask for up to 15 minutes or according to the manufacturer's directions.

Step 12: Apply a hydrating serum using light effleurage movements.
Step 13: Apply a finishing cream and sunscreen.

Your Protocol:

_____

_____

_____

_____

_____

_____

_____

_____

_____

TIP Remember to fully remove any cream or talc from the electrode and electrode holder. This will keep electricity from going astray and giving you accidental shocks.

■ YOUR EQUIPMENT INFORMATION

Manufacturer info:

Name/phone number: _____

Web site: _____

Date purchased: _____   Registration: _____

Warranty info: _____

Replacement parts info: _____

TROUBLESHOOTING

Electrode does not turn on.

Check the fuse on the back of the machine; clean the electrode tips and the inside of the electrode handle with alcohol. Check for cracks in the glass of the electrode. Check wires connecting the electrode handle to the machine; if these are cracked or broken, replace them. Never patch wires. The electrode handle may have worn out. If the electrode holder is over two years old, you will need to replace it.

Sparks cause small shocks when the unit is turned on.

The electrode handle has probably been contaminated with lotion or talc. Clean well with alcohol. If this does not work, check for separation at the end of the electrode between the glass and metal conductor.

The machine will not turn on at all.

If your machine is not an eight-in-one system, check the outlet to see if the fuse has blown. If you have a multiple-unit machine, check that the main power switch is on; make sure you are using a surge protector, and check all fuses in the machine. When one unit blows a fuse, it is possible for the whole machine to be affected.

Q & A

What are the pros and cons of HF equipment?

Pros

Effective results: This modality has been used for over 50 years with good results.
Cost: HF equipment is inexpensive.
Ease of use: This modality is simple to use with a minimum of training.

Cons

High maintenance: These machines must be carefully wiped down after every service to lessen the risk of errant shocks.
Client discomfort: Some clients find the sound and application of fulguration uncomfortable.
Client contraindications: This modality is not for use on all clients. A thorough client intake form must be completed and reviewed.

Can I achieve results without HF equipment?

Yes, but you will not get the same results as you would with the machine. For example, sparking is a highly effective way to reduce inflamed papules and pustules. Acne products cannot duplicate the effects, though you will still need to recommend an at-home acne product for your client to use.

Should I buy or lease my machine?

This decision must be based on your own financial situation. In general, a single HF unit is such a low-dollar purchase that a leasing company would not finance it unless you grouped it with other equipment.

Can HF treatments make a difference in my practice?

Yes, but they are not a necessity. High frequency is a versatile and simple tool. As an esthetician, you definitely need to know how to use this modality, but it is not mandatory. There are many product lines that do not require the use of machines.

Is less expensive equipment just as good as more expensive units?

No. The chances of errant sparks in a poorly made machine are high. Be careful when you purchase, and test the equipment first if possible.

What does the FDA say about high-frequency treatments?

The FDA has not listed HF machines. This means that they are exempt from FDA classification.

REFERENCES

1. D'Angelo, J., Dean, P., Dietz, S., Hinds, C., Lees, M., Miller, E., & Zani, A. (2003). *Milady's Standard Comprehensive Training for Estheticians.* New York: Thomson Delmar Learning.
2. Simmons, J. V. (1989, 1995). *Science and the Beauty Business: The Beauty Salon and its Equipment* (2nd ed.). United Kingdom: Macmillan Press Ltd.
3. Lees, M. (2001). *Skin Care: Beyond the Basics.* New York: Thomson Delmar Learning.
4. Nordman, L. (2005). *Professional Beauty Therapy, The Official Guide to Level 3* (2nd ed.). London: Thomson Learning.

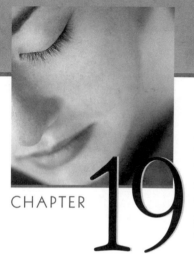

Galvanic Therapy

Galvanic therapy is one of the most effective and misunderstood esthetic modalities, even though it has been used for over 70 years in the esthetic industry. It is affordable and easy to use once you understand the basic applications. Galvanic therapy is also used in the medical profession to penetrate various drugs into localized areas of the body. In this chapter we will explore the basic electrical principles relative to the galvanic current machine. We will explore how to use galvanic therapy, why it works, and protocols for its use and safety.

■ FUNCTIONS

Galvanic therapy is used to deep-clean the skin, increase absorption of water-soluble products, reduce superficial swelling and puffiness, increase microcirculation in the cells, and improve skin texture. It is also used in body treatments for the effect of increased cell metabolism and penetration of products. Figure 19-1 shows an example of a galvanic current machine.

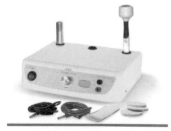

Figure 19-1 Galvanic current machine.

■ ELECTRICAL CURRENT INTENSITY

An ampere is the unit of measurement of current flowing along the path of a circuit. It is named after the French physicist, André-Marie Ampère. The greater the electrical current flowing through the circuit, the higher the amperage. A low-intensity direct current is used in galvanic therapy, and it is measured in milliamps. A **milliamp** (mA) equals 1/1000 of an ampere, measured by a milliammeter; the strength of the current is regulated by a **rheostat.** To keep the electric current at a safe and consistent level, an electronic circuit is used. Galvanic current uses a maximum of 3 mA for the face and 8 mA for the body.

The galvanic current machine uses a direct current at up to 100 volts. The current is 220 volts from the main, but it is converted to 100 volts by the **transformer.** A **rectifier** then changes the alternating current to a direct current, and a capacitor smoothes out any irregularities in the current; these three parts—the transformer, rectifier, and capacitor—are the major components of a galvanic current machine.

The transformer is responsible for changing the voltage of alternating current from the main. For example, a 220-volt alternating current from the main would be reduced to 100 volts inside the machine; this is called a **step-down,** or **reducing the current.** A transformer can also increase the voltage, or **step-up** the current. For the purpose of galvanic therapy, the transformer performs a step-down.

The rectifier changes the alternating current to a direct current by using **diodes,** which allow current to flow through in one direction but not in reverse. This creates direct current, which is the kind that causes chemical changes within the skin.

A capacitor is responsible for smoothing out the "bumps" in the electrical current; they function much the same as shocks on an automobile. Another name for a capacitor is a **condenser.** *Active* and *indifferent* electrodes are used to apply current to the area being treated; the electrical current flowing through the skin between the electrodes completes the electrical circuit. Figure 19-2 provides examples and descriptions of electrodes.

■ HOW IT WORKS

A direct current is passed through an **ionized solution** into the skin; this solution is water-based, which creates a chemical response within the epidermis that can be regulated to target specific nerve endings. The chemical effects caused by galvanic current are used to improve the condition of the skin. Two reactions are created in the skin: under the **positive pole,** an acid reaction is created that is **vasoconstrictive;** it is soothing to nerve endings and firms tissues. The **negative pole** creates an alkaline reaction that is **vasodilative;** this increases microcirculation, stimulates nerve tissues, causes **saponification,** and softens tissues.

Electrode	Illustration	Use
Indifferent metal bar		Held by client to complete electrical circuit. Must be wrapped in with damp sponge. Facial use
Indifferent metal plate	electrode fits into viscose cover	Placed firmly in contact with skin behind shoulder to complete electrical circuit. Facial use
Ball electrode		Used to treat small areas of face
Roller electrode		Used for face and upper body
Mushroom electrode		Used for face and upper body. Has holder for dampened sponge in head of holder
Tweezer electrode		Tips are wrapped in cotton or lint soaked in disincrustation solution
Carbon electrodes		Used in pairs for treatment of the body
Metal plate electrodes		Used in pairs covered with damp sponge for treatment of the body
Mask		Used on face to assist absorption of products

Figure 19-2 Electrodes and their uses.

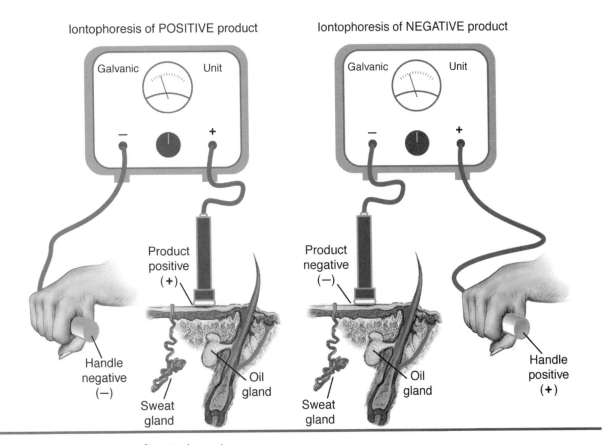

Iontophoresis of POSITIVE product   Iontophoresis of NEGATIVE product

Figure 19-3 Illustration of iontophoresis.

Ionized solutions are used under the electrodes to facilitate absorption into the epidermis, a process known as **iontophoresis.** Ionized solutions are called **electrolytes,** and they are conductors of electricity. Electrolytes contain salts and acids, which increase conductivity. When electrolytes are dissolved in water, they split and form ions that carry either a positive or negative charge. A positively charged ion is called a **cation,** and a negatively charged ion is called an **anion.** Figure 19-3 provides an illustration of iontophoresis.

When galvanic current is introduced into the electrolyte solution, the ions begin to move to either the positive pole, called the **anode,** or the negative pole, called the **cathode.** Because the fluids in the body have electrolytic properties, they allow the current to pass through the tissue, thus creating chemical effects in the skin. Figure 19-4 shows an example of a cathode and anode.

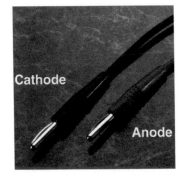

Figure 19-4 Cathode and anode.

TIP Galvanic therapy works on the electrical principle that like charges repel and opposite charges attract.

PRODUCT ABSORPTION AND THE SKIN

To fully understand how galvanic therapy affects the skin, you need to understand the process of dermal absorption, which is a controversial subject. Here are some basic scientific facts about absorption:

- Absorption is directly affected by the concentration of the substance and the area over which it is applied. For example, lidocaine applied to small areas of the skin is safe; however, applied to large areas, such as legs (especially with occlusion) can lead to overdose.
- The thickness of the stratum corneum determines the degree of absorption. Areas where this layer of skin is thin, such as the genitals, are much more receptive to absorption than, say, the soles of the feet, where this layer is thicker.
- A damaged skin barrier will facilitate absorption at a faster rate. This is why estheticians should always exfoliate before applying serums and massage; this is also why the lipid barrier is removed before performing a chemical peel.
- Occlusion of the skin enhances product penetration. Occlusion means applying some substance to the skin that air cannot penetrate. You can purchase specific plastic masks that create an occlusive environment in the skin.
- The composition of the product affects penetration of the product. It is not one certain ingredient that makes the difference, but rather the molecular weight and how the ingredient is carried. If the ingredient carrier damages the lipid barrier, then absorption will occur at a faster rate.
- Lipid-soluble products will absorb better than others. Any product that is similar to the intercellular "cement" will be readily accepted by the stratum corneum. Below the stratum corneum, the epidermis is hydrophilic. The challenge is to find a carrier that will benefit the lipophilic stratum corneum and also the hydrophilic epidermis.
- Increasing the temperature of the skin aids absorption. This why high-frequency can indirectly affect how a product is absorbed: warmer skin will generally absorb product at a faster rate.

WHAT IT DOES TO THE SKIN

There are two kinds of effects with galvanic therapy: physical and chemical. The chemical effect occurs at the site of the electrode and is called the **polar effect.** The physical effect is the movement of ions within the body; it is called the **interpolar effect.** The polar effects of the electrode are based on whether it is positive (an anode) or negative (a cathode). The cathode produces an alkaline effect, and the anode produces an acid effect. When performing a treatment, we are concentrating on the polar effect.

Effects of the Positive Pole (Anode)

- Soothing of nerve response
- Constriction of blood vessels
- Reduced blood flow
- Tightening and firming of tissues
- Astringent action
- Germicidal action

Effects of the Negative Pole (Cathode)

- Stimulation of nerve response
- Dilation of blood vessels and increased blood flow
- Softening and even desquamation of tissues
- Emulsification and removal of grease (desincrustation)

TIP Two electrical leads come with galvanic current machines; they are color-coded. Red indicates the positive (anode), and black indicates the negative (cathode).

■ HOW TO USE IT

Galvanic therapy has two applications: *iontophoresis,* which we covered earlier, and **desincrustation,** or **disincrustation.** Iontophoresis is the process of propelling ions into the skin through water based lotions and gels. Desincrustation is also called saponification, which is the process of emulsifying the sebum within the skin. Usually a desincrustation solution is used, but a standard baking soda and water combination will work. Refer to Figure 19-1.

During treatment, a client will hold an indifferent electrode wrapped in a wet sponge or will have it placed behind their shoulder. The active electrode is then used to create the chemical effects. Desincrustation is used on the cathode (-), and iontophoresis is used on the anode (+), depending on the polarity of the product. A polarity switch can usually be found on the machine, usually on the front, although now there are even machines that will digitally change polarity for you.

■ IONIZATION AND PRODUCTS

Many manufacturers have products that are classified as either negative or positive to be penetrated with galvanic therapy. Deciding which polarity to use can be confusing. Polarity of the products used is important for

TIP If the cathode (negative) and anode (positive) are not clearly marked, use the following to test the polarity: Put the tips of both electrodes into a cup of water, and add a teaspoon of salt to each. Turn on the galvanic current without the two electrodes touching. The negative electrode will produce more bubbles.

the esthetician to know before setting the polarity on the galvanic current machine. For example, if the manufacturer states that the product has a negative polarity, then the galvanic current must be set on negative to penetrate the product. The polarity is determined by the pH of the product, which is the measurement of *potential hydrogen* in a substance on a scale numbered from 0 to 14. Figure 19-5 shows an example.

The lower the number on the pH scale, the more acidic the product. The product would be considered an **acid** if it fell below 7 on the pH scale. Products higher than 7 on the scale are considered **alkaline;** these are often referred to as **bases.** Skin is in a slightly acidic state and usually measures from 4.5 to 6.2 on the pH scale.

The **acid mantle** is the barrier on the skin created by sweat and sebum. This is the skin's first line of defense. The acid mantle is fragile; it is impacted by the environment, products, and internal stress. When the acid mantle is exposed to acid or alkaline products, inflammation and irritation can occur—which is why it is so important to make sure that galvanic therapy uses both poles to balance the acid mantle.

Acidic products are considered positive in polarity, and products with an alkaline pH are considered negative in polarity. Products used for galvanic current must be water-based. Oil-based products do not carry the current well and generally have a higher molecular weight. When in doubt about the polarity of a product, start the treatment at negative for 3 to 5 minutes, then switch polarity to positive for 3 to 5 minutes. Many manufacturers have products that are dual polarity, so use this technique unless the manufacturer indicated the correct polarity of the product. Figure 19-6 shows an ionization chart you can use.

During iontophoresis, your clients may have a slight metallic taste in their mouths; this is due to the current interacting with metal fillings.

TIP To remember which polarity to use, think of it this way: negative takes out, and positive pushes in.

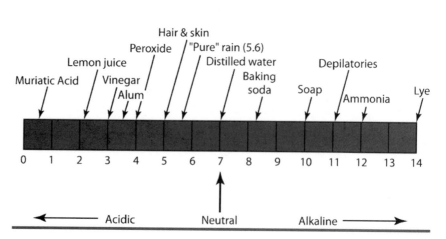

Figure 19-5 The pH scale.

If product is	Polarity used	Benefits
Acid based or +	Positive pole 1.5 mA max 5-7 minutes	Constrict pores, reduce redness, facilitate absorption
Alkaline or −	Negative pole 1.5 mA max 3-5 minutes	Desincrustation, improve circulation, remove surface cells
Both − and + or unknown polarity	First negative 3 minutes then positive 5-7 minutes	Facilitate absorption of water-based product

Figure 19-6 Products and iontophoresis.

TIP Underwriters Laboratory (UL) is the U.S. organization responsible for testing products for consumer safety. Many international products are not UL certified, although UL has recently started an international section of certification. Alternatives to UL listing are CE or CSA certification. The UL mark on a product tells you that the machine has been thoroughly tested and investigated by a team of product safety professionals.

Excessive dental work may be a contraindication, but some fillings will not be a problem.

■ HOW TO BUY

Galvanic current machines come in two forms: as an individual unit or in a combination machine that has other equipment built in with it. Figure 19-7 shows an example of a combination machine.

The approximate price for an individual machine is about $200 to $450. Combination machines start at $1,000 and can go as high as $3,500. All machines have the same technology; the differences in price relate to the quality of materials and the level of support the manufacturer offers. Make sure your equipment has a safety certification, such as a UL listing or a CSA, CE, or ISO certification. UL, CE, and CSA listings indicate that the equipment has been tested for safety. ISO certification indicates that the unit has been manufactured per international standards and that the manufacturer is tested twice a year.

Buyer's Checklist

- What is the price?
- Do you have an instruction manual, DVD, on-site training, or technical support?
- Is the machine UL listed, ISO certified, or CE or CSA tested?
- Does the unit come with electrodes, or do those have to be purchased separately?
- Can I buy replacement parts?
- If so, what parts are available, and how much do they cost?

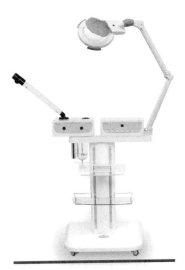

Figure 19-7 Cirrus combination machine.

Galvanic current	UL listed or CE mark
	Automatic polarity
	Multiple electrodes
	Clear electrical output display
	Metal casing
	Replacement parts available
	Warranty

Figure 19-8 Features to look for.

- What is covered under the warranty, and for how long?
- Do you have a loaner program if my machine breaks?
- Where is the equipment manufactured?

See Figure 19-8 for a chart of features to look for when you buy.

■ SAFETY

In general, galvanic current is a very safe modality to use. The situations that increase the potential for minor electric shocks and galvanic burns are lack of proper machine upkeep, a poorly grounded plug, broken wires, damaged electrodes or electrode holders, and a poorly made machine.

All electrical equipment in the United States must meet the National Electrical Code, and equipment should be UL listed. UL listing is important, because it shows that an independent agency has certified that the equipment has been tested as safe. CSA is another independent testing agency that many North American manufacturers use. Theirs is also a very good certification to have, and it is one alternative to a UL listing. CE listing is another alternative; it is used in the European Union. Unfortunately, there is no governing body that inspects esthetic machines, unless they are classified by the FDA. See Chapter 1 for more information on FDA regulations and UL listing.

Wall outlets should be the three-prong, grounded-wire type. Make sure that you do not overload the outlet. A ground fault circuit interrupter (GCFI) is required on all outlets within six feet of a water source. For the purposes of a facial room, it is a good idea to have them.

■ MAINTENANCE

Maintenance is one of the most important aspects of owning esthetic machines, and upkeep on a galvanic current machine is very easy. Manufacturers will also have their own protocols, so be sure to follow their directions. In general, use these guidelines:

- Clean electrodes and the electrode holder after each use.
- Use isopropyl alcohol on a saturated cotton tip to clean inside the electrode holder once or twice a month.
- Do not store electrodes in a UV sterilizer.
- Check all wires before use. Do not use the unit if wires appear worn or if loose wires are visible.
- Check sponges monthly and replace as needed.

■ DISINFECTION AND SANITIZATION

- Wash all gels and lotions off the electrodes with soap and water.
- Disinfect electrodes by saturating them with a state-approved disinfectant, but do not submerge electrodes in disinfectant solution.
- Place electrodes in a UV sanitizer for 20 minutes for additional disinfection, but do not store them in the sanitizer.
- Store electrodes in the container that came with your machine. They may also be stored in surgical envelopes, which are available from medical and esthetic suppliers.

See Figure 19-9 for a chart of maintenance and disinfection.

Disinfection	Maintenance
Disinfect electrodes and sponges in EPA-approved disinfectant – saturate; do not submerge	Check all wires before use
Store in clean, closed container	Clean electrode holder once a month with 70% alcohol
Wipe down exterior after each use with EPA-approved disinfectant	Check sponges monthly; replace as needed

Figure 19-9 Disinfection and maintenance steps.

CONTRAINDICATIONS AND CAUTIONS

The consultation is extremely important to determine contraindications or special needs your client may have. Do not rely exclusively on the intake form; it is also important to verbally get information and clarification from your client.

- Metal implements in the body or pacemakers: Electricity will concentrate in those areas containing metal, because the metal acts as a conductor. Pacemakers will be interrupted. IUDs are considered a metal implement for the purpose of galvanic body treatments.
- Pregnancy: Electrotherapy treatments should not be used on pregnant clients.
- Heart problems: A heart in a compromised condition is unable to cope with an increased constriction or dilation of blood vessels; this can lead to fainting or a heart attack.
- Blood vessel disorders: Arteriosclerosis, or hardening of the arteries, affects the arteries' ability to handle increased blood flow. Fainting can result when increased dilation of the blood vessels occurs during heat treatments.
- Skin inflammation: Most electrical treatments increase circulation, which can make inflammation worse.
- Skin disorders or diseases: These may be aggravated by treatment.
- Very sensitive skin: Clients with this skin type may be very uncomfortable during treatment.
- Migraines or severe headaches: Treatment may cause worsening of an existing headache but is not known to cause them.
- Lack of tactile sensation (e.g., numbness due to stroke): Clients with diminished sensitivity will not be able to gauge the intensity of the current, which could cause injury.
- Nervous clients: Treatment will be ineffective if the client cannot relax.
- Excessive metal dental work: Current will concentrate around metal but not around porcelain veneers. Clients with braces will be very uncomfortable.
- Metal piercings anywhere in the body: These will concentrate the current around the metal. Have the client remove jewelry prior to treatment.
- Botox: No treatment should be performed until 72 hours after injection.
- Epilepsy: Unknown how the electrical current will affect a client with epilepsy. Could possibly cause a seizure.

- Cuts and abrasions: Electrical current will concentrate in the area, because bodily fluids act as a conductor.
- Severe bruising: Bruising will make treatment uncomfortable for the client.
- High or low blood pressure: These conditions could be made worse due to the increase in circulation. Even if the condition is being treated and is under control, use caution. Never leave the client alone, and help them on and off the treatment bed.
- Recent scar tissue: Scarred skin is very sensitive and less resistant; proceed with caution when using electrotherapy. Galvanic current therapy is okay if it has been six weeks since the injury or surgery and there is no pulling of the skin during treatment.
- HIV.
- History of blood clots (thrombosis) or embolism: Treatment could aggravate the condition and cause a heart attack or stroke.
- Malignant melanoma: Treatment for the malignancy must be completed, and the client must be in remission. Obtain physician approval. Do not apply treatment when in doubt about a possible abnormality; instead, refer the client to a dermatologist.
- One possible side effect of galvanic current therapy is **galvanic burn**, which is caused by a concentration of alkali on the skin.

To minimize the potential for galvanic burn, follow these guidelines:

- Reduce the current when going over thinner areas of the face and body.
- Make sure sponges are evenly saturated with water.
- Always clean sponges thoroughly after use to remove residue.
- Communicate frequently with your client about the sensation the current is producing; do not perform treatment on a client with lack of sensation.

Some clients may have noticeable redness after treatment. This is due to increased microcirculation; such redness is normal and will go away in a few hours. To minimize redness, reduce the level of the current, reverse the polarity, and apply a cool gel to the skin. Aloe vera is especially soothing.

■ PREPARATION FOR TREATMENT

- Have your client fill out an assessment form.
- Check for contraindications.
- Have your client change into a treatment gown and remove all jewelry and contact lenses.
- Analyze the skin using a magnifying lamp.

TIP What do you do when a client has a contraindication? Explain that you would not want to make an existing condition worse, and make it clear that the treatment may do just that. Offer an optional service if one is available. Treatment may also be possible with a modification. For example, do not go over the area of a severe bruise, or ask your client to remove her piercings. When in doubt, refer to a physician.

- Explain the procedure. Your clients may become uncomfortable if they do not understand that the tingling or slight metallic taste in their mouths is normal.
- Make sure to test all equipment before applying treatment to your client.
- Inspect all wires and electrodes.
- Follow manufacturer's instructions for the setup of your galvanic current machine.

TIP Always remember to check for contraindications with any electrotherapy treatment. Client comfort and safety should be top priorities.

■ PROTOCOLS

Listed below is a basic galvanic current protocol.

Iontophoresis

Check client contraindications before performing treatment, as shown in Figure 19-10.

> *Step 1:* Skin should be clean and slightly moist.
> *Step 2:* Apply ampoule or treatment gel in a medium thickness around the face. See Figure 19-11.
> *Step 3:* Apply a wet sponge to the active electrode; if using a metal roller, apply gauze.
> *Step 4:* Have your client hold the inactive electrode, as shown in Figure 19-12.
> *Step 5:* Place the electrode on the client's forehead, as shown in Figure 19-13.

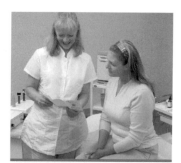

Figure 19-10 Check for contraindications.

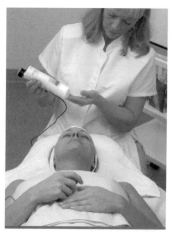

Figure 19-11 Apply ampoule or treatment gel.

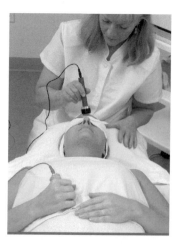

Figure 19-12 Apply electrode to forehead.

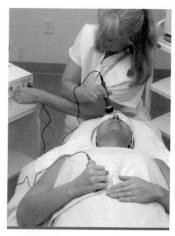

Figure 19-13 Adjust amperage.

Step 6: Turn on the machine, and select the positive polarity (+) anode; milliamps should start at .3 with a maximum of 1.5 mA. See Figure 19-14.

Step 7: Move the electrode in a circular motion over the skin's surface. Figure 19-15 shows the correct pattern. Do not exceed 1.5 milliamps. See Figure 19-16.

Treatment should last approximately 5 to 7 minutes.

Desincrustation and Cataphoresis

Step 1: Have the client hold the indifferent electrode wrapped in a wet sponge or lint.

Step 2: Apply desincrustation solution with sponge to the active electrode, or apply it directly to the skin if in gel form. Apply desincrustation only in the areas of congestion. See Figure 19-18 for an example.

Step 3: While touching the client's skin with the active electrode, turn on the machine.

Step 4: Increase the current until the client feels a warm tingling sensation.

Step 5: Move the electrode over the skin's surface, and gradually increase current to 1.5 mA. See Figure 19-17.

Step 6: Perform desincrustation for 3 to 5 minutes.

Step 7: When finished, maintain contact with client's skin with the electrode until you turn the unit off.

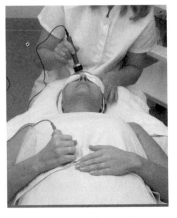

Figure 19-14 Have client hold inactive electrode.

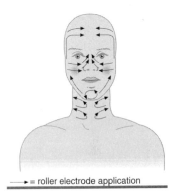

—▸ = roller electrode application

Figure 19-15 Pattern of electrode application.

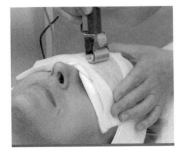

Figure 19-16 Apply electrode in circular movements.

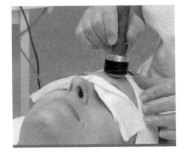

Figure 19-17 Move electrode over face.

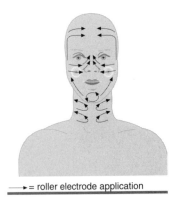

—▸ = roller electrode application

Figure 19-18 Desincrustation application: use only in oily areas.

Step 8: Take the electrode from the client.

Step 9: Remove remaining residue from the client's skin.

Galvanic Body Application

Step 1: Place electrodes on the bed in the proper position. Figure 19-19 shows body electrode placement.

Step 2: Saturate sponge electrode sleeves, and secure all electrodes to electrical leads.

Step 3: Apply active solution under the negative electrode; this treatment is usually for cellulite.

Step 4: Apply conducting gel under the positive electrode.

Step 5: Firmly strap electrodes in place.

Step 6: Turn the machine on. Turn on the negative pole.

Step 7: Proceed to turn the dial up until the client feels a slight tingling sensation.

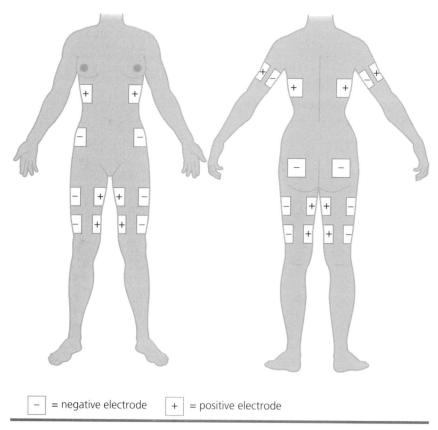

$\boxed{-}$ = negative electrode $\boxed{+}$ = positive electrode

Figure 19-19 Placement of body electrodes.

Step 8: Increase amperage up to 4.25 mA for 10 minutes. Subsequent treatments should last 20 minutes.

Step 9: Reverse polarity for 2 to 3 minutes to neutralize chemical reactions and soothe the skin.

Step 10: Slowly reduce current, and turn the machine off. A slight redness is normal.

Step 11: Remove electrodes, and remove any solution residue.

Step 12: Apply appropriate body product.

Your Protocol:

_____

_____

_____

_____

_____

_____

_____

_____

TIP For effective results with galvanic current, make sure that the current is used at the right intensity and duration. Check with your client often about the sensations they feel, and watch for skin sensitivity to avoid galvanic burns.

YOUR EQUIPMENT INFORMATION

Manufacturer info:

Name/phone number: _____

Web site: _____

Date purchased: _____ Registration: _____

Warranty info: _____

Replacement parts info: _____

TROUBLESHOOTING

Electrode does not turn on.

Check electrical leads and clean electrode tips. Check wires that connect the machine to the mains; if these are cracked or broken, replace them. Never patch wires. Electrode handles may have worn out. If the electrode is over two years old, you will need to replace it.

Client experiences a strong sensitizing reaction.

This is caused when the skin releases histamine. Reverse current polarity and apply a soothing, cooling mask.

The machine will not turn on at all.

If your machine is not an eight-in-one system, check the outlet to see if the fuse has blown. If you have a multiple-unit machine, check that the main power switch is on; make sure you are using a surge protector, and check all fuses in the machine. When one unit blows a fuse, it is possible for the whole machine to be effected.

Q & A

What are the pros and cons of galvanic equipment?

Pros

Effectiveness: Galvanic current has been used for many years in the esthetic profession. It has a safe track record with visible benefits.
Cost: This is a very cost-effective and inexpensive machine.
Ease of use: Galvanic current therapy is an easy modality to use when estheticians are correctly trained.
Safety: This is a very safe machine; however, shocks can result from poorly maintained machines or operator misuse.

Cons

Training: Use of galvanic current therapy requires in-depth training in electrotherapy and contraindications to this modality. Some esthetic schools provide this, but training may not be as in-depth as it could be.
Maintenance: This equipment requires consistent and through cleaning to avoid errant shocks.

Can I achieve results without galvanic equipment?

No. You will not get the same results with another modality as you would with the galvanic current machine. There are other modalities that can be used instead of galvanic current, but the actual iontophoresis process is unique to galvanic treatment.

Should I buy or lease the equipment?

This should be based on your financial situation. In general, a single galvanic current unit is so inexpensive that a leasing company would not finance it unless you grouped it with other equipment.

Can galvanic current therapy make a difference in my practice?

Yes. Galvanic current is an easy tool to use, and now manufacturers have developed safe and shockproof units. One uses a pulsating current that digitally reverses polarity for you. As an esthetician, it is good to know how to use this modality, but it is not mandatory. There are many product lines that do not require the use of machines.

Is less expensive equipment a better bargain?

No. The chances of galvanic burn in a poorly made machine are a possibility. Be careful when you purchase. Test it first if possible.

What does the FDA say about galvanic current?

Medical galvanic current machines are used to penetrate medication into the dermal layer and are Class II devices. Models used for esthetic applications are not listed in the classification, but it is a requirement that a manufacturer be registered with the FDA if they are manufacturing medical equipment. See Chapter 3 for more information.

REFERENCES

1. D'Angelo, J., Dean, P., Dietz, S., Hinds, C., Lees, M., Miller, E., & Zani, A. (2003). *Milady's Standard Comprehensive Training for Estheticians*. New York: Thomson Delmar Learning.
2. Simmons, J. V. (1989, 1995). *Science and the Beauty Business, The Beauty Salon and its Equipment* (2nd ed.). United Kingdom: Macmillan Press Ltd.
3. Lees, M. (2001). *Skin Care: Beyond the Basics*. New York: Thomson Delmar Learning.
4. Nordman, L. (2005). *Professional Beauty Therapy, The Official Guide to Level 3* (2nd ed.). London: Thomson Learning.
5. Gerson, J. (2004). *Milady's Standard Fundamentals for Estheticians*. New York: Thomson Delmar Learning.
6. Pivot Point (2004). *Salon Fundamentals: Esthetics*. Evanston, Illinois: Pivot Point International.

Microcurrent

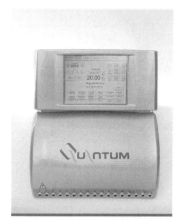

CHAPTER 20

Microcurrent is one of the most popular antiaging technologies used by estheticians. It is used by alternative medicine practitioners for healing injury, and estheticians use it for firming and toning the skin. Results are reported to be immediate and continue to improve with each subsequent use. In this chapter you will learn the theory of how it works, what it does, and protocols for use and safety. The theory of electrotherapy, covered in Chapter 18, is also important for the esthetician to understand to fully grasp the effectiveness of microcurrent.

■ FUNCTIONS

Microcurrent rejuvenates facial muscles, increases cellular functioning, improves skin tone and texture, improves lymphatic circulation, and increases circulation. Figure 20-1 shows a microcurrent machine.

■ HOW IT WORKS

To better understand how microcurrent works, it is helpful to understand the nature of our cells. Much research has been done to learn how **adenosine triphosphate (ATP)** in the cell increases with microcurrent use. To see how important this is to the esthetic use of microcurrent, let us look at how our cells function.

Cells are the basic building blocks of the human body. There are trillions of cells in the human body, and they are always moving, working, and dying. Cells perform many functions. Some are chemical functions, such as the creation of proteins; other functions are communication and recognizing other cells as friends or foes.

Groups of cells in the body specialize in particular functions. Those cells that share function, shape, and size are called *tissues*. In turn, these

Figure 20-1 CACI Quantum.

216

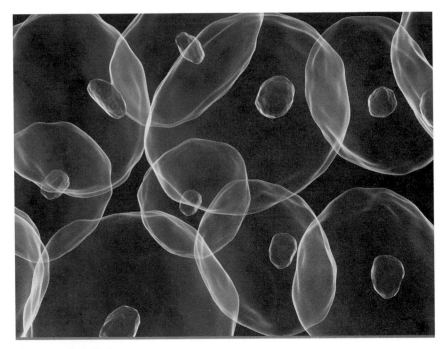

Figure 20-2 Cells.

tissues can be grouped to form organs. The tissues with which we are most concerned in regard to microcurrent are epithelial and muscle tissues. Figure 20-2 shows cells.

Each cell has a cell membrane that is the barrier between the cell and its environment. The cell membrane is porous, and it allows nutrients to enter and waste to exit the cell. The membrane is made up of proteins and fats, also called *lipids.* It has what is known as *selective permeability;* this allows some substances in and keeps others out, which is how membranes allow nutrients to enter the cell. These nutrients come from food that has been broken down in the intestinal tract and passed into the bloodstream. This nutrition is delivered to the cells: blood brings nutrients, oxygen, and water to the cells, and removes waste products from the cell, such as carbon dioxide. Lymph fluid assists the lymphatic system by removing waste and filtering it into the bloodstream. Impacting lymph movement is an important component of microcurrent therapy.

The cell membrane has another important feature, and these are the *receptor sites;* these receive signals from the body in the form of hormones and other biochemicals. These sites accept only specific types of signals, and they are influenced by certain drugs and hormones. See Figure 20-3 for an illustration of a cell membrane.

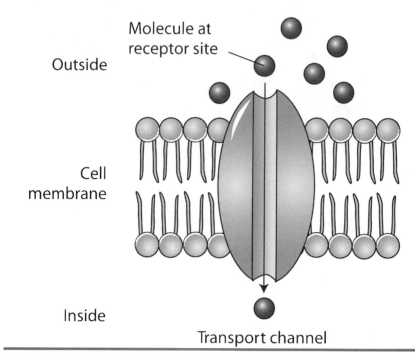

Outside

Molecule at
receptor site

Cell
membrane

Inside

Transport channel

Figure 20-3 Cell transport.

The liquid in the cell is called the **cytoplasm.** Scattered throughout the membrane are very small parts, called **organelles,** which are responsible for specific functions of the cell. **Mitochondria** are the organelles responsible for producing the energy for the cell; these organelles break nutrients down into smaller units that are used for the manufacture of ATP, the substance that ultimately provides energy to the cell. This process is important for the health of every cell and will directly affect the health of the skin and the entire body. Without energy, cells cannot reproduce and function in a healthy manner. Other organelles within the cytoplasm are **ribosomes,** lysosomes, and the **Golgi apparatus.** See Figure 20-4 for an illustration of a cell.

The cell cycle contains four phases. The first growth phase is known as *G1,* when the cell grows and increases in size. The next phase is the *S* phase. This is when the DNA synthesis occurs and chromosomes are formed. The second growth phase of the cell is known as *G2.* At this phase, energy gained is used for the next phase of cell mitosis, or cell division. This is also the phase in which cytokinesis happens, which is the splitting off of the daughter cell. Throughout this process, the use of energy in the cell cycle is essential, so this is when ATP is important. See Figure 20-5 for a picture of cells dividing.

TIP Ribosomes are responsible for the building of proteins for different cell functions. Lysosomes are sacs that produce enzymes that break down the cell when it dies, as well as breaking down large molecules of nutrients and killing bacteria.

TIP The Golgi apparatus was discovered in 1898 by **Camillo Golgi.** It functions as a storage organelle, holding protein for further use.

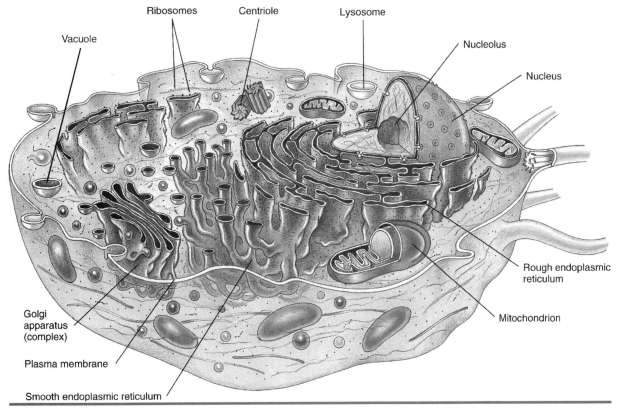

Figure 20-4 Illustration of a cell.

■ ELECTRICAL EFFECTS ON CELLS

At the cellular level, electricity is abundant. A large portion of the cell's energy is used for the separation of ions. When positively and negatively charged ions separate, a voltage is created. This charge is an important source of energy for the cell; it creates a force that moves ions across the cell membrane, which transports molecules that are necessary for healthy cell function.

The mitochondrion is where metabolism takes place, with the help of special enzymes called **cytochromes.** As the ions are then allowed to move across the cell membrane, they power the production of ATP, the major source of energy for the cell. The energy of the cell can be estimated chemically by the amount of ATP available; it can also be measured electrically based on total ionic charge separation.

If an electrical current of the appropriate size were to be applied to the cell, it would cross the membrane barrier and increase the energy

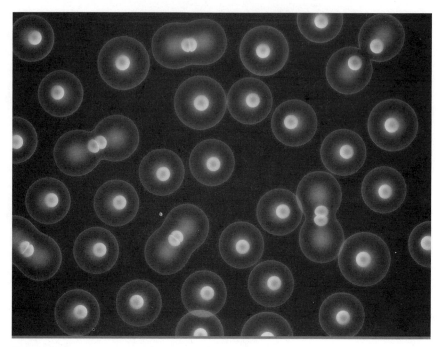

Figure 20-5 Dividing cells.

available to the cell. This means that any cell impairment that could be positively affected by an influx of energy would be improved by a supply of electrical current. This energy influx leads to increased cell growth, synthesis of DNA, **protein metabolism,** and ATP synthesis.

■ WHY IT WORKS

Microcurrent is microamperage stimulation, which is insufficient to activate motor nerves that would cause muscle movement. Microcurrent works with the body's own electrical impulses to increase cellular reactions that slow down as we age, get injured, have an illness, or experience an increase in stress. Microcurrent assists the body by mimicking the body's bioelelectric currents. This leads to the repairing of tissue and increased cellular metabolism, activity, and exchange.

Microcurrent uses direct electric currents ranging from 10 mA to 500 mA at varied waveforms and frequencies. Some manufacturers include a faradic current, which is an interrupted AC current. Technology is rapidly changing; a new addition to the microcurrent market is the use

MICROCURRENT **221**

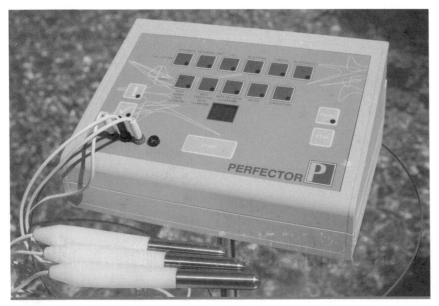

Figure 20-6 Perfector.

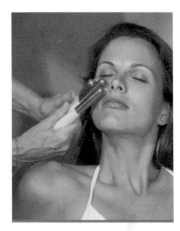

Figure 20-7 Perfector.

of nanotechnology. The theory is that nanocurrent—current in the range of one-billionth of an ampere—is more readily recognized by the cells; these currents have been shown to even produce amperage in the pico range, or one-trillionth of an ampere. Figures 20-6 and 20-7 show examples.

Most manufacturers have their own proprietary information about how their machine produces currents and waveforms. The different waveforms used are *square, sine, rectangle,* and *pulsed.* These are standard waveforms recognized within electrical engineering; how a company chooses to modify and market them is the key to selling their machine. Also used are low- and high-frequency currents that also are proprietary to certain manufacturers.

When direct microcurrent is used, it does not only affect the skin tissue; the correct movements that the esthetician uses will also lengthen or shorten various muscle groups. It is very important to understand the muscles of the face and where the insertion and origin of each muscle is. For example, to firm the nasal labial folds, you would shorten the muscle with a specific movement.

Microcurrent will reprogram the muscle fiber, allowing it to be lengthened or shortened, depending on the direction of the application. When a muscle contracts and shortens, one of its attachments usually remains fixed, and the other one moves. Figure 20-8 shows a microcurrent application.

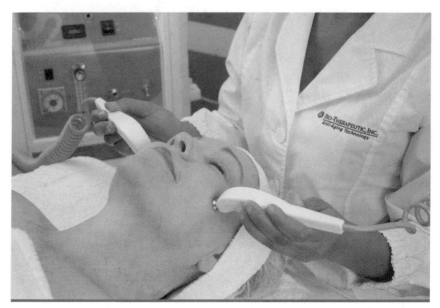

Figure 20-8 Biotherapeutic application.

■ WRINKLE FORMATION

Understanding the basic process of wrinkle formation will assist the esthetician when using microcurrent. The process is complex, with many factors that affect the skin. Muscles play a part in the process by pulling down on the fiber matrix of the skin, which includes collagen and elastin. Wrinkles form across muscle in an up-and-down or perpendicular pattern. See Figure 20-9 for an example.

When the skin loses collagen and elastin, it cannot stay firm, and a wrinkle will develop. The muscles of the face are attached to the skin via **fascia,** where the collagen and elastin are. When these become weak, they are no longer able to resist the pull of gravity or muscle contraction. When muscle contraction is lessened or stopped, as with the use of **Botox,** the skin will not form deep wrinkles. There are different types of wrinkles:

- **Atrophic crinkling rhytids:** These are fine horizontal and parallel wrinkles that tend to form later in life. They can occur anywhere on the face and body. Figure 20-10 shows an example.
- **Permanent elastotic creases,** or **static rhytids**: These wrinkles occur in a crisscross pattern and are generally seen on the cheeks and neck. They gradually become permanent. Figures 20-11 and 20-12 show examples.

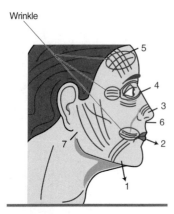

Figure 20-9 Wrinkles form across the muscle.

- **Dynamic expression lines**: These are the typical frown lines, laugh lines, and crows' feet. These wrinkles (as shown in Figure 20-13) respond well to Botox, as shown in Figure 20-14.
- **Gravitational fold,** or **deep wrinkle**: This is a deep groove that is long and straight. It can occur anywhere on the face. See Figure 20-15.

Aging skin is complex, and science is making new discoveries every day. It is important for the esthetician to get further education in this subject. It takes a multimodality approach to treat aging skin effectively.

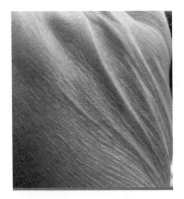

Figure 20-10 Crinkling wrinkles.

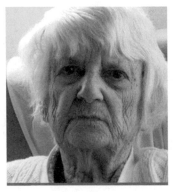

Figure 20-11 Static wrinkles.

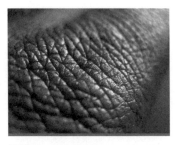

Figure 20-12 Permanent elastic, or static, wrinkles.

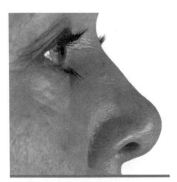

Figure 20-13 Dynamic expression lines.

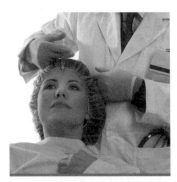

Figure 20-14 Dynamic expression lines respond well to Botox.

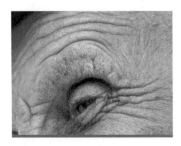

Figure 20-15 Gravitational folds.

■ WHAT IT DOES TO THE SKIN

Microcurrent causes multiple effects in the skin and body:

- **Increases ATP**: This molecule is involved in the cell to provide cellular energy transport and enzyme regulation. Microcurrent has been reported to increase ATP as much as 500% based on a study done by Cheng and colleagues (1982). When ATP metabolism is reduced in the cell, the aging process is accelerated, and the signs of aging appear at a faster rate.
- **Increases fibroblast activity**: Fibroblast cells are large oval cells found in connective tissue. They are responsible for producing collagen and elastin in the skin. Collagen and elastin are some of the most important parts of our skin; when we age, they deteriorate and cause a loss of firmness.
- **Increases protein synthesis**: Muscles are largely influenced by proteins that also act as part of antioxidant defenses. Elastin and collagen are also proteins.
- **Increases cell permeability**: When the body ages, cells become less permeable, so various functions in the body slow down. **Transepidermal water loss (TEWL)** is reduced by microcurrent, so the skin stays hydrated, which creates the correct pH for **homeostasis** in the skin. This is important in order for the cells to absorb more nutrients, oxygen, and water; it also helps the cells excrete toxins to the lymph and blood system.

■ HOW TO BUY

Purchasing a microcurrent machine is a capital investment and requires a substantial amount of research. It is always a good idea to try the machine first before purchasing. Prices range from $4,500 to $18,000. Each manufacturer has a different system for delivering current. This is a type of machine that may work well on one person and not have the same effect on another, although technology is improving quickly. See Figure 20-16 for an example of a small microcurrent unit.

Another option in equipment is the multiple modality machine. These machines combine microcurrent with LED light therapy, microdermabrasion, and ultrasound. The different combinations depend on the manufacturer. See Figure 20-17 for an example.

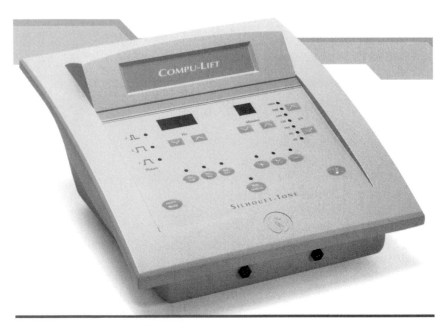

Figure 20-16 Compulift.

Buyer's Checklist

- What is the price?
- What is the cost of shipping?
- Do you have an instruction manual, DVD, or on-site training?
- Is the machine UL listed, ISO certified, or CE or CSA tested?
- Does it come with all the accessories, or do those have to be purchased separately?
- Can I buy replacement parts?
- What is covered under the warranty, and for how long?
- Is the manufacturer FDA-registered?
- Who will service the machine if repairs are needed?

See Figure 20-18 for a chart of features to look for when you buy.

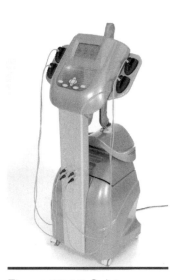

Figure 20-17 Soli tone.

■ HOW TO USE IT

Each machine manufacturer has a proprietary system for using their machine. When purchasing a microcurrent machine, it is important to receive the proper training on the use and maintenance of the equipment. In general, accessories such as probes or electric gloves are used to physically

Microcurrent	UL listed or CE mark
	Manufacturer FDA-registered
	Results based on clinical research
	Clear electrical output display
	Training included in purchase
	Replacement parts available
	Warranty

Figure 20-18 Features to look for.

TIP Water is a good conductor of electricity, so you will see better results with a client who is hydrated than one who is dehydrated. Create a preservice protocol for your client that includes internal and external hydration.

move the muscle into the desired position to perform what is known as **muscle reeducation,** the process of lengthening or shortening muscles. Most machines have one to five phases preprogrammed into the equipment. A clear digital face that is easy to use is an important feature to look for. See Figure 20-19. Each protocol is different based on manufacturer instructions, but most are fairly easy to use. See the microcurrent protocols that appear later in this section for a general step-by-step outline.

Working a muscle from the "belly" outward will have a lengthening effect that is necessary on muscles that have become increasingly contracted through many years of facial expressions. Working a muscle from the origin and insertion point inward will have a shortening effect that is

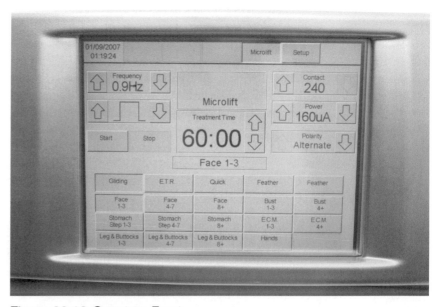

Figure 20-19 Quantum Front.

necessary for the majority of the facial muscles, which become elongated over many years of age and gravity.

▪ SAFETY

The possibility of injury using a microcurrent machine is very slight. Situations that increase potential problems are lack of proper machine upkeep, a poorly grounded plug, broken wires, damaged probes, and a poorly made machine.

All electrical equipment in the U.S. should meet the National Electrical Code, and equipment should be UL listed. UL listing is significant due to the fact that an independent agency has certified that the equipment has been tested as safe. CSA is another independent testing agency that many North American manufacturers use, and CE certification is used in the European Union. These are also good certifications to look for, and they can offer an alternative to UL listing. Unfortunately, there is no governing body that inspects esthetic machines unless they are classified by the FDA. See Chapter 1 for more information on FDA regulations and UL listing.

Wall outlets should be the three-prong, grounded-wire type. Make sure that you do not overload the outlet. A ground fault circuit interrupter (GCFI) is required on all outlets within six feet of a water source. For the purposes of a facial room, it is a good idea to have them.

▪ MAINTENANCE

Maintenance is one of the most important aspects of owning esthetic machines, and for a microcurrent machine, it is very easy. Manufacturers will also have their own protocols, so be sure to follow their directions. In general, you can use these guidelines:

- Clean the electrode holder after each use.
- If the holder uses cotton swabs, discard them after use.
- Do not store electrodes in a UV sterilizer.
- Wipe down the exterior of your machine after each use.
- Check all wires before use. Do not use when wires are cracked or loose wires are visible.

▪ DISINFECTION AND SANITIZATION

Most microcurrent machines use disposable tips in the electrode holder. Dispose of the tips after each use.

Disinfection	Maintenance
Disinfect electrodes in EPA-approved disinfectant – saturate; do not submerge (metal only)	Check all wires before use
Any part of the machine in contact with the client should be saturated with EPA-approved disinfectant	Clean electrode holder once a month with 70% alcohol
Wipe down exterior after each use with EPA-approved disinfectant	Discard cotton swabs after use

Figure 20-20 Chart of disinfection and maintenance.

- If metal electrodes are used, disinfect the electrode by saturating the portion that contacts skin with an EPA-approved high-level disinfectant.
- Do not submerge metal ends in the solution.
- Place electrodes in a UV sanitizer for 20 minutes for additional disinfection. Do not store electrodes in a UV sanitizer.
- Store electrodes in the container that came with your machine or in surgical envelopes (available from medical and esthetic suppliers).

See Figure 20-20 for a chart of disinfection and maintenance steps.

■ CONTRAINDICATIONS AND CAUTIONS

Because microcurrent is considered an electrotherapy treatment, the consultation is extremely important to determine contraindications or special needs that your client may have. Microcurrent is known to be very healing with no side effects, but use your best judgment when determining how to proceed with your client. Do not rely exclusively on the intake form; it is also important to verbally get information and clarification from your client.

- Metal implements in body and pacemakers: Electricity will concentrate in the areas with a metal conductor, and pacemakers will be interrupted.
- Pregnancy: Use caution when using microcurrent on pregnant clients. Seek medical approval first.
- Heart problems: Use caution when using microcurrent on clients with heart problems. It is unknown how the micro amperage will affect them; it is generally safe.
- Skin inflammation: Most electrical treatments increase circulation, which can make inflammation worse.

- Skin disorders or diseases: These may be aggravated by treatment.
- Very sensitive skin: Clients with this skin type may be very uncomfortable.
- Lack of tactile sensation (e.g., numbness due to stroke): The client will not be able to gauge the intensity of the current, which could result in injury.
- Nervous clients: Treatment will be ineffective if the client cannot relax.
- Excessive metal dental work: Current will concentrate around metal but not porcelain veneers. Clients with braces will be very uncomfortable.
- Metal piercings in the body: Current will concentrate around the metal.
- Botox: No treatment should be applied until 72 hours after injection. The treatment paralyzes muscle, so any treatment to stimulate muscle would be ineffective.
- Epilepsy: Electrotherapy should not be performed on clients with epilepsy. It could cause a seizure.
- Cuts and abrasions: Electrical current will concentrate in the area, because bodily fluids act as a conductor.
- Severe bruising: Clients with bruising will be uncomfortable.
- High or low blood pressure: Either condition could be made worse due to the increase in circulation. Even if it is treated and under control, use caution. Never leave a client with blood pressure issues alone, and help them on and off the treatment bed.
- Recent scar tissue: Scarred skin is very sensitive and less resistant. Use caution when using electrotherapy.
- HIV.
- History of blood clots (thrombosis) or embolism: These could aggravate the condition and cause a heart attack or stroke.
- Malignant melanoma: Treatment must be completed, and client must be in remission. Obtain physician approval. Do not apply treatment when in doubt about a possible abnormality; instead, refer client to a dermatologist.

■ PREPARATION FOR TREATMENT

- Have your client fill out an assessment form.
- Check for contraindications.
- Have your client change into a treatment gown and remove all jewelry.
- Analyze the skin using a magnifying lamp.
- Explain the procedure.

TIP What do you do when you have a contraindication? Explain that you would not want to make an existing condition worse and that the treatment may do that. Offer another service if possible. Treatment may also be possible with a modification; for example, do not go over the area of a severe bruise, or you may ask your client to remove any piercings. When in doubt refer to a physician.

TIP Always remember to check for contraindications with any electrotherapy treatment. Client comfort and safety are top priorities.

- Make sure to test all equipment before applying treatment. After testing your electrode, disinfect the surface before applying it to the client's skin.
- Inspect all wires and electrodes.
- Follow manufacturer's instructions for the setup and preparation of your microcurrent machine.

▪ PROTOCOLS

Listed below is a general microcurrent protocol.

Basic Microcurrent Protocol

Manufacturers will have their own protocol, so be sure to check before using this one.

Step 1: Perform first and second cleanse.
Step 2: Exfoliate.
Step 3: Apply a gel recommended by the manufacturer.
Step 4: Saturate the probes with a conductor, or use metal probes if recommended by the manufacturer.
Step 5: Start at the base of the neck; hold both probes a half-inch apart for a count of six, working toward the ear. Apply to both sides of the neck. See Figures 20-21a through 20-21e.
Step 6: Place one probe on the center of the chin; slowly move the second probe vertically. Hold each point for a count of six. Move from the center of the mouth to the corner on both sides. See Figure 20-22.

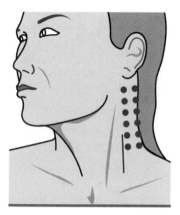

Figure 20-21a Step 5.

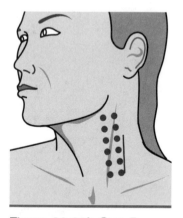

Figure 20-21b Step 5.

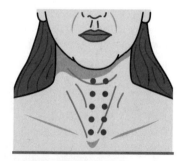

Figure 20-21c Step 5.

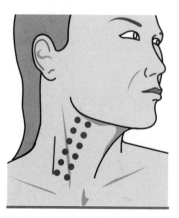

Figure 20-21d Step 5.

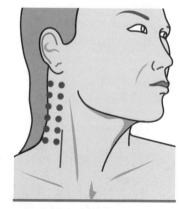

Figure 20-21e Step 5.

Step 7: Place one probe in the center of the upper lip; with the second probe, scoop and lift the muscle toward the probe on the upper lip. Hold for a count of six. See Figure 20-23.

Step 8: Place one probe at the jawline; pinch the muscle and hold for a count of six. Move the second probe toward the ear, not higher than the cheekbone. This technique is used to shorten the masseter. See Figure 20-24.

Step 9: Place one probe just under the lower edge of the cheekbone, and place the second probe under the edge of the jawbone. Lift the muscle up with a pinch, and work toward the ear; hold each movement for a count of six. See Figure 20-25.

Step 10: Place one probe below the corner of the mouth; lift up with a pinch, and move the second probe up the side of the nose with three separate movements, ending at the inner corner of the eye. See Figure 20-26.

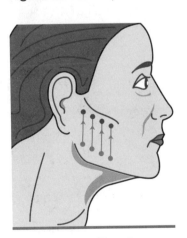

Figure 20-22 Step 6.

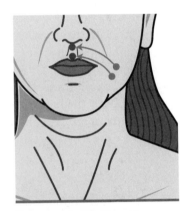

Figure 20-23 Step 7.

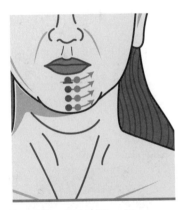

Figure 20-24 Step 8.

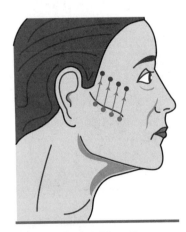

Figure 20-25 Step 9.

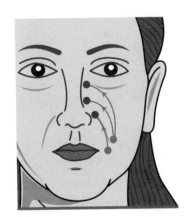

Figure 20-26 Step 10.

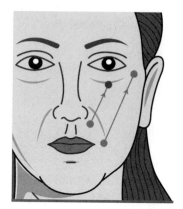

Figure 20-27 Step 11.

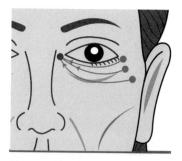

Figure 20-28a Step 12.

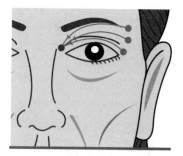

Figure 20-28b Step12.

Step 11: Place one probe at the lower rim of the eye muscle, and place the second probe just under the cheekbone. Push the muscle up with a pinch, and work from the center of the face outward toward the ear. Hold each movement for a count of six. See Figure 20-27.

Step 12: Place one probe at the inner corner of the eye; move the second probe slowly toward the first probe, and repeat with three to four strokes. Repeat on the upper eye, working only on the **orbital area,** not directly on the eye. See Figures 20-28a and 20-28b.

Step 13: Place one probe above the eyebrow; lift with the second probe, starting at the inner edge of the brow and working toward the outer edge. Hold for a count of six with each movement. See Figure 20-29.

Step 14: Put both probes together in between the brows, and slowly pull them away from each other; repeat two to three times. See Figure 20-30.

Step 15: Place one probe an inch from the hairline; place the second probe in the middle of the forehead; lift the muscle upward, and hold for a count of six. Work out to the sides of the forehead. See Figure 20-31.

Step 16: Place one probe an inch inside the hairline and another probe at the hairline; lift the muscle upward, and hold for a count of six. See Figure 20-32.

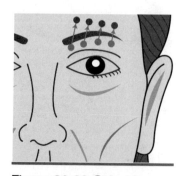

Figure 20-29 Step 13.

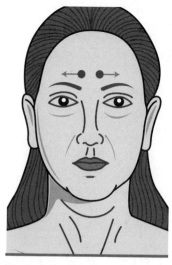

Figure 20-30 Step 14.

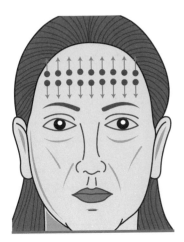

Figure 20-31 Step 15.

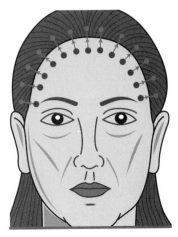

Figure 20-32 Step 16.

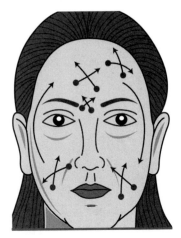

Figure 20-33 Step 17.

Step 17: Apply serum specified by manufacturer, or use a water-based serum and perform the feathering technique; this is done with a crisscross pattern over the face and around the eyes, as shown in Figure 20-33.

Treatment should last approximately 30 to 45 minutes. To create a luxurious antiaging treatment, you can follow with this collagen mask treatment:

Step 18: Apply a marine collagen mask for 20 minutes.
Step 19: Apply a hydrating cream using light effleurage movements.
Step 20: Apply SPF if you are finishing the treatment in the daytime.

Your Protocol:

_____

_____

_____

_____

_____

_____

_____

_____

_____

■ YOUR EQUIPMENT INFORMATION

Manufacturer info:

Name/phone number: _____

Web site: _____

Date purchased: _____   Registration: _____

Warranty info: _____

Replacement parts info: _____

TROUBLESHOOTING

All troubleshooting with this type of advanced machine should be addressed by the manufacturer. If no technical support is available, reevaluate purchasing from this manufacturer or vendor.

Q & A

Can I achieve the same results without a microcurrent machine?

No. This machine is designed to perform a specific function at the cellular level within the skin. You do not need it to provide an effective antiaging treatment, but the same specific results provided by the machine cannot be duplicated with skin care products alone.

Should I buy or lease the equipment?

This should be based on your financial situation. It is a higher priced piece of equipment that may be purchased via a lease, so it might be wise to get professional financial advice before purchasing.

Can microcurrent therapy make a difference in my practice?

Yes, but it is not a necessity. As an esthetician, you definitely need to know how to use microcurrent, but its use is not mandatory. Expertise with massage modalities, such as lymphatic drainage and a professional skin care line that supports your client's goals, can be very effective.

Is less expensive better?

No. Quality manufacturing is important when purchasing a machine of this caliber. Do your research well.

What does the FDA say about microcurrent?

This is a Class I exempt machine. The manufacturer must register, but the distributor does not have to.

REFERENCES

1. D'Angelo, J., Dean, P., Dietz, S., Hinds, C., Lees, M., Miller, E., & Zani, A. (2003). *Milady's Standard Comprehensive Training for Estheticians*. New York: Thomson Delmar Learning.

2. Simmons, J. V. (1989, 1995). *Science and the Beauty Business, The Beauty Salon and its Equipment* (2nd ed.). United Kingdom: Macmillan Press Ltd.

3. Lees, M. (2001). *Skin Care: Beyond the Basics*. New York: Thomson Delmar Learning.

4. Nordman, L. (2005). *Professional Beauty Therapy, The Official Guide to Level 3* (2nd ed.). London: Thomson Learning.

5. Becker, R. O., & Selden, G. (1985). *The Body Electric*. New York: William Morrow.

6. Sofra-Weiss, X. (2007). "The Effects of Nanocurrent on Cellular Life." Available online at http://www.arasysperfector.com.

7. Cheng, N., Van Hoof, H., Bockx, E., Hoogmartens, M. J., Mulier, J. C., De Dijcker, F. J., Sansen, W. M., & De Loecker, W. (1982). "The Effects of Electric Currents on ATP Generation, Protein Synthesis, and Membrane Transport in Rat Skin." *Clinical Orthopaedics and Related Research*, Nov–Dec (171): 264–272.

8. Quatresooz, P., Thirion, L., Piérard-Franchimont, C., & Piérard, G. E. (2006). "The Riddle of Genuine Skin Microrelief and Wrinkles." *International Journal of Cosmetic Science* Dec 28 (6): 389–395.

Advanced Technological Equipment

SECTION

5

Oxygen Machines

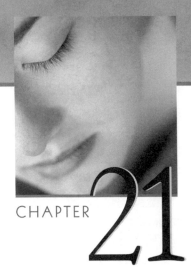

The theory of applying oxygen to the skin is controversial, and no peer-reviewed independent studies have been published to prove that it works. Still, many estheticians use this equipment and stand by the results they see. The oxygen therapy provided by estheticians using oxygen machines is not to be confused with **hyperbaric oxygen therapy,** which is used by doctors to help heal damaged skin, to treat compression sickness, and to kill bacteria. That therapy uses a medical unit that controls the atmospheric pressure.

CHAPTER 21

FUNCTIONS

Oxygen machines assist in the penetration of skin care products, create an antibacterial environment on the skin, increase cellular respiration, and improve the texture of the skin.

HOW IT WORKS

Oxygen is filtered from the air into a compressor, which is then applied to the skin via a mask or handheld applicator, much like an airbrush. Usually a product or mask is applied first to enhance the results. Another method for application is a nebulizer that takes an active ingredient and infuses atmospheric oxygen into it, producing a liquid that is then dispensed much like the mist from a Lucas spray.

WHAT IT DOES TO THE SKIN

The use of oxygen on the skin is reported to increase cell metabolism and microcirculation; it also kills anaerobic pathogens, increases the skin's ability to heal, and may enhance collagen production.

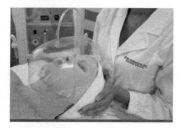

Figure 21-1 Bio-Therapeutic oxygen mask application.

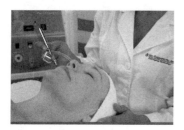

Figure 21-2 Bio-Therapeutic oxygen treatment.

This is where the controversy begins: ninety percent of the metabolic processes of the skin are anaerobic. For oxygen to have a biological effect, it must reach the basal layer. On the surface, however, it is an effective bleaching agent and gentle germicide; this is where the possible benefits are seen by estheticians.

HOW TO USE IT

Use of oxygen depends on the type of machine purchased, and each manufacturer will have a specific procedure to follow. One of the options for application is a mask applied over the face. See Figure 21-1 for an example.

Other applications use a unit with a nebulizer. Active ingredients are placed in the nebulizer, and an oxygen concentrator pulls the oxygen from the room and mixes it with the active ingredients, which are sprayed in a fine mist over the skin. See Figure 21-2 for an example.

HOW TO BUY

This is a controversial subject, so how and whether you buy may depend on how much you know about cellular biology. A liquid applied to the skin has the opportunity to be absorbed, but there is no evidence that oxygen will penetrate products into the dermis. On a clinical level, some estheticians who use this system say that they see an improvement in the look and texture of the skin.

If you are considering purchasing an oxygen system, here are a few guidelines:

- Look for manufacturers that have been in business for at least three years.
- Ask for studies to back up their claims.
- Be cautious of claims that state product penetration to the dermal level. This is outside the scope of an esthetics practice.
- Always ask for a demonstration first.
- Do not purchase a system that requires 100% tanked oxygen. This is medical equipment and can be very hazardous.
- Look for an output of at least 25 pounds of pressure.
- Volume of airflow is not as important as quality. Look for an output of at least 95% oxygen.

Buyer's Checklist

- What is the price?
- What is the cost of shipping?
- Do you have an instruction manual, DVD, or on-site training?
- Is the machine UL listed, ISO certified, or CE or CSA tested?
- Does it come with all the accessories, or do those have to be purchased separately?
- Can I buy replacement parts?
- What is covered under the warranty, and for how long?
- Is the manufacturer FDA registered?
- Who will service the machine if repairs are needed?

See Figure 21-3 for features to look for when you buy.

■ SAFETY

Do not use a system that requires 100% tanked oxygen that requires re-filling. This can be *very dangerous* and most states will not allow you to do this without medical supervision. It is a fire hazard.

■ MAINTENANCE

Maintenance must be followed per your manufacturer's directions. As with all esthetic equipment, you can also follow these general guidelines:

- Wipe down exterior of machine after each use.
- Check all wires before use. Do not use if cracked or loose wires are visible.

Microcurrent	UL listed or CE mark
	Manufacturer FDA-registered
	Results based on clinical research
	Output of 25 PSI
	Outflow of at least 95% oxygen
	Training included in purchase
	Replacement parts available
	Warranty

Figure 21-3 Chart of features to look for.

■ DISINFECTION AND SANITIZATION

Any part of the machine that touches the client must be disinfected. Use an EPA-approved disinfectant to clean all surfaces, including the inside of the oxygen mask.

See Figure 21-4 for a chart of maintenance and disinfection.

■ CONTRAINDICATIONS AND CAUTIONS

Most manufacturers state that there are no contraindications to using an oxygen machine. Here are some general guidelines:

- Skin inflammation: Increased circulation could make inflammation worse.
- Skin disorders or diseases: These may be aggravated by treatment.
- Very sensitive skin: Treatment may be very uncomfortable for the client.
- Botox: Apply no treatments until 72 hours after injection. Botox paralyzes muscle, so any treatment to stimulate muscle would be ineffective.
- High or low blood pressure: Either condition could be made worse by an increase in circulation. Even if the condition is treated and under control, use caution. Never leave such clients alone, and help them on and off the treatment bed.
- HIV.
- Malignant melanoma: Treatment for the cancer must be complete, and the client must be in remission. Obtain physician approval and ask

Disinfection	Maintenance
Disinfect mask in EPA-approved disinfectant	Check all wires before use
Any part of the machine in contact with the client should be saturated with EPA-approved disinfectant	Do not use tanked oxygen
Wipe down exterior after each use with EPA-approved disinfectant	

Figure 21-4 Chart of maintenance and disinfection.

the client for a waiver. Do not apply treatment when in doubt about a possible abnormality; instead, refer the client to a dermatologist.

■ PREPARATION FOR TREATMENT

- Have your client fill out an assessment form.
- Check for contraindications.
- Have your client change into a treatment gown and remove all jewelry and contact lenses.
- Analyze the skin using a magnifying lamp.
- Explain the procedure.
- Make sure to test all equipment before applying treatment.
- Inspect all hoses, wires, and plugs.
- Follow the manufacturer's instructions for the setup of your oxygen machine.

■ PROTOCOLS

Protocols are specific to your manufacturer's instructions. Here is a basic facial treatment protocol.

Step 1: Look at the skin through a magnifying lamp for initial skin analysis.

Step 2: Remove makeup with appropriate makeup remover.

Step 3: Cleanse skin with appropriate cleanser.

Step 4: Remove cleanser with sponges or a warm towel.

Step 5: Apply toner.

Step 6: Perform a skin analysis with a magnifying lamp and a Woods lamp. Turn the steamer on.

Step 7: Apply a proteolytic enzyme exfoliant and steam for 10 to 15 minutes, depending on the manufacturer's instructions.

Optional Step: Use brush machine under steam for a deep cleanse.

Step 8: Remove exfoliant with sponges or a warm towel.

Step 9: Massage skin 15 to 20 minutes.

Step 10: Apply serum.

Step 11: Apply marine collagen mask; wet the surface with activator or distilled water.

Step 12: Place the oxygen mask on the client's face, and turn on the machine per the manufacturer's instructions.

Step 13: Remove the mask after 10 minutes.

Step 14: Apply toner, appropriate moisturizer, and sunscreen.

■ YOUR EQUIPMENT INFORMATION

Manufacturer info:

Name/phone number: _____

Web site: _____

Date purchased: _____   Registration: _____

Warranty info: _____

Replacement parts info: _____

TROUBLESHOOTING

This is high-tech equipment that should only be serviced by the manufacturer. Refer to your vendor or manufacturer instructions.

REFERENCES

1. Pugliese, P. (2001). *Physiology of the Skin II*. Carol Stream, Illinois: Allured Publishing.
2. Wenburg, C. (2006). *The Esthetic Benefits of Oxygen Skin Care*. Carol Stream, Illinois: Allured Publishing.

Theory of Light

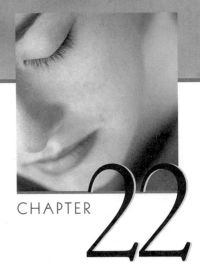

It is important to have a general understanding of light to appreciate the advanced technological equipment in the esthetic market. In this chapter we will look at the fundamentals of light.

Light therapy is used with laser, intense pulsed light (IPL), and LED technology. Some of these machines can be used by estheticians, but others are restricted. Most states do not allow estheticians to use lasers or IPL. Refer to the index for a state-by-state listing. It is still important to understand how light works, the types of machines available, and light's effects on the skin.

Light-based machines are primarily used for skin rejuvenation and correction of disorders such as acne. Laser hair removal is also one of the most popular uses of this technology and one that the public is most familiar with; Figure 22-1 shows an example. LED light therapy is gaining in popularity and is currently the subject of many studies.

■ WHAT IS LIGHT?

This question has been pondered by minds as great as Einstein's. Light is defined as visible electromagnetic radiation of various wavelengths that travels at approximately 186,282,397 miles per second in a vacuum. Physics defines light as a form of energy in which the elementary particle that defines it is the **photon;** to create light, electrons need to emit photons. When higher-energy electrons orbiting an atom drop to a lower orbit, the photon is released to get rid of the additional energy that the electron had at the higher orbit; this release is seen as light. Light as a form of energy can be converted to other forms of energy, such as electricity. See Figure 22-2.

The two scientific theories of light are the **wave theory** and the *particle theory.* In wave-particle duality, light comprises particles called photons, but the movement of the photon is considered a wave. Light is electromagnetic radiation that travels in a vacuum. It does not need a

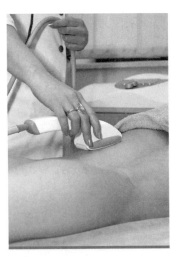

Figure 22-1 Laser hair removal is very popular.

245

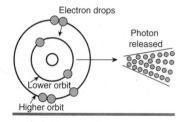

Figure 22-2 Photons are created when an electron at a higher orbit drops to a lower orbit.

medium to travel through, such as a wave in the water; it can travel independent of any matter.

The three basic dimensions of light that we are concerned with in esthetics are *amplitude, wavelength,* and *frequency.*

- **Amplitude** is the intensity or strength of the wavelength.
- **Wavelength** is the measurement of light from the distance between two corresponding points. Wavelengths travel in a 360-degree direction.
- **Frequency** is the measurement of the number of waves that cycle over a single point per second. It can be measured in hertz (Hz), or 100 cycles per second; kilohertz (kHz), or 1,000 cycles per second; or **megahertz** (MHz), or 1,000,000 cycles per second.

■ LIGHT FORMS

Light comes in different forms: monochromatic, coherent, traditional, and collimated.

- Monochromatic light is a single wavelength of light.
- Coherent light waves travel in a single direction and do not lose energy as they move away.
- Traditional light waves are polychromatic, which means that all colors and wavelengths are included. This is the visible light that we see from day to day. A broad spectrum of colors comprises visible light, and a prism will display these colors. See Figure 22-3.
- Collimated light moves in one small, parallel direction.

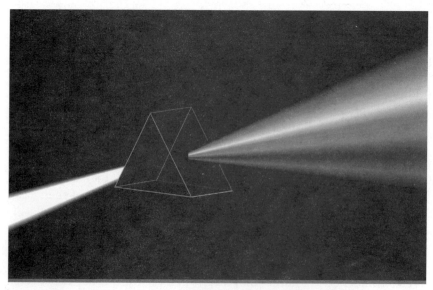

Figure 22-3 Visible light refracted through a prism.

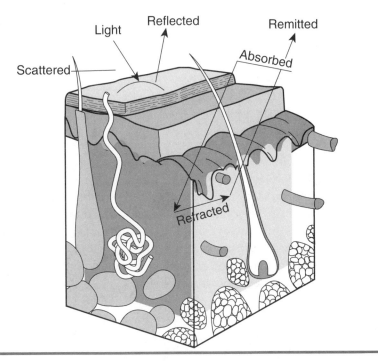

Figure 22-4 How light reacts upon hitting the skin.

Light in its various forms can be *scattered, reflected, absorbed, refracted,* and *remitted.* In regard to the skin, this is how it works:

- Depending on the angle of incidence, light striking the skin is first scattered, then reflected, then absorbed.
- After being absorbed, the light is then bent (refracted) depending on the changes in tissue density. When the photon is absorbed, it transfers its energy to a specific molecule.[1]
- After the light reaches the depth it is able to penetrate, it is then remitted; this is the light being reflected back toward the surface of the skin. Figure 22-4 provides an illustration.
- Specific wavelengths perform different actions on the skin; for example, red light will penetrate deeply.

One of the ways light affects the skin depends on the refractive index. All matter has a refractive index, which is the measure of how much the speed of light is reduced by hitting it. For example, skin has a refractive index of 1.55, and glass has a refractive index of 1.33.[2] If you apply a medium to the skin that is close to the refractive index of the skin, such as water, the light will penetrate the skin deeply. A sunburn is a good example of the end

[1]Fundamentals of Laser Science, Part 1, Skin Inc., July 2004
[2]Fundamentals of Laser Science, Part 1, Skin Inc., July 2004

result of this action. Sunscreen should have a higher refractive index than the skin to help scatter and reflect light.

■ THE ELECTROMAGNETIC SPECTRUM

The electromagnetic spectrum comprises a wide range of wavelengths. Some are visible to the human eye, but many are invisible, such as microwaves and ultraviolet light. Wavelengths of light are measured in nanometers (nm).

Electromagnetic radiation that is considered visible light is within the 400 to 700 nm range. The optical spectrum also includes infrared and ultraviolet light, but these are not visible to the human eye. Also included in the electromagnetic spectrum are higher energy gamma rays and x-rays and lower energy microwaves, radiowaves, and TV waves. Figure 22-5 shows the electromagnetic spectrum.

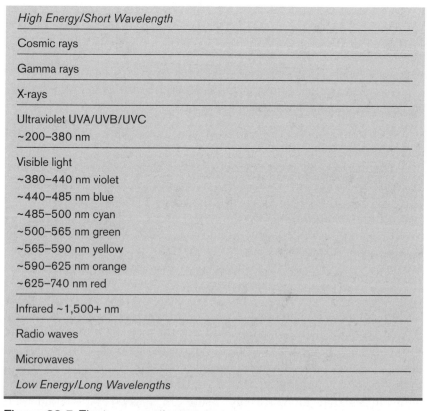

High Energy/Short Wavelength

Cosmic rays

Gamma rays

X-rays

Ultraviolet UVA/UVB/UVC
~200–380 nm

Visible light
~380–440 nm violet
~440–485 nm blue
~485–500 nm cyan
~500–565 nm green
~565–590 nm yellow
~590–625 nm orange
~625–740 nm red

Infrared ~1,500+ nm

Radio waves

Microwaves

Low Energy/Long Wavelengths

Figure 22-5 Electromagnetic spectrum.

The different wavelengths visible to the human eye are:

- Red: the longest wavelength, about 700 nm
- Violet: the shortest wavelength, about 400 nm
- Orange: 590 to 620 nm
- Yellow: 565 to 590 nm
- Green: 500 to 565 nm
- Blue: 440 to 485 nm

Wavelengths outside the range of visible light are called **ultraviolet;** they have a short wavelength. **Infrared** waves have a long wavelength. See Figure 22-6 for an example of the electromagnetic spectrum of visible light.

ENERGY AND POWER

The shorter the wavelength, the greater the energy in the photon; however, the shorter wavelength will not penetrate as deeply into the skin. The opposite is true with a longer wavelength, which has less energy but will penetrate deeply. See Figure 22-7 for a diagram of wavelengths.

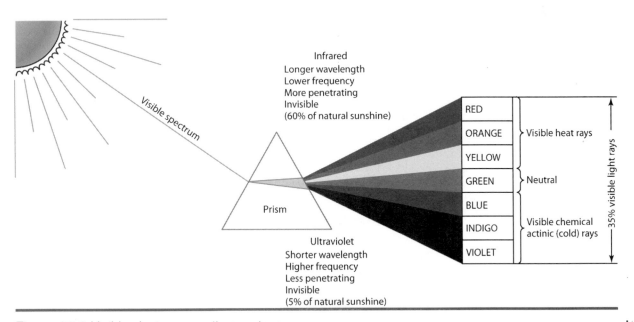

Figure 22-6 Visible electromagnetic spectrum.

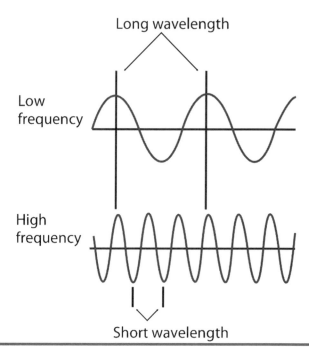

Figure 22-7 Wavelengths.

In physics it is important to understand the measurements and descriptions of *energy, work,* and *power.* This is important for esthetics, too, because it helps explain the strength of the laser, LED, or IPL machine.

- *Energy* is the ability to perform a force over distance.
- *Work* is the application of a force over distance.
- *Power* is how fast the application of force is performed or how fast energy is transferred over distance.

In physics, energy and work have the same measurement: **joules.** This is a measurement much used—and misused—in light therapy devices. Power is measured in watts, which you see in electric devices. A watt is one joule per second. The effective measurement of energy and power for laser, LED, and IPL equipment varies and is different depending on the manufacturer.

The strength of the light, or **luminous intensity,** is the rate at which light energy falls on a surface. This is measured in lumens with a light meter. Light meters are frequently used by photographers; see Figure 22-8 for an example.

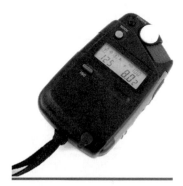

Figure 22-8 A light meter is used to measure light.

■ PHOTOBIOLOGY

Photobiology is the science of the interaction of light with biological living matter.[3] There are many subspecialties within this field. The fundamentals of photobiology state that for a substance to create a chemical or physical change, the light must be absorbed.

Each substance has a unique absorption spectrum, which is the probability that light will be absorbed at a given wavelength. When the light is absorbed at the correct wavelength, a photobiological effect will occur. One aspect of photobiology is to study the correct wavelengths that will produce photobiological responses and standardize the requirements. These standardized requirements are much like drug dosing; the correct dosage, time frame, and instructions must be followed for the therapy to be effective. This is a field that is always evolving and particularly relates to LED therapy.

[3]Physiology of the Skin II (2001)

REFERENCES

1. Simmons, J. V. (1989, 1995). *Science and the Beauty Business: The Beauty Salon and its Equipment* (2nd ed.). United Kingdom: Macmillan Press Ltd.
2. Lees, M. (2001). *Skin Care: Beyond the Basics.* New York: Thomson Delmar Learning.
3. Becker, R. O., & Selden, G. (1985). *The Body Electric.* New York: William Morrow.
4. Pugliese, P. (2004). *Fundamentals of Laser Science, Part I.* Carol Stream, Illinois: Allured Publishing. 52–60.
5. Dennis, J. & Moring, G. (2006). *The Complete Idiot's Guide to Physics* (2nd ed.). New York: Penguin Group, Inc.
6. Freudenrich, C. "How Light Works". Available online at http://science.howstuffworks.com.
7. Pugliese, P. (2001). *Physiology of the Skin II.* Carol Stream, Illinois: Allured Publishing.
8. Smith, K. (2007). *Laser and LED Therapy Is Phototherapy.* American Society of Phototherapy. Available online at http://www.pol-us.net.

LED Light Therapy

LED light therapy is also known as *photorejuvenation* and *phototherapy*. LED light therapy is considered a nonlaser light source and is available to estheticians. It is primarily used for antiaging treatments and acne treatments.

LED is considered a low-power, nonthermal light device, unlike lasers, which use high-power coherent light. LED light therapy uses noncoherent light in various wavelengths, generally in the red, infrared, and blue spectrums. Light therapy remains controversial within the medical and scientific community, because not enough studies have been done for widely accepted peer-reviewed journals. We will take a look at the purported functions of LED light therapy for the beauty industry, with the understanding that they have not been truly scientifically proven but are only reported observations within the esthetics community.

■ FUNCTIONS

LED therapy appears to reduce static and dynamic rhytids (lines and wrinkles), increase collagen production, reduce rough skin texture, reduce uneven pigmentation, improve lymphatic flow, increase microcirculation, assist in tissue repair, and increase the production of ATP. Figure 23-1 shows an LED machine.

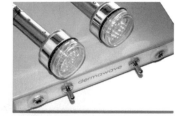

Figure 23-1 Dermawave LED.

■ THE NASA STUDY

One study that is frequently quoted by LED light-therapy manufacturers is the Whelan study by NASA's Marshall Space Flight Center as part of their Small Business Innovation Research (SBIR) program. It is important to note that the objective of the study was to assess the effects of hyperbaric oxygen and near-infrared light therapy on wound healing. LED light therapy was originally developed by NASA for plant growth studies for the space program. The study took that technology and did **in vivo** and **in vitro** studies on animal and human tissues, as well as on human subjects with acute and chronic wounds. Various LED wavelengths and strengths were used.

The researchers found that LED produced in vitro increases of cell growth in mouse-derived fibroblasts, rat-derived osteoblasts, and rat-derived skeletal muscle cells. Researchers also found a growth increase of between 155% and 171% in normal human epithelial cells; cell growth increased by 155% percent in human epithelial cells with a wavelength of 670 nm, 4 j/cm^2 energy density. Collagen synthesis was doubled when compared to the control cells, which were treated with 670 nm at 8j/cm^2. Wound healing on human subjects was also conducted daily at 670 nm, 4j/cm^2, and subjects showed improvement.

From this study we can interpret that there are definite positive effects of this treatment modality. However, we must note the following:

- Multiple wavelengths were not used together because of the physics law of destructive interference.
- The study was not testing for skin rejuvenation; it studied wound healing and plant photosynthesis in a hyperbaric oxygen environment.

■ HOW IT WORKS

An LED machine produces noncoherent light in a specific color or wavelength, at a specific strength (measured in joules), with multiple frequencies. It uses light-emitting diodes (LEDs) applied by handheld probes in a pattern, or by a faceplate set about an inch from the face, for a certain length of time. Figure 23-2 shows an example of the handheld wands used in LED therapy.

The electrical components of the light are encased by a clear epoxy, and a metallurgic compound is applied over the electrical junction of the LED light bulb. These compounds are known as **inorganic semiconductor materials.** When excited by an electrical voltage, particular colors are emitted. See Figure 23-3 for a chart of inorganic semiconductor materials used.

Different colors, such as red and blue, are used to activate different cellular responses in the skin, much like a plant grows under the sun. The greatest cellular reaction happens closest to the light source.

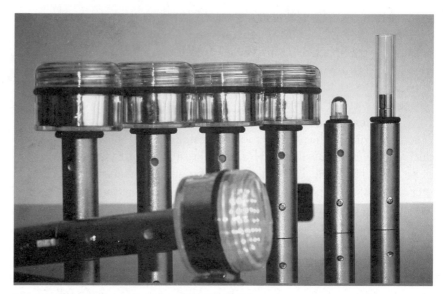

Figure 23-2 Dermawave handheld wands.

Semiconductor materials	Color wavelength created
AigAaS	Red and infrared
AlGaP	Green
AlGaInP	High bright orange, red, yellow, green
GaAsP	Red, orange-red, orange, yellow
GaP – gallium phosphide	Red, yellow, green
GaN	Green, emerald green, blue
InGaN	Near ultraviolet, blue green, blue
SiC – silicon carbide	Blue
Si – silicon	Blue
$A_{12}O_3$ – sapphire	Blue
ZnSe – zinc selenide	Blue
C – diamond	Ultraviolet
AIN – aluminium nitride	Near to far ultraviolet
AlGaN	Near to far ultraviolet
AlGaInN	Near to far ultraviolet

Figure 23-3 Inorganic semiconductors.

WHAT IT DOES TO THE SKIN

In order to understand what LED therapy can do to the skin, we need to take a look at the science of photobiology. **Photobiology** is the study of light interactions with living organisms. The first law of photochemistry is that light must be absorbed in order to create a biological reaction within a cell. Each wavelength has a different effect on the cellular pathways. Light particles called photons must be absorbed by receptors in the cells to be effective. Not every wavelength will be absorbed to create a biological reaction; however, the longer the wavelength, the deeper the penetration. Shorter wavelengths do not penetrate as far. Deeper penetration of light does not always mean that the light will be more effective. Figure 23-4 illustrates wavelength penetration in the skin.

The theory is that when light is absorbed by photoreceptors in the cell mitochondria, a short respiratory chain reaction occurs that leads to enhanced synthesis of ATP. In particular, the cytochromes, which are the parts of the cell that respond to light and color, are activated, and their energy increases. This leads to increased cell proliferation, tissue growth, and regeneration.

The most important thing to remember about light-therapy devices is this: all we know about how light actually affects the cell is only a theory, but it would appear that the light must be the correct wavelength and

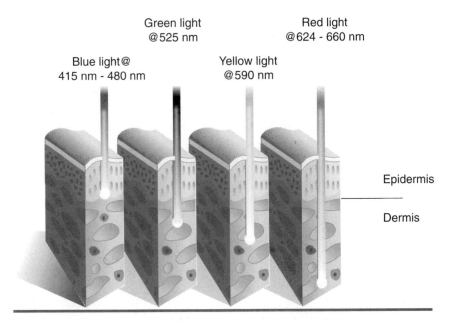

Figure 23-4 Wavelength penetration.

strength to get results. This is where it gets complicated, depending on who you talk to. The NASA study used 660 to 880 nm, but other studies have been done focusing on skin rejuvenation at the high 500 nm and low 600 nm ranges. There are really three parts to the effectiveness of light therapy: *wavelength*, *pulse frequency*, and *pulse width*. A good design will utilize all three to treat a desired target.

It is interesting to note that in many studies, the energy output is measured in a cumulative manner. This means that a certain wavelength and strength were applied on a daily basis over a certain time frame. This is not a modality that is driven by immediate results; clients must be committed to multiple sessions to see a difference.

Effects of Red Light

Many machines produce red light at 624 nm, 633 nm, and 660 nm; each is considered the optimal wavelength for various treatments. Many benefits have been suggested.

- Increases circulation: Speeds up the healing process by supplying additional oxygen and nutrients to the cell.
- Stimulates collagen production: Collagen is an essential protein that holds cells together and gives firmness to the skin.
- Stimulates ATP: Adenosine triphosphate is the major carrier of energy to all cells. It increases the energy level of cells, which leads to increased cell production. One theory of aging is that the ability for cells to produce energy is reduced, which leads to many symptoms of aging.
- Increases lymphatic flow: Lymph removes toxins from the body.
- Increases RNA and DNA synthesis: Damaged cells are replaced more quickly.
- Stimulates fibroblastic activity: This aids in the repair process and helps form collagen.
- Increases **phagocytosis:** This process of finding and ingesting dead or dying cells by the phagocytic cells helps reduce inflammation.
- Increases thermal effects: Treatment increases the temperature of the cells without heating the surface of the skin. This may lead to better product penetration.

Effects of Blue Light

This wavelength (415 nm to 480 nm) was recently studied as a treatment for acne. The finding was that blue light at 415 nm and red light at 660 nm was more effective than blue light alone. This combination produces **singlet oxygen,** which kills the *p. acnes* bacteria.

Color	Effect
Red	Increased circulation, stimulation of fibroblasts, stimulation of ATP, increased lymphatic flow, increased cell rejuvenation and metabolism
Amber	Same effects as red when used at 590 nm
Yellow	Increased lymphatic flow
Green	Decreased melanin production
Blue	Kills *p. acnes* bacteria
Infrared	Increased circulation and heat in tissues which helps with pain relief

Figure 23-5 Colors and their biological effects.

Effects of Yellow Light

Yellow light at 590 nm is used for its healing, draining, and detoxifying properties. It is absorbed by the body fluids in the lymph and blood circulatory systems and promotes wound healing. It increases lymphatic flow to evacuate more waste products and boosts cellular activity.

Effects of Green Light

Green light at 525 nm decreases melanin production, reduces pigmentation, and eliminates the redness associated with the use of chemical peels and bleaching products.

Figure 23-5 shows a chart of colors and their biological effects.

■ HOW TO USE IT

Every LED manufacturer has a protocol for you to follow. Many have proprietary skin care products to be used during the treatment. In general, a LED wand is applied over the face in sections. The LED wand is in contact with the skin and is held for up to four minutes in each area, depending on the machine. Some LED machines have a freestanding arm that can be positioned over the face and set on a timer. See the general protocol for step-by-step instructions.

The body can also be treated with light therapy, and many manufacturers have machines specifically designed for this. Also popular are multimodality machines that combine different equipment, such as microcurrent, microdermabrasion, and vacuum massage.

■ HOW TO BUY

The complicated part of utilizing this technology is deciding what to buy. Many machines have been relabeled as photorejuvenation machines, from their original use for pain relief, without modifications in wavelength. Prices can range from $3,000 to $35,000; the machine marketed to physicians can range upwards of $35,000.

Buyer's Checklist

Based on many studies, here are some general guidelines for purchase:

- Make sure your manufacturer is FDA-registered.
- Make sure they have research that proves their machine works.
- Check that they are using the latest LED technology. Is their device a relabeled pain device that utilizes red and infrared together?
- Does the unit have sensors or a manual control knob that can adjust for Fitzpatrick skin types? In order for the light to affect the cell receptors it must be absorbed. The blue light is the only light that does not need adjustment. Each Fitzpatrick skin type has its own reflectance and light-absorption properties. Suffice it to say that LED light therapy may not work for every client, depending on how well-made the machine is. A machine that has the capacity to optimize output based on melanin in the skin is ideal.
- What is the price?
- Do you have an instruction manual or DVD?
- Is the machine UL listed, ISO certified, or CE or CSA tested?

TIP Before and after photos can be very deceiving. This is a definite buyer-beware machine at this point in time.

LED light therapy	UL listed or CE mark Automatic Fitzpatrick type adjustment
	FDA-registered manufacturer
	Proof to support claims
	Training with purchase
	Replacement parts available
	Warranty
	Red and infrared not on at the same time (destructive interference)
	Short treatment time

Figure 23-6 Features to look for.

- How many LED heads does it come with?
- Can I buy replacement parts?
- What is covered under the warranty, and for how long?
- Do you have a return policy?

See Figure 23-6 for a chart of features to look for.

■ SAFETY

LED light therapy is a very safe modality, although it is important to protect the eyes from direct exposure to the light. Have your client wear eye pads or tanning goggles when applying treatment.

This is an electrical appliance, so make sure that wall outlets are the grounded, three-prong type. Make sure that you do not overload the outlet. A ground fault circuit interrupter (GFCI) is required on all outlets within six feet of a water source. For the purposes of a facial room, it is a good idea to have them.

■ MAINTENANCE

Maintenance is the same as for other esthetic machines and is one of the most important aspects of owning such machines. Maintenance for a LED light therapy machine is very easy. Manufacturers will also have their own protocols, so be sure to follow their directions. In general, use these guidelines:

- Wipe the machine clean after each use with a clean, soft cloth.
- Use isopropyl alcohol on a saturated cotton tip to clean LED heads as needed.
- Do not store LED heads in a UV sterilizer.
- Check all wires before use. Do not use the unit if cracked or loose wires are visible.

■ DISINFECTION AND SANITIZATION

- Disinfect the LED head by spraying the glass portion in contact with the skin with state-approved high-level disinfectant. Recommended leave-on time is 10 to 15 minutes, depending on the manufacturer.
- Do not submerge the LED head in high-level solution.
- Do not store the LED head in a UV sanitizer.

Disinfection	Maintenance
Disinfect any probe or part of machine in contact with client with an EPA-approved disinfectant	Check all wires before use
Store in clean, closed container	After each use, clean probe with 70% alcohol and soft cloth
After each use, wipe down exterior with EPA-approved disinfectant	Check that all bulbs are working daily

Figure 23-7 Chart of disinfection and maintenance.

- Store in LED head in the container that came with your machine or in another clean, closed container.

See Figure 23-7 chart of disinfection and maintenance.

■ CONTRAINDICATIONS AND CAUTIONS

LED therapy is very safe to use, but there are some health cautions to take into consideration when applying LED treatments. The consultation is extremely important to determine contraindications or special needs that your client may have. Do not rely exclusively on the intake form; it is also important to verbally get information and clarification from your client.

- Pregnancy: Use caution when working on pregnant clients; they are very sensitive.
- Skin disorders or diseases: These may be aggravated by treatment.
- Botox: No treatment can be applied until 72 hours after injection.
- Epilepsy.
- Severe bruising: Bruised areas will be uncomfortable for the client.
- High or low blood pressure: These conditions could be made worse due to the increase in circulation. Even if the condition is treated and under control, use caution. Never leave such a client alone, and help them on and off the treatment bed.
- Malignant melanoma: Treatment for the malignancy must be complete, and the client must be in remission. Obtain physician approval. Do not apply treatment when in doubt about a possible abnormality; instead, refer the client to a dermatologist.
- Use of photosensitizing drugs: Accutane use must have stopped at least six months prior to treatment.

- Autoimmune disorders or connective tissue disease.
- Herpes simplex.

■ PREPARATION FOR TREATMENT

- Have your client fill out an assessment form.
- Check for contraindications.
- Have your client change into a treatment gown and remove all jewelry and contact lenses.
- Analyze the skin using a magnifying lamp.
- Explain the procedure and the skin type analysis.
- Make sure to test all equipment before applying treatment.
- Inspect all wires and LED heads.
- Follow manufacturer's instructions for use.

■ PROTOCOLS

Every machine manufacturer has a specific protocol for use. Here are some general guidelines.

General Light Therapy with Handheld Wands

See Figure 23-8 for an example.

Step 1: Perform first and second cleanse.

Step 2: Exfoliate (microdermabrasion is a perfect complement; see Chapter 26).

Step 3: Apply serum for specific skin condition. Some manufacturers recommend that you not use any product on the skin.

Step 4: Divide the face into six sections; start with left and right halves, and then partition out three horizontal areas, starting at the forehead.

Step 5: Start at the first section, and apply the LED light wand very slowly—about an inch every 10 seconds over the area for 2 minutes (most machines have a timer). The LED light wand should be in contact with the skin.

Step 6: Move to the second section in a clockwise manner, and repeat for two minutes, moving into the third area. Repeat movements into all six areas, ending up back at the first section.

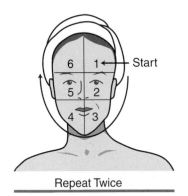

Figure 23-8 Divide the face into six parts and apply in clockwise motion.

Step 7: Repeat over all six areas again. With some machines, a higher frequency can be used for the second pass.

Step 8: Use the LED wand over any areas of concern for the client (i.e. crow's feet, nasolabial folds). Move slowly for two minutes in each area.

Step 9: Apply appropriate moisturizer and sunscreen.

■ YOUR EQUIPMENT INFORMATION

Manufacturer info:

Name/phone number: _____

Web site: _____

Date purchased: _____ Registration: _____

Warranty info: _____

Replacement parts info: _____

TROUBLESHOOTING

All troubleshooting with this type of advanced machine should be addressed by the machine manufacturer. If there is no technical support available, reevaluate purchasing from this manufacturer or vendor.

Q & A

What are the pros and cons of LED equipment?

Pros

Effectiveness: The results are promising.
Ease of use: LED is an easy modality to use with minimal training.
Training: Training to use the machine is very easy. A basic knowledge of the physics of light is needed to effectively understand why the treatment works.
Safety: LED units are very safe with no possibility of thermal damage to the skin.

Cons

Cost: Equipment can be very expensive, and engineering varies widely between manufacturers.
Maintenance: Unit requires consistent cleaning and careful handling.

What does the FDA say about LED therapy?

LED is considered a Class II medical device. Still a gray area for this therapy, it is equivalent to an LED flash lamp, which can be classified either as an infrared lamp or in the laser category, which is divided into several more categories. The only concern with this type of equipment is overexposure to the eyes.

REFERENCES

1. Simmons, J. V. (1989, 1995). *Science and the Beauty Business, The Beauty Salon and its Equipment* (2nd ed.). United Kingdom: Macmillan Press Ltd.
2. Lees, M. (2001). *Skin Care: Beyond the Basics.* New York: Thomson Delmar Learning.
3. Papageorgiou, P., Katsaambus, A., & Chu, A. (2000) "Phototherapy with blue (415 nm) and red (660 nm) light in the treatment of acne vulgaris." *British Journal of Dermatology* (142): 973–978.
4. Schindl, A., Heinze, G., Schindl, M., Pernerstorfer-Schon, H., & Schindl, L. (2002). "Systemic effects of low intensity laser irradiation on skin microcirculation in patients with diabetic microangiopathy." *Microvascular Research* 64: 240–246.
5. Whelan, H. T., Buchmann, E. V., Whelan, N. T., Turner, S. G., Cevenini, V., Stinson, H., Ignatius, R., Martin, T., Cwiklinski, J., Meyer, G. A., Hodgson, B., Gould, L., Kane, M., Chen, G., & Caviness, J. (2001). *NASA Light Emitting Diode Medical Applications from Deep Space to Deep Sea.* CP552, Space Technology and Applications International Forum, American Institute of Physics.

WEB SITES

Photobiology
http://www.wikipedia.com

Society of Phototherapy
http://www.pol-us.net

Ultrasound

Ultrasound is one of the modalities more recently introduced into the esthetics industry, and it is very controversial. The type of ultrasound used is the therapeutic type, usually used for pain management and for healing injury by physical therapists and other allied health professionals. This equipment is considered a Class II prescriptive device, which means it must come with a label. See Figure 24-1 for an example of an ultrasonic device. Many states consider this device outside the scope of esthetics practice, and it may be hard to get liability insurance to cover its use, because it can cause harm to the body if not used correctly. But it has also shown some very promising results in the care of aging skin.

■ FUNCTIONS

Ultrasound provides epidermal penetration of specific **cosmeceuticals** formulated for use with ultrasound, treats hyperpigmentation, reduces fine lines and wrinkles, increases microcirculation, stimulates production of collagen, speeds up the skin's repair process, and removes dead skin.

■ HOW IT WORKS

Ultrasound works by using sound waves at specific frequencies to create physical changes at the cellular level. The frequencies are measured in megahertz (MHz), and ultrasound works at a range exceeding 20,000 cycles per second. See Figure 24-2 for a chart of sound waves.

Ultrasound energy is created by a crystal contained in the sound head; the crystal converts normal 110-volt energy from the outlet using a transformer. The conversion of energy to ultrasound occurs through

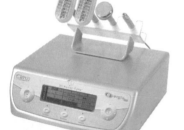

Figure 24-1 A Cirrus 900, from Silhouet-Tone Ltd.

infrasound	acoustic		ultrasound		
	20 kHz		1 MHz 2 MHz 3 MHz		
20 Hz		200 MHz			
Notes	Low Bass		Medical & tissue destructive	Therapeutic range	

Figure 24-2 Sound waves.

a scientific principle called the **piezoelectric effect.** This is when an electrical charge is delivered to the crystal , creating mechanical pressure and causing the crystal to vibrate and produce sound waves.

The ultrasonic waves are delivered through tissue via a coupling medium. This medium is a specifically created glycerin or water-based gel that allows the ultrasound energy to pass through it. The tissue density also effects how the ultrasound is delivered into the tissue. Tissue with the highest protein content will absorb most effectively.

Therapeutic ultrasound has a frequency range of 1 MHz to 3 MHz. The lower the frequency, the deeper it penetrates. For example, 1 MHz can penetrate bone. This is not to be confused with the commonly called *ultrasonic machine,* which creates high-frequency mechanical oscillations in the range of 25,000 to 28,000 vibrations per second. This ultrasonic machine uses a metal spatula to exfoliate the skin in a process called **cavitation**, which creates bubbles in water or an ultrasound gel that implode when the ultrasound energy creates compression and refraction in the medium. Unstable cavitation places stress on thinner structures, which could cause rupture and cell or tissue destruction. Unstable cavitation is when the bubbles created by sound waves explode under pressure. This can be caused by continuous high-frequency ultrasound application. Figure 24-3 shows an ultrasonic application.

■ WHAT IT DOES TO THE SKIN

Therapeutic ultrasound for esthetic purposes primarily uses **sonophoresis,** which is a means of penetrating a special ultrasonic gel with active ingredients deep into the skin. This process is most beneficial at a range of 20 to 25 KHz with the waveform pulsed on and off every second. Sonophoresis is effective at creating microscopic channels, called **lacunae**, in the intercellular layers of the skin. This opens up the intercellular pathways that allow products with a high molecular weight a better degree of penetration.

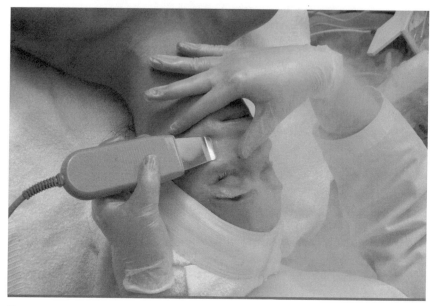

Figure 24-3 Ultrasonic application.

Therapeutic ultrasound also has the following benefits:

- Increases temperature within the skin, which stimulates circulation, lymph drainage, and cell metabolism.
- Increases cell permeability.
- Increases intracellular calcium, a messenger for cell function.
- Helps speed up the inflammatory healing response.

HOW TO USE IT

Therapeutic ultrasound requires specific training that must be supported by the manufacturer. Each machine functions differently, so it is imperative to refer to the manufacturer's guidelines for safe and effective treatment.

HOW TO BUY

Therapeutic ultrasound is considered a Class II prescriptive device. Before purchasing a unit, make sure your state regulations will allow you to use it; also check with your liability insurance carrier to make sure your policy covers ultrasound.

Buyer's Checklist

- What is the price?
- What is the cost of shipping?
- Do you have an instruction manual, DVD, on-site training, or technical support?
- Is the machine UL listed, ISO certified, or CE or CSA tested?
- Does it come with sound heads, or do those have to be purchased separately?
- Can I buy replacement parts?
- What is covered under the warranty, and for how long?
- Do you have a loaner program if my machine breaks?
- Where is the equipment manufactured?
- Do you have FDA 501k clearance?
- Do you have clinical studies to prove this machine works?

See Figure 24-4 for a chart of features to look for when you buy.

■ SAFETY

There are many safety issues connected with ultrasound:

- The lowest frequency recognized in therapeutic ultrasound penetrates the deepest, and this frequency can cause deep bone burn.
- Low-energy, low-frequency devices can still produce harmful effects if the treatment is not delivered in the correct manner. The sound head must be moved constantly.
- Cavitation of aqueous fluid in the eyes can lead to cataract formation on the lens of the eye.
- Treatment can cause a release of plaque associated with heart attack or stroke.

Ultrasound	UL listed or CE mark
	3 MHz low power low frequency
	FDA-registered manufacturer
	Proof to support claims
	Training with purchase
	Replacement parts available
	Warranty
	Sound heads included

Figure 24-4 Features to look for.

■ MAINTENANCE

Maintenance of ultrasound machines must be directed by the manufacturer; this is one of the most important aspects of owning an ultrasound machine. In general, follow these guidelines:

- Clean sound heads and machine after each use with a clean, soft cloth.
- Use isopropyl alcohol on a saturated cotton swab tip to clean the sound head after each use.
- Do not store sound heads in a UV sterilizer.
- Check all wires before use. Do not use the unit if cracked or loose wires are visible.
- Follow the manufacturer's directions.

■ DISINFECTION AND SANITIZATION

- Disinfect the sound head by spraying the portion in contact with the skin with an EPA-approved high-level disinfectant. Recommended leave-on time is 10 to 15 minutes, depending on the manufacturer.
- Do not submerge the sound head in high-level solution.
- Do not store the sound head in a UV sanitizer.
- Store the sound head in the container that came with your machine or in another clean, closed container.

See Figure 24-5 for a chart of disinfection and maintenance steps.

■ CONTRAINDICATIONS AND CAUTIONS

The consultation is extremely important to determine contraindications or special needs that your client may have. Do not rely exclusively on the intake form; it is also important to verbally get information and clarification from your client.

- Pregnancy.
- Heart problems: A heart in a compromised condition is unable to cope with an increased constriction or dilation of blood vessels. This can lead to fainting or heart attack.
- Blood vessel disorders: Arteriosclerosis, or hardening of the arteries, affects the arteries' ability to handle increased blood flow. Ultra-

Disinfection	Maintenance
Disinfect any sound head or part of machine in contact with client with EPA-approved disinfectant	Check all wires before use
Store in clean, closed container; do not store in UV sanitizer	After each use, clean heads with 70% alcohol and soft cloth
After each use, wipe down exterior with EPA-approved disinfectant	

Figure 24-5 Disinfection and maintenance.

sound can possibly loosen plaque that forms in the arteries and may lead to a heart attack or stroke.

- Skin inflammation: Ultrasound will cause an increase in circulation, which would make inflammation worse.
- Skin disorders or diseases: These may be aggravated by treatment.
- Very sensitive skin: Treatment may be very uncomfortable for the client.
- Nervous clients: Treatment will be ineffective if the client cannot relax.
- Botox: Administer no treatment until 72 hours after injection. The treatment paralyzes muscle, so any treatment to stimulate muscle would be ineffective.
- Epilepsy.
- Cuts and abrasions: Do not perform any facial treatment on open cuts and abrasions.
- Severe bruising: Bruised areas will be uncomfortable for the client.
- High or low blood pressure: Such conditions could be made worse due to the increase in circulation. Even if these conditions are treated and under control, use caution. Never leave such clients alone, and help them on and off the treatment bed.
- Recent scar tissue: Scarred skin is very sensitive and less resistant. Use caution when using electrotherapy. Ultrasound is okay if applied more than six weeks after an injury or surgery, if there is no pulling of the skin.
- HIV.
- History of blood clots (thrombosis) or embolism: Treatment could aggravate the condition and cause a heart attack or stroke.
- Malignant melanoma: Treatment for the malignancy must be complete, and client must be in remission. Obtain physician approval. Do not apply treatment when in doubt about a possible abnormality; instead, refer the client to a dermatologist.

PREPARATION FOR TREATMENT

- Have your client fill out an assessment form.
- Check for contraindications.
- Have your client change into a treatment gown and remove all jewelry and contact lenses.
- Analyze the skin using a magnifying lamp.
- Explain the procedure. Your client may become uncomfortable if they do not understand how the machine will affect them.
- Make sure to test all equipment before applying treatment.
- Inspect all wires and electrodes.
- Follow manufacturer's instructions for the setup of your ultrasound machine.

TIP Before using ultrasound make sure that your state board will allow it.

PROTOCOLS

Basic Ultrasound Protocol

Step 1: Perform first and second cleanse.

Step 2: Exfoliate; microdermabrasion is a good method.

Step 3: Remove crystals and completely dry the skin.

Step 4: Apply a hydrating mask with an occlusive plastic mask over top. Let penetrate for 10 minutes.

Step 5: Apply specific ultrasound gel.

Step 6: Use only 3 MHz on the face in the pulsed mode or per manufacturer directions.

Step 7: Divide the face into three areas. Starting at the forehead, move right to left down the face for five minutes or as directed by machine manufacturer. See Figure 24-6.

Step 8: Use a continuous, slow circular movement at all times.

Step 9: Remove excess product and finish treatment.

Always follow the manufacturer's instructions, and get as much ultrasound education as possible before attempting to use this equipment.

YOUR EQUIPMENT INFORMATION

Manufacturer info:

Name/phone number: _____

Web site: _____

Date purchased: _____ Registration: _____

Warranty info: _____

Replacement parts info: _____

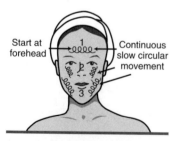

Figure 24-6 Start at the forehead and move in a continuous, slow manner.

TROUBLESHOOTING

All troubleshooting with this type of advanced machine should be addressed by the machine manufacturer. If there is no technical support available, reevaluate purchasing from this manufacturer or vendor.

Q & A

What are the pros and cons of using ultrasound equipment?

Pros

Effectiveness: There is evidence that ultrasound works.
Maintenance: Equipment is fairly easy to maintain when manufacturer directions are followed.

Cons

Cost: These are expensive machines.
Ease of use: Equipment can be very technical; to use, you must follow directions closely.
Safety: Safety is an issue regarding many aspects of use. Ultrasound is a Class II prescriptive device.
Training: Use requires in-depth training in ultrasound theory and contraindications to this modality, but not much education exists.

Can I achieve the same results without ultrasound equipment?

No. The same results cannot be obtained with another machine. There are other modalities that can be used, such as galvanic current, but the sonophoresis process is unique to this machine.

Should I buy or lease my machine?

This should be based on your financial situation. It is a machine that would qualify for a lease.

What does the FDA say about ultrasound?

Ultrasound is considered a Class II prescriptive device. This means that it must have 510k clearance, and the manufacturer must be registered. See Chapter 3 for more information.

REFERENCES

1. Simmons, J. V. (1989, 1995). *Science and the Beauty Business: The Beauty Salon and its Equipment* (2nd ed.). United Kingdom: Macmillan Press Ltd.

2. Bunting, A. & Root, L. (2002). *Ultrasound and Electrotherapy: Applications, Techniques, and Technology for Medical Aesthetics.* Bunting and Root.

3. Bunting, A. (2004). *Background of Ultrasound Devices Used for Aesthetic Applications.* Florida, prepared for the NCEA annual meeting.

4. Mah, A. (2007). *Breaking the Sound Barrier.* Skin, Inc. 88–96.

Microdermabrasion

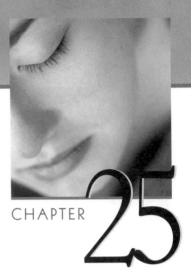

Microdermabrasion is one of most effective treatment modalities an esthetician can use. It is a simple technology with clinical studies to prove its efficacy, but it requires adequate training to provide optimal benefits. It is an operator-dependent technology, which means that outcomes can be different with each operator. It is wonderful for the treatment of **rhytids, dyschromia, hyperpigmentation,** and **keratinized** skin.

CHAPTER **25**

It facilitates the exfoliation of the **stratum corneum,** which enhances product penetration and improves the appearance of the skin. It is a quick, effective procedure with no downtime for the client. The client can go back to normal everyday activities right away and can even wear (appropriate) makeup. This is the true "lunchtime" peel. It is also one of the modalities used by estheticians that has current and ongoing independent clinical studies to prove its efficacy.

▪ FUNCTIONS

- Increased desquamation of the skin due to the exfoliation of the stratum corneum. This smoothes coarse skin, softens fine lines and wrinkles, decreases the appearance of scarring, decreases pore size, and reduces superficial hyperpigmentation.
- Increased microcirculation in the skin improves the transport of oxygen and nutrients to the cells.
- Multiple uses are theorized to stimulate cellular functions of the dermal and epidermal layers, which can cause an increase in collagen production.
- Increased lymphatic drainage reduces puffiness and eliminates accumulated wastes.

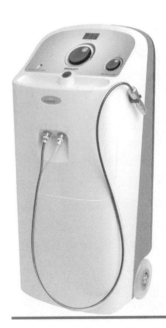

Figure 25-1 Dermaglow II.

HOW IT WORKS

A vacuum, which is created by a compressor that draws air from the atmosphere, is created when the handpiece is applied to the skin. This causes the aluminum oxide crystals to be moved to the handpiece by negative pressure, which then flows to the surface of the skin, exfoliating it in the process. The epidermal debris and crystals are returned via a separate tube to a disposal canister or filter bag. The depth of exfoliation is controlled by the strength of the vacuum and the crystal flow.

Another popular alternative is the diamond-encrusted tip; it uses the same vacuum technology but has no crystals flowing through the system. It provides exfoliation by moving different handpieces with various diamond-grit types over the surface of the skin. See Figure 25-2 for an example.

The removed skin is then returned to a disposable filter to be discarded after each use. Most machines have a larger HEPA filter as a secondary filtration system, and they use a single tube. See Figure 25-3 for an example of a diamond-peel system.

CRYSTALS

Aluminum oxide crystals, also known as **corundum,** have generated some controversy. Corundum is the second-hardest mineral next to diamonds. It is insoluble in water and has a high melting point.

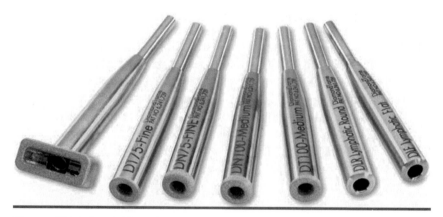

Figure 25-2 A peel handpiece.

It is an inert mineral, which means that there is no adverse reaction to it; OSHA has determined that it is nontoxic and is not a known carcinogen. There has been no correlation established between aluminum oxide and Alzheimer's disease, and it has been shown that the crystals used in microdermabrasion are too large to penetrate the alveoli of the lungs.

Aluminum oxide has been used in the dental industry for more than 60 years. The studies that support the possible toxicity of aluminum oxide focused on mine workers who also smoked and had been exposed to significant amounts of particulate dust. This is not a risk factor for estheticians. We will talk about particulate dust in greater detail in the Safety section.

There are other types of crystals that may be used, such as **sodium chloride** (salt) and **sodium bicarbonate** (baking soda). Both of these are not inert but are water-soluble. Their abrasive power is 25% less than aluminum oxide crystals. These compounds are also lighter in weight, which may cause more discomfort in treatment. Not all machine manufacturers have the option to use these other alternatives.

Another important aspect of a microdermabrasion machine is dual control. The ability to control the level of exfoliation (crystal flow or diamond-tip grit) and vacuum strength is very important to treat different areas of the face.

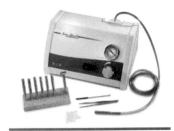

Figure 25-3 A diamond-peel microdermabrasion machine.

> **TIP** The usual size of aluminum oxide crystals used in microdermabrasion is between 100 and 200 microns. Particles must be less than 5 microns to be damaging to the lungs.

■ HOW TO USE IT

Proper use of each machine should be taught by the machine manufacturer, because each unit will have its own selling points. Technique is very important with any microdermabrasion treatment, regardless of the type of equipment used. Consistent pattern technique, holding the skin tight, the workspace setup, an easy-to-use handpiece, dual vacuum-crystal control, and correct skin analysis are all very important. With this modality, practice truly makes the difference. See Figure 25-4 for an example.

It is important to note certain vital safety precautions. This modality must include the use of safety glasses, gloves, and a face mask. The safety glasses do not need to be laser-grade, but they do need to provide a shield for the eyes in case crystals become airborne. Good technique and a high-quality machine reduce this risk significantly. Gloves are standard for several reasons and should be used with all esthetic services. Use of gloves follows the OSHA universal precautions and keeps bacteria on the esthetician's hands from contaminating the client. Exfoliation always

Skin condition/type	Machine Settings–initial treatment *Always hold skin tight with thumb and middle finger while working.*	Products to use during treatment
Normal skin	Balanced crystal and vacuum flow	Hydrating cream mask
Oily skin	High crystal flow: 3 passes	Hydrating gel mask
Dry skin	Low crystal flow: 2 passes hydrating soothing mask	Lipid repairing and hydrating mask, ceramide serum, hylauronic acid
Sensitive skin	Low crystal-low vacuum: 1–2 passes	Azulene, aloe vera, gel mask, 1% hydrocortisone, colloidal oatmeal mask Ceramide serum, hylauronic acid
Hyperpigmentation	High crystal and low vacuum: 3 passes	Melanin suppressant, multi acid peel (pre-treat) gentle enzyme mask
Noninflamed acne	High crystal and high vacuum: 2–3 passes	Enzyme mask, multi acid peel (pre-treat)
Fine lines and wrinkles	High crystal and high vacuum: 2–3 passes	Multi acid peel (pre-treat) enzyme peel, hydrating mask, ceramide-hylauronic acid serum

Figure 25-4 Chart of techniques to use.

TIP Used crystals are considered medical waste by the EPA, which requires the use of red bagging for such material in a clearly marked biohazard receptacle, in this case a bag that can be sealed. A sharps container is also an example of this. The companies that provide the biohazard receptacles usually will also provide for disposal. It is very important for estheticians to use this system and to be clear about the requirements. Check with your state board and the EPA for specifics.

disrupts the acid mantle, even if it is light exfoliation, so gloves are very important to use. Latex allergies are more common than ever, and an esthetician really should only use non-latex gloves. A mask is important due to the possibility of breathing airborne crystals, and a mask should always be used when disposing of used crystals. Figure 25-5 shows the proper outfitting for a microdermabrasion treatment.

Protocols

Step 1: Prepare your client for the service.
Step 2: Remove all makeup and debris from skin.
Step 3: Remove all oil from skin with any substance that will completely dehydrate the skin; for example, 70% alcohol or non-oily makeup remover.
Step 4: Make sure skin is completely dry.

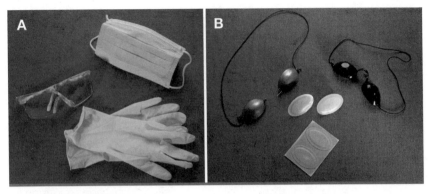

Figure 25-5 Use gloves, mask, and eye protection during microdermabrasion.

Step 5: After determining proper skin type and condition, set correct vacuum level and crystal flow. Divide face into three areas: forehead, mid face, and lower face.

Step 6: Start first-pass application horizontally; see Figure 25-6. Start at the forehead and work down. Evaluate skin: if no adverse reaction, then continue with a second pass.

Step 7: Continue second pass vertically, starting at the forehead and working down, as shown in Figure 25-7.

Step 8: If the client's skin can handle it, continue with a third pass diagonally, starting at the brow line, as shown in Figure 25-8.

Step 9: Move to the second section of the face; lower the crystal and vacuum flows, then move around the eye area. Increase crystal and vacuum flow and repeat first two passes after moving to second section (horizontal and vertical); complete a third pass (diagonal) if the client's skin can handle it. See Figures 25-9a through 25-9d.

1st Pass

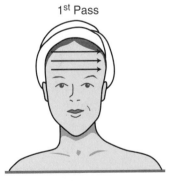

Figure 25-6 First pass, first section (forehead to brow).

2nd Pass

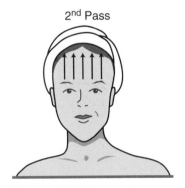

Figure 25-7 Second pass, first section.

3rd Pass

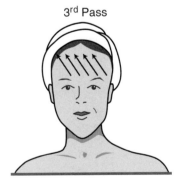

Figure 25-8 Third pass, first section.

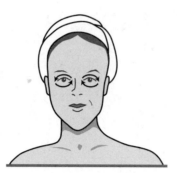

Figure 25-9a Lower crystal and vacuum flow, then move around the eye area.

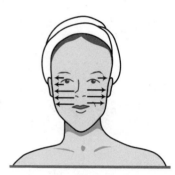

Figure 25-9b First pass, second section (mid face to lip).

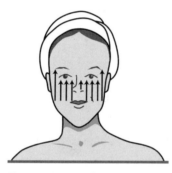

Figure 25-9c Second pass, second section.

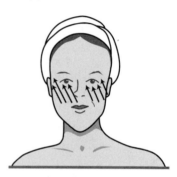

Figure 25-9d Third pass, second section.

TIP It is always advisable to check in with your client frequently. A good line of questioning would be, "On a scale of 1 to 10, 10 being the most uncomfortable, how do you feel?" If your client responds with a number above 6, lower your settings.

Step 10: Move to the third section of the face and make two passes (horizontal and vertical); move to a third pass (diagonal) if indicated. See Figures 25-10a through 25-10c.

Step 11: Move to the neck and use a horizontal pass followed by a vertical pass. Work into décolleté if indicated. A third pass is generally too abrasive. See Figures 25-11a and 25-11b.

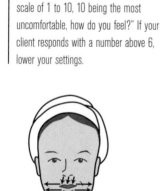

Figure 25-10a First pass, third section (lip to chin).

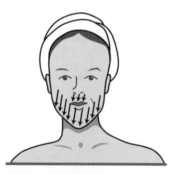

Figure 25-10b Second pass, third section.

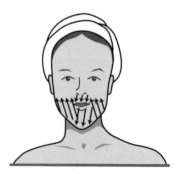

Figure 25-10c Third pass, third section.

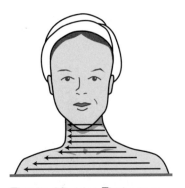 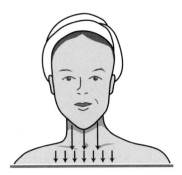

Figure 25-11a First pass (neck).

Figure 25-11b Second pass (neck).

With some skin types and conditions, you may want to proceed with additional passes. Repeat the three-pass pattern for consistency. Watch carefully for excess redness and verbally check with your client about discomfort level.

> *Step 12*: Apply vacuum-only setting and remove excess crystals. You should not have an extreme excess of crystals if your machine is working properly and you are controlling crystal flow.
>
> *Step 13*: Apply a mild cream cleanser to remove excess crystals.
>
> *Step 14*: Proceed with the rest of the protocol chosen for the skin type.

With a diamond microdermabrasion system, follow the pattern listed above but use your manufacturer recommended handpieces as indicated.

■ CORRECT SKIN ANALYSIS

Regardless of what type of machine you use, every good microdermabrasion treatment is dependent upon a correct skin analysis. This is very important due to the pigmentation problems that can occur with any advanced resurfacing technique; see Chapter 1 for a thorough and effective system. Figure 25-12 provides a chart that will give you an idea of what makes someone a good candidate for microdermabrasion.

■ HOW TO BUY

There are many factors to consider when considering purchasing a microdermabrasion machine. All manufacturers have their own unique selling position, and each should be looked at carefully. Most machines run anywhere from $3,500 to $13,000. It is a costly investment that must

Skin Types	Conditions
Dry	• Fine lines & wrinkles
	• Superficial hyper pigmentation
	• Loss of elasticity
Combination	• Poor circulation
	• Large pores
	• Congested skin
	• Uneven texture
Oily	• Blackheads
	• Milia
	• Congested skin

Figure 25-12 Indications for microdermabrasion.

be supported by the vendor. Microdermabrasion is included in some multiple modality units. Here are some issues to consider before you buy:

- Method of disposal and filtering of used crystals and biological debris
- Control of both vacuum strength and crystal flow or exfoliation strength
- Size, comfort, and effectiveness of the handpiece
- Size of the machine
- Consistent performance of the machine and handpiece
- Warranty and loaner program
- Price per use

Method of Exfoliation: Crystals vs. Diamond Tips

The method of exfoliation is really a matter of personal preference, cost, and ability to effectively sanitize equipment. Many crystal machine manufacturers offer additional diamond-tip modifications to your existing crystal machine. Diamond tip works for some skins but not for others. More sensitive skin is better suited to the diamond tip, but when using this type of equipment, it is very important to have a reliable protocol and to apply consistent pressure.

Training

On-site training is very important. Videos and DVDs are great, but most estheticians need hands-on training to fully grasp—literally—all of the knowledge needed to be effective. If you are spending thousands of dollars on equipment, insist on training. Many states also require certification of training for the esthetician before he or she is allowed to perform the service.

FDA Registration and Other Listings

Microdermabrasion is a Class I exempt machine, so the manufacturer must be registered with the FDA. If your vendor is a reseller, they do not need to be listed, but the original manufacturer does. Certain listings (UL, CE, and CSA) are important for safety. See Chapter 3 for details on the significance of the various listings.

Buyer's Checklist

- What is the price?
- Do you have an instruction manual, DVD, or on-site training?
- Is the machine UL listed, ISO certified, or CE or CSA tested?
- Are you a manufacturer or reseller?
- Is the manufacturer FDA-registered?
- Does the unit come with supplies to start treatments, or do those have to be purchased separately?
- Can I buy replacement parts?
- What is covered under the warranty, and for how long?
- Do I need to buy crystals from the manufacturer for the warranty to be valid?
- Where is this machine manufactured?

See Figure 25-13 for a chart of features to look for when you buy.

Microdermabrasion	UL listed or CE mark
	Closed crystal system
	FDA-registered manufacturer
	Dual control (crystal and vacuum)
	Training with purchase
	Replacement parts available
	Warranty

Figure 25-13 Chart of features to look for.

TIP Always check your manufacturer's directions first.

SAFETY

It is important to be conscientious when performing microdermabrasion. Safety must be paramount in the esthetician's mind. Here are some guidelines to follow:

- Always check electrical cord and plugs, and do not use a unit with cracked or worn wires.
- Make sure that tubes are securely inserted, that no cracks are evident, and that no debris is trapped inside.
- Make sure tips have no cracks or irregular surfaces that could scratch the skin.
- If using a diamond tip, make sure that the tip is inserted tightly into the tube and filters are tight.
- Always check vacuum strength before applying it to the client's skin.
- Make sure you have adequate eye protection for your client.
- Never reuse crystals.

For your protection, use gloves, disposable masks, and goggles. The same goes for a diamond-tip machine, because biological debris could be released into the air.

MAINTENANCE

Every manufacturer has a specific protocol for machine maintenance. This protocol is very important to follow, because many warranties depend on following directions for the warranty to remain valid. In general, here are some valuable guidelines:

- Wipe down the exterior of the machine after each use.
- Always use the correct disinfection protocol for your tips.
- Test the strength of the vacuum daily before use.
- Do not store a machine with crystals in it.
- Do not leave used disposable filters in the diamond-tip machine.
- Replace tubes as soon as they get a milky look to them or as the manufacturer directs.
- Purchase the highest-quality crystals with the least amount of dust.
- Purchase high-quality diamond tips to avoid excessive and uneven abrasion on skin. The best tips are usually the most expensive.

DISINFECTION AND SANITIZATION

The debris created by microdermabrasion can be considered a medical waste. All applicable state and federal regulations regarding disposal must be followed. Check with your state medical and cosmetology board and the EPA.

Crystal Machine

- Use a closed system, and do not open a used crystal container. Place in a separate bag and dispose of per state biological waste guidelines.
- Use an enzyme cleaner to clean tips, then soak tips in EPA-approved high-level disinfectant per manufacturer and state instructions.
- Use reusable tips only as directed by the manufacturer.
- Use an EPA-approved high-level disinfectant on every surface touched.

Diamond-Tip Machine

- Clean diamond tips with enzyme cleaner and autoclave if possible. If no autoclave is available, use ultrasonic cleaner to remove all biological debris from small crevices.
- Do not open used prefilter without proper personal protection.

■ CONTRAINDICATIONS AND CAUTIONS

The consultation is extremely important to determine contraindications or special needs that your client may have. Do not rely exclusively on the intake form; it is also important to verbally get information and clarification from your client. See Figure 25-13 for a list of indications for microdermabrasion.

- Diabetes: If uncontrolled, the skin is not able to heal effectively.
- Vascular conditions, such as rosacea and telangiectasia: In some cases, microdermabrasion can make the appearance of telangiectasia worse by removing layers of stratum corneum. It is not making the condition worse; it is only exposing what is already there.
- Skin inflammation: Microdermabrasion treatments increase circulation, which could make inflammation worse.
- Bacterial infections: These may be aggravated by treatment. Examples include cellulitis, impetigo, and folliculitis.
- Very sensitive skin: Clients with this skin type may be very uncomfortable.
- Lack of tactile sensation (e.g., numbness due to stroke): When the client cannot gauge the intensity of exfoliation, injury can result.

- Botox: Administer no treatment until 72 hours after injection. Use this treatment preferably before Botox injection.
- Cuts and abrasions: Skin that has trauma will not respond well to microdermabrasion and condition can be made worse.
- Anticoagulation drugs: These interfere with blood coagulation, which can slow healing.
- High or low blood pressure: Such conditions could be made worse due to the increase in circulation. Even if the condition is treated and under control, use caution. Never leave such a client alone, and help them on and off the treatment bed.
- Keloid scarring: Microdermabrasion could make this condition worse.
- Pigmentation disorders.
- HIV, Hepatitis B, AIDS: must use OSHA bloodborne pathogen guidelines for safety of client and technician
- History of blood clots (thrombosis) or embolism: Treatment could aggravate the condition and cause a heart attack or stroke.
- Malignant melanoma: Cancer treatment must be completed, and client must be in remission. Obtain physician approval. Do not apply treatment when in doubt about a possible abnormality; instead, refer the client to a dermatologist.
- Fungal infections (e.g., ringworm, yeast infection).
- Viral infections, active herpes simplex: Some exfoliation procedures can increase the likelihood of an outbreak. With shingles and facial warts, microdermabrasion will cause the virus to spread.
- Sunburn: Advise your client not use an indoor tanning bed within 72 hours of service. Any deliberate UV exposure is strongly advised against. Inform your client fully of the damage UV exposure causes to the skin before proceeding.
- Grade II through IV Acne: Inflamed pustules will increase, but closed comedones and milia will not be affected.
- Use of isotretinoin: This drug shrinks the sebaceous glands, which causes a slowing of the skin's healing process. Clients must wait a full year after stopping treatment before attempting microdermabrasion.
- Smoking: A smoker's skin heals more slowly and is more dehydrated; this can result in fissures in the skin. Proceed with extreme caution. It is important to know your clients' daily smoking habits, and explain that they will not get the full benefits of treatment if they smoke. At-home compliance during posttreatment care is a must.

Possible Posttreatment Complications

It is very important to have written posttreatment care instructions to avoid complications. Although rare, there can be complications; these are usually caused by poor technique or insufficient safety procedures. If clients experience any complications, they must come in for an evaluation and possible referral to a doctor. Make sure to document all complications; it is also wise to take pictures.

Corneal Abrasions

These occur when proper eye protection is not used. Make sure that the eye area is completely covered throughout the treatment. This includes the crystal removal stage. Always have a saline eye wash on hand to irrigate the client's eyes if needed.

Infections and Skin Abrasions

Infections are related to technique and improper client selection; abrasions can happen with a technique that is too aggressive or from using tips that have sharp edges. Reused tips that have been improperly disinfected will introduce bacteria onto the skin. There is no need for an esthetician to be aggressive with microdermabrasion to see results. Pinpoint bleeding and abrasions are signs of a poor treatment; see Figure 25-14. Should infection result, a doctor must treat it.

Sun Sensitivity

It is important to provide clear instructions for posttreatment care that include lifestyle instructions. A client who receives microdermabrasion must understand that the skin is in a very vulnerable state after treatment and must be protected. It is a good idea to recommend no sun exposure for at least two days after treatment, and a full-spectrum sunscreen must be used. If the client disregards the instructions and does receive a sunburn, they must come in to see the esthetician for treatment. This would include a deep hydrating facial, home care that will rebuild the lipid barrier, and light exfoliation when the sunburn is healed. If the client is inclined to disregard posttreatment instructions, it is wise to reevaluate whether treatment should be continued.

■ PREPARATION FOR TREATMENT

- Have your client fill out an assessment form and microdermabrasion waiver.
- Ask about any changes in skin condition or new medications started.

TIP **What do you do when you have a contraindication?** Explain that you would not want to make an existing condition worse, and make it clear that the treatment may do just that. Offer an optional service if possible. Microdermabrasion is very safe, but do not modify treatment if your client has any of the contraindications listed. Make sure your client has signed a waiver, and verbally go over the waiver with your client. When in doubt, refer client to a physician.

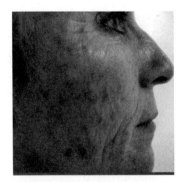

Figure 25-14 Abrasions and pinpoint bleeding can happen when treatment is too aggressive.

- Check for contraindications.
- Have your client change into a treatment gown and remove all jewelry and contact lenses.
- Apply a headband and hair covering.
- Analyze the skin using a magnifying lamp and a Woods lamp.
- Explain the procedure. Your client may become uncomfortable if they do not understand what you are doing.
- Test all equipment before applying treatment.
- Inspect the handpiece, tubes, and crystal container or diamond tip.
- Follow manufacturer's instructions for the setup and priming of your microdermabrasion machine.
- Apply goggles or eye pads. No crystals or debris should go into the eye area.
- Make sure the client is comfortable, warm, and well-covered.
- Wear protective eye covering, gloves, and a mask.

Posttreatment Instructions

Posttreatment care is as important as the pretreatment protocol. The skin is going through a superficial wound healing process and must be treated gently. Reepithelialization starts within 12 hours of injury and takes 7 days to complete in healthy skin. A disrupted lipid barrier impairs efficient cell migration, which is why it is very important to keep the client's skin optimally hydrated after treatment. There are different types of wounds, and the esthetician should become educated about them and about the wound healing process. The three stages of wound healing are as follows:

1. **Inflammatory stage:** immune response, increased cellular response
2. **Proliferative stage:** increased vascularity in wound, scar tissue begins to build, increased collagen production
3. **Remodeling stage,** or **maturation:** increased tissue strength without additional collagen, scar tissue is broken down

Posttreatment products help assist the skin through the healing process. Most skin care lines now have postpeel kits, which are a good idea to include in the price of the first microdermabrasion treatment. See Figure 25-15 for a chart on the stages of superficial wound healing.

General Instructions

- Use a gentle cleanser with a neutral to slightly acidic pH.
- Hydrate with a hydrating serum as needed throughout the day.
- Apply a hydrating cream or lotion based on skin type twice a day.

Time	Result
Injury	Damage occurs to epidermis
12 hours	Epithelial cells start to migrate to repair damage
7 days	Epithelialization is complete

Figure 25-15 Microdermabrasion causes a superficial wound that heals in stages.

- Sun protection is mandatory, even on days with little sun exposure. Many clients are very sensitive to chemical sun protection after microdermabrasion. Find a very gentle physical sun block, such as titanium dioxide, and mineral makeup with an SPF rating of 15 or higher.
- A gentle, at-home exfoliation is recommended 5 to 7 days after treatment. This can be an enzyme mask or very gentle scrub.
- Make sure to call your client within 48 hours to follow up.

■ PROTOCOLS

Microdermabrasion for Dry Skin

Step 1: Cleanse skin; do not use a milky cleanser.

Step 2: Analyze the skin.

Step 3: Prepare the skin with an oil remover or alcohol or a makeup remover with no residue.

Step 4: Dry the skin completely.

Step 5: Start the first pass on the low vacuum/crystal setting. If using a diamond tip, use a low vacuum and a low-grit tip. Refer to your manufacturer's recommendations for directions on settings.

Step 6: Start the second pass on a medium setting.

Step 7: Make the third pass on a medium setting, and gently work areas of hyperpigmentation. If deciding to do additional passes with a diamond tip, change your filter.

Step 8: Use the vacuum-only setting to remove crystal residue, and apply cream cleanser to pick up any crystals left on the skin. When using a diamond tip, omit this step.

Step 9: Remove with warm—not hot—towels or sponges if allowed by your state cosmetology board.

Step 10: Apply a gentle toner.

TIP Always remember to check for contraindications with any microdermabrasion treatment. Client comfort and safety are top priorities.

Step 11: Apply a gently hydrating cooling or marine collagen mask. Leave on 10 to 15 minutes. Perform additional massage to hands, feet, or scalp.

Step 12: Remove with a cool towel.

Step 13: Apply a hydrating serum, moisturizer, and nonchemical sun protection. Sun protection can be omitted if treatment is performed at night.

Microdermabrasion for Combination/Oily Skin

Step 1: Cleanse the skin with a gel cleanser.

Step 2: Analyze the skin.

Step 3: Prepare the skin with an oil remover, alcohol, or makeup remover (with no residue).

Step 4: Dry the skin completely.

Step 5: Start the first pass on a low vacuum/crystal setting. If using a diamond tip, use a low vacuum and a low-grit tip. Refer to your manufacturer's guidelines for directions on settings.

Step 6: Start the second pass on a medium setting.

Step 7: Begin the third pass on a medium setting, and gently work areas of hyperpigmentation. Most oilier skins can handle multiple passes; proceed with the three-pass pattern to maintain consistency while raising vacuum and crystal settings. When using the diamond tip, increase the grit and vacuum strength.

Step 8: Use vacuum-only setting to remove crystal residue, and apply cream cleanser to pick up any crystals left behind. When using a diamond tip, omit this step.

Step 9: Remove excess product with warm—not hot—towels or sponges (if allowed by your state cosmetology board.)

Step 10: Apply a gentle toner.

Step 11: Apply a serum (e.g., vitamin C, melanin suppressant, or hydration) to treat specific conditions.

Step 12: Apply a gentle hydrating cooling mask. Leave on 10 to 15 minutes. Perform additional massage to hands, feet, and scalp.

Step 13: Remove cooling mask with a cool towel.

Step 14: Apply a hydrating serum, moisturizer, and nonchemical sun protection. Sun protection can be omitted if treatment is performed at night.

Advanced Microdermabrasion Protocol

Step 1: Clean skin with an appropriate cleanser.

Step 2: Remove additional oil with a defatting agent.

Step 3: Steam skin with proteolytic enzyme mask for up to 10 minutes, or perform a gentle chemical peel (30% blend of different acids, 3.0 to 3.5 pH). To reduce liability, higher acid peels should be used in combination with microdermabrasion only under a physician's supervision. Follow manufacturer's instructions.

Step 4: Remove excess product with a warm towel; dry skin thoroughly.

Step 5: Proceed with microdermabrasion treatment based on skin type.

Step 6: Apply a gentle cooling and hydrating or marine collagen mask for 10 to 15 minutes. Massage hands, feet, and scalp.

Step 7: Apply a hydrating serum.

Step 8: Apply a hydrating cream that is more emollient than the one the client currently uses (i.e., if a client has oily skin and uses a gel, apply a lotion).

Step 9: Apply a gentle, nonchemical sunscreen, unless treatment is performed at night.

Your Protocol:

_____

_____

_____

_____

_____

_____

_____

_____

_____

_____

_____

■ YOUR EQUIPMENT INFORMATION

Manufacturer info:

Name/phone number: _____

Web site: _____

Date purchased: _____   Registration: _____

Warranty info: _____

Replacement parts info: _____

TROUBLESHOOTING

All troubleshooting with this type of advanced machine should be addressed by the machine manufacturer. If there is no technical support available, reevaluate purchasing from this manufacturer or vendor.

Machine will not turn on.

Check the plug and the fuse on the machine. Some machines require that the HEPA filter cartridge be closed tightly for the machine to turn on. Empty the crystal filter bag and replace it. If the machine still will not start, contact the manufacturer.

Q & A

What are the pros and cons of using microdermabrasion?

Pros

Immediate results: Smoother, softer skin will result.
Effective clinical results: Treatment has been proven to improve the look of fine lines, to improve the general tone and texture of skin, and to alleviate acne and pigmentation problems.
Client recognition: Microdermabrasion has been marketed heavily, so the general public is aware of the procedure. It is a treatment that is often marketed to the large baby-boomer population.
Cost: Cost per treatment is relatively low.
Safety: Equipment is safe to operate when used effectively.

Cons

Very operator-dependent: An esthetician must go through practical training to provide consistent, safe results. This includes training on the machine provided by the manufacturer, as well as adequate training in all aspects of skin analysis, diseases, disorders, and correct treatment procedures.
Price: Microdermabrasion can be a costly investment for a small practice.
Complications: If misused, treatment can cause overexfoliation, pinpoint bleeding, and the spread of infection if skin conditions are not recognized correctly.
Maintenance: Machines can clog if not well made or maintained.

Should I buy or lease my equipment?

This decision must be based on your financial situation. Most machines have a price high enough to warrant a lease.

Can microdermabrasion make a difference in my practice?

Yes, but this modality is not a necessity.

What does the FDA say about microdermabrasion?

The FDA considers it a Class I exempt device, which means that the manufacturer must be registered.

REFERENCES

1. D'Angelo, J., Dean, P., Dietz, S., Hinds, C., Lees, M., Miller, E., & Zani, A. (2003). *Milady's Standard Comprehensive Training for Estheticians.* New York: Thomson Delmar Learning.
2. Simmons, J. V. (1989, 1995). *Science and the Beauty Business: The Beauty Salon and its Equipment* (2nd ed.). United Kingdom: Macmillan Press Ltd.
3. Lees, M. (2001). *Skin Care: Beyond the Basics.* New York: Thomson Delmar Learning.
4. Nordman, L. (2005). *Professional Beauty Therapy, The Official Guide to Level 3* (2nd ed.). London: Thomson Learning.
5. Root, L. (2004). *A Complete Guide to Microdermabrasion Treatment, Technique, and Technology.* Scottsdale, AZ: Esthetician Education Resource.
6. Jones, G. M., & Jones, R. (2003). *Guide to Medical Microdermabrasion.* Ridgewood, NJ: Paramedical Consultants, Inc.
7. Hill, P. (2006). *Milady's Aesthetician Series: Microdermabrasion.* New York: Thomson Delmar Learning.
8. Arroyave, E. (2006). *Understanding Cosmetic Procedures: Surgical and Nonsurgical.* New York: Thomson Delmar Learning.

CHAPTER 26

Electrical Desiccation

Electrical desiccation, also known as **electrocoagulation,** is used in the treatment of minor, superficial skin conditions. This technology enables rapid and precise removal of minor epidermal irregularities that are benign in nature but that contribute to a rough skin texture. These skin conditions are seen by estheticians on a daily basis, and they are found in all skin types and ages but are more prevalent in aging skin. Figures 26-1 and 26-2 show examples of desiccation equipment.

FUNCTIONS

Electrical desiccation treats a wide range of superficial skin irregularities, including sebaceous, vascular, and keratin disorders.

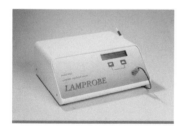

Figure 26-1 Lam probe.

HOW IT WORKS

Electrical desiccation works on the principles of radio and high-frequency technology, and it utilizes various sizes of disposable probes. The tip of the probe is placed as close as possible to the skin condition under treatment, but it does not necessarily have to touch the skin. The current is emitted at the tip of the probe and attracts liquids placed on the skin's surface. If the irregularity does not already contain fluids such as blood or sebum, a water-based conductive medium used for electrotherapy can be used instead. When electrical energy is emitted by the probes, it heats up and cauterizes the irregularity to remove it from the epidermis. See Figure 26-3 for an example.

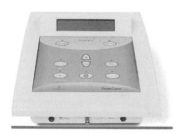

Figure 26-2 Vasculyse.

WHAT IT DOES TO THE SKIN

As a skin-resurfacing tool, electrical desiccation is used in conjunction with microdermabrasion, chemical peels, and regular skin treatments to achieve a smoother skin texture. It is designed to treat a wide range of minor skin irregularities including sebaceous, vascular, and keratin disorders. Keratin disorders include skin tags, fibromas, actinic and seborrheic lesions, vascular disorders (telangiectasia, hemangiomas), and sebaceous deposits (clogged pores, milias, pimples, cysts, xanthelasma, cholesterol deposits). These can all be treated in a few seconds, and treatment is fast (with minor discomfort). See Figures 26-4a through 26-4c for examples of superficial irregularities that can be treated.

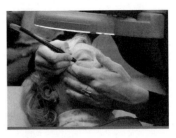

Figure 26-3 Electrocoagulation. Always remember to wear gloves.

HOW TO USE IT

This equipment is very manufacturer-dependent; all directions for use and on-site training should be supplied by the manufacturer. Be sure to check with your state board before operating electrical desiccation equipment. All treatment is superficial, which is within most states' scope of practice, but this is a technology unknown to most state boards. Also, do not use the word "desiccation" when advertising this service; that term is used to imply a medical application.

HOW TO BUY

The cost of most electrical desiccation units ranges from $4,500 to $6,000. This is a controversial modality and is under review by state boards.

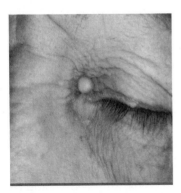

Figure 26-4a Cholesterol deposit.

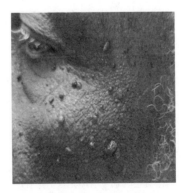

Figure 26-4b Fibromas.

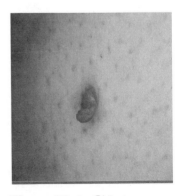

Figure 26-4c Skin tag.

The FDA has recently been involved in the removal of some machines from the market pending approval.

The best way to determine if this modality is within your scope of practice is to contact your state board and your insurance agent. If you cannot get liability insurance for this equipment, you will not be able to perform the treatment.

■ SAFETY

Electrical desiccation is a safe modality. It is completely noninvasive and works rapidly. Treatment only takes 3 to 5 seconds and requires no anesthesia; by comparison, waxing is more painful. The tips are disposable, which reduces the chance of cross-contamination, but in-depth education is required with purchase.

■ MAINTENANCE

Electrical desiccation equipment requires little or no maintenance. Follow these general guidelines for electrical equipment:

* Clean electrode holder after each use.
* Dispose of tips after each use.
* Do not store electrodes in a UV sterilizer.
* Check all wires before use. Do not use equipment if cracked or loose wires are visible.

■ DISINFECTION AND SANITIZATION

Electrical desiccation uses disposable probes for each treatment. There is some concern regarding disposal of irregularities removed from the skin, such as skin tags. Skin debris is considered a biohazard, so both state and federal regulations must be followed. Removed surface irregularities are considered medical waste by the EPA, which requires the use of red bagging and a clearly marked biohazard receptacle, in this case a bag that can be sealed. A sharps container is an example of a biohazard receptacle, and the companies that provide these receptacles usually will provide for disposal. It is very important for estheticians to use this system and be clear about the requirements. Check with your state board and the EPA for specifics.

■ CONTRAINDICATIONS AND CAUTIONS

Like any other procedure, do not treat skin diseases, open wounds, or any suspicious lesions. Pregnant women should not be treated using electrical desiccation. Training is essential for this modality, and it is usually included in the purchase price of the unit.

The consultation is extremely important to determine contraindications or special needs that your client may have. Do not rely exclusively on the intake form; it is also important to verbally get information and clarification from your client.

- Metal implements in the body and pacemakers: Electricity will concentrate in areas with a conductor, and pacemakers will be interrupted. IUDs are considered metal implements for the purpose of electrical desiccation.
- Pregnancy.
- Heart problems: A heart in a compromised condition is unable to cope with an increased constriction or dilation of blood vessels. This can lead to fainting or a heart attack.
- Blood vessel disorders: Arteriosclerosis, or hardening of the arteries, affects the arteries' ability to handle increased blood flow. Fainting can occur when increased dilation of the blood vessels results from heat treatments.
- Skin inflammation: Most electrical treatments increase circulation, which could make inflammation worse.
- Skin disorders or diseases: These may be aggravated by treatment.
- Very sensitive skin: This may be very uncomfortable for the client.
- Migraines or severe headaches: Treatment may cause worsening of existing headaches but is not known to cause them.
- Lack of tactile sensation (e.g., numbness due to stroke): A client impaired in this way will not be able to gauge the intensity of the current, which could cause injury.
- Nervous clients: Treatment will be ineffective if the client cannot relax.
- Botox: Administer no treatment until 72 hours after injection. Botox treatment paralyzes muscle, so any treatment to stimulate muscle would be ineffective.
- Epilepsy.
- Cuts and abrasions: Electrical current will concentrate in the area, because bodily fluids act as a conductor.
- Severe bruising: Bruised areas will be uncomfortable for the client.

- High or low blood pressure: These could be made worse due to the increase in circulation. Even if these conditions are treated and under control, use caution. Never leave such a client alone, and help them on and off the treatment bed.
- Recent scar tissue: Scarred skin is very sensitive and less resistant. Use caution when using electrotherapy. Treatment is allowable after six weeks of injury or surgery if there is no pulling of the skin.
- HIV.
- History of blood clots (thrombosis) or embolism: Treatment could aggravate these conditions and cause a heart attack or stroke.
- Malignant melanoma: Cancer treatment must be completed, and client must be in remission. Obtain physician approval. Do not apply treatment when in doubt about a possible abnormality; instead, refer the client to a dermatologist.

■ PREPARATION FOR TREATMENT

- Have your client fill out an assessment form.
- Check for contraindications.
- Have your client change into a treatment gown and remove all jewelry and contact lenses.
- Analyze the skin using a magnifying lamp.
- Explain the procedure.
- Make sure to test all equipment before applying treatment to your client.
- Inspect all wires and electrodes.
- Follow manufacturer's instructions for the setup of your electrical desiccation equipment.

■ PROTOCOLS

The protocol for use is specific to each manufacturer. To perform treatment, the esthetician must be fully trained by the manufacturer.

▪ YOUR EQUIPMENT INFORMATION

Manufacturer info:

Name/phone number: _____

Web site: _____

Date purchased: _____   Registration: _____

Warranty info: _____

Replacement parts info: _____

TROUBLESHOOTING

This equipment should only be serviced by the manufacturer to avoid injury to the client. To avoid liability, do not try to troubleshoot the equipment yourself.

Q & A

What are the pros and cons of using electrical desiccation therapy?

Pros

Immediate results: Desiccation removes surface irregularities quickly.
Effective results: Results are seen immediately after treatment.
Cost: Cost per treatment is relatively low.
Safety: Equipment is safe to operate when used effectively by trained personnel.

Cons

Requires intensive training: This equipment must come with in-depth training for the esthetician.
Scope of practice issues: State boards may not allow the use of this equipment.
Price: This modality can require a costly investment for a small practice.

Should I buy or lease the equipment?

This decision should be based on your financial situation. Most machines have a price high enough to warrant a lease.

Can desiccation therapy make a difference in my practice?

Yes, but it is not a necessity.

REFERENCES

1. D'Angelo, J., Dean, P., Dietz, S., Hinds, C., Lees, M., Miller, E., & Zani, A. (2003). *Milady's Standard Comprehensive Training for Estheticians*. New York: Thomson Delmar Learning.

2. Lees, M. (2001). *Skin Care: Beyond the Basics*. New York: Thomson Delmar Learning.

3. Nordman, L. (2005). *Professional Beauty Therapy, The Official Guide to Level 3* (2nd ed.). London: Thomson Learning.

4. Simmons, J. V. (1989, 1995). *Science and the Beauty Business: The Beauty Salon and Its Equipment* (2nd ed.). United Kingdom: Macmillan Press Ltd.

5. Lam, P. (2004). *Nutrition: The Healthy Aging Solution*. Carol Stream, IL: Allured Publishing.

Esthetic Equipment for a Medical Practice

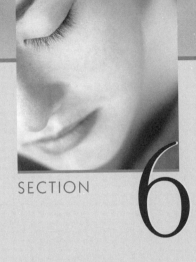

SECTION

6

299

Lasers, Intense Pulsed Light, and Other Technology

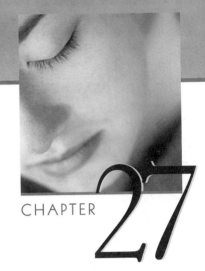

Lasers and intense pulsed light (IPL) technology offer some of the most exciting and effective treatments for skin that have ever been used. Lasers have been used in medical treatments since the early 1960s.

Laser surgery is definitely in the medical realm and outside the esthetician's scope of practice unless supervised by a physician. The exciting part of laser technology is that it is getting safer and less invasive. Currently, some states allow IPL technology for use in non-doctor-supervised clinics, but this is controversial and is being reviewed by many regulating boards.

■ WHAT IS A LASER?

Laser is actually an acronym that stands for *light amplification by the stimulated emission of radiation.* This technology is based on the theories of **Max Planck** and **Albert Einstein.** Planck's theory states that the nucleus of an atom is positively charged and that the orbit is negatively charged. The closer the electron is to the nucleus of an atom, the lower the energy; this is called the **ground state.** When energy is introduced to the atom, it will cause negatively charged electrons to jump farther from the nucleus and create an excited state. The electron wants to return to the ground state, so it must give off the extra energy in the form of photons. Refer to Chapter 22 for more information.

Einstein's theory expands on Planck's and states that when the photons created crash into an excited system, they create multiple photons of the same wavelength, building a large amount of light energy in one wavelength. The substance that these photons reflect off of determines the wavelength. For example, the mineral alexandrite will create wavelengths of 755 nm.

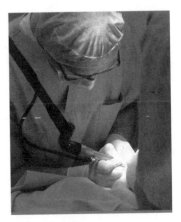

Figure 27-1 Lasers are used in surgery.

TIP The NCEA is an organization of esthetic professionals, associations, schools, and manufacturers. Their mission is to represent the esthetic profession by defining and conveying standards of practice, while educating the industry and the public. The NCEA statement on laser and light therapy follows:

- Skin care professionals shall be permitted to use FDA-approved energy-based devices and therapies for esthetic procedures.
- Such use shall be within the scope of practice as defined by the regulations of individual states, where such regulations exist.
- Skin care professionals shall meet the training requirements for the use of such devices as defined by their individual licensing board or other regulatory agency.

■ HOW DOES IT WORK?

Laser technology emits photons in a coherent beam. A laser has three parts: *energy source, active medium,* and *optical cavity.*

Energy Source: This is the energy that excites the active medium; usually, this is electricity.

Active Medium: This is a solid, gas, or liquid that is excited by the energy source, releasing photons that determine wavelength.

Optical Cavity: This is also called a *resonator,* an area equipped with a high-reflectance mirror and a partial-reflectance mirror. A photon cascade bounces off the mirrors and gains strength until it pushes through the partial-reflectance mirror.

Laser light is monochromatic and is emitted in a narrow beam created by energizing the lasing medium (e.g., ruby, alexandrite, CO_2) in the laser's optical cavity then bouncing the beam off two mirrors. One mirror is fully reflective, the other is partially reflective. This allows the partially reflective mirror to shutter open and close to release the photons, thus producing a laser beam. *Q-switching* is a method of providing intense laser pulses by utilizing a mechanical or electrical q-switch. How this energy is produced and applied to the skin makes a difference in the type of results you will get. See Figure 27-2 for an illustration of components of a laser. This is a simplified explanation; the esthetician should get advanced training as recommended by the National Coalition of Esthetic Associations (NCEA).

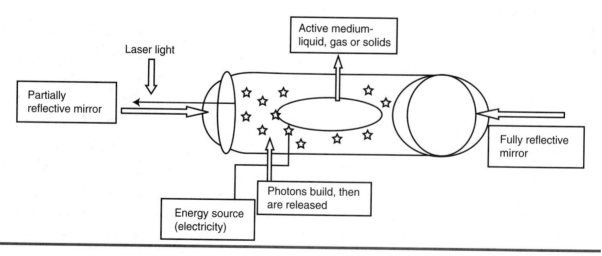

Figure 27-2 Components of a laser.

■ WHAT IT DOES TO THE SKIN

Different lasers target different components in the skin. This is accomplished by a process called **selective photothermolysis,** in which laser wavelengths heat the skin and are absorbed by the target **chromophore,** which is the part of the molecule that absorbs or detects light energy. For example, oxyhemoglobin (blood), melanin, or water have specific chromophores which will attract a certain wavelength. See Figure 27-3 for a chart of wavelengths and their targets.

When lasers generate enough heat, they can **vaporize** or destroy tissues. Pulses of power measured in milliseconds help protect the surrounding tissue. This allows for a controlled cool-down period. There is no one laser that will produce results for all skin conditions. Lasers are classified by the medium used to produce the specific wavelengths; these classes are *solid state, semiconductor, gas,* and *dye.*

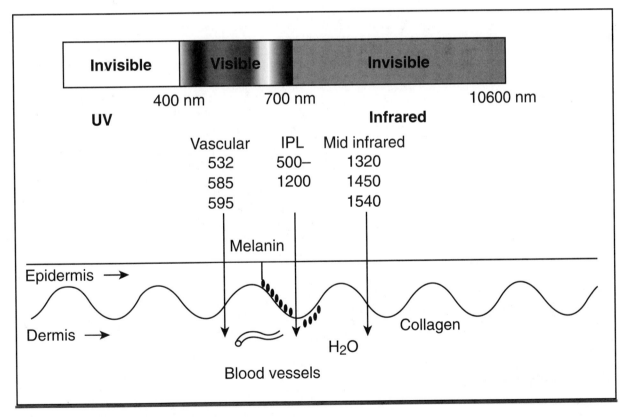

Figure 27-3 Chart of wavelengths and their targets.

■ LASER SAFETY

Laser safety is not an area in which ignorance can be accepted. Estheticians must be fully trained in laser safety. The American National Standards Institute (ANSI) has created standards for the safe use of lasers in health care facilities. This standard is used by OSHA, and every facility—no matter how small—must comply. Also established is a laser hazard classification that is used by the FDA and ANSI. See Figure 27-4 for laser hazard classifications and Figure 27-5 for an outline of ANSI safety requirements.

The design of the laser room is an important part of the safe use of lasers. The room should be set up with a well-grounded outlet, a separate circuit breaker, proper ventilation, nonreflective surfaces, either no windows or windows blocked with protective covering, and a door that can be locked during the service. Also, the treatment room should provide access to eye protection before entering the room and a danger sign on the exterior of the door. See Figures 27-6 and 27-7 for some examples.

TIP New lasers are being developed and sold frequently with more advanced safety features. Always use the safety recommendations of the laser manufacturer which include proper room design.

Type	Hazard
Class 1	Considered safe, no hazard label needed, do not inflict harm
Class 2	Emit a visible laser beam 400–780 nm, cannot stare into beam without eye protection
Class 3A	Special training to operate, hazard to eyes, protective goggles must be worn, output of .5mW or less
Class 3B	Special training to operate, hazard to eyes protective goggles must be worn, output of .5W or less
Class 4	Hazardous emissions to eyes and skin, protected wavelength safety glasses must be worn, special training to operate, control measures (ANSI) must be followed.

Figure 27-4 All lasers are considered to be FDA Class III prescriptive devices. They are classified by hazard.

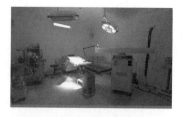

Figure 27-6 A laser treatment room should have standard laser safety provisions and no reflective surfaces.

Requirements	Safety Training and Education
ANSI Standards	Employ Laser Safety Officer
	Follow state & federal regulations for use
	Develop standards of care
	Assure safety to clients and staff
	Provide equipment safety and maintenance

Figure 27-5 ANSI safety requirements.

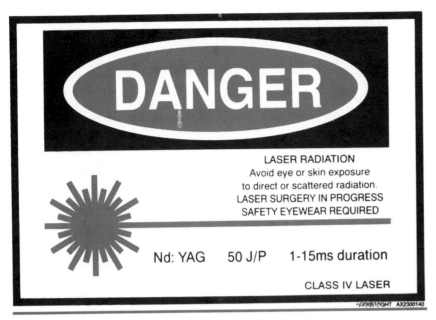

Figure 27-7 A danger sign must be placed on the outside of the laser room door.

WHAT AN ESTHETICIAN MUST KNOW

Different Fitzpatrick types respond differently to laser hair removal and laser resurfacing treatments. See Figure 27-8 for a chart of Fitzpatrick skin types and laser hair removal indications. An esthetician must be fully trained before using a laser, even under the supervision of a physician.

Fully understanding spot size, fluence, wavelength, thermal storage coefficient, pulse duration, and thermal relaxation time is important for the esthetician. Most lasers have preprogrammed parameters that eliminate "much" of the guesswork, but it is still important to understand why the laser works the way it does. See Figure 27-9 for a chart of defined terms.

When it comes to laser resurfacing, estheticians will mainly be involved with pretreatment and posttreatment care. To create effective treatments, it is important to understand the wound-healing process, wound care, basic chemistry, cellular biology, and basic pharmaceuticals. For example, a client may be taking a **nonsteroidal anti-inflammatory drug (NSAID)** and the herb St. John's Wort, either of which can impair wound healing. This information is included in the advanced clinical training available to estheticians after graduation or in a highly skilled primary training program.

Fitzpatrick Skin Type	Description	Laser Hair Removal Considerations
Type I	Very fair skin accompanied by blond or light-red hair and blue or green eyes. Never tans, always burns.	May not be good candidates because of lack of contrast between hair and skin color.
Type II	Fair skin accompanied by light-brown or red hair and green or brown eyes. Occasionally tans, always burns.	Good candidates for laser hair removal.
Type III	Medium skin accompanied by brown hair and brown eyes. Often tans, sometimes burns.	Good candidates for laser hair removal.
Type IV	Olive skin, accompanied by brown or black hair and dark-brown or black eyes. Always tans, rarely burns.	Good candidates for laser hair removal. Best done by experienced practitioners.
Type V	Dark-brown skin accompanied by black hair and black eyes. Rarely burns.	May not be good candidates because of lack of contrast between hair and skin color. If performed, use only YAG lasers. Best done by experienced practitioners.
Type VI	Black skin accompanied by black hair and black eyes. Rarely burns.	May not be good candidates because of lack of contrast between hair and skin color. If performed, use only YAG lasers. Best done by experienced practitioners.

Figure 27-8 Fitzpatrick skin types and laser hair removal indications.

■ INTENSE PULSED LIGHT (IPL)

IPL is a **nonablative** laser that uses a broad spectrum of light (non-coherent) instead of a single collimated beam at a specific wavelength. Intense pulsed light (IPL) can deliver multiple color combinations of light at a time. Pulsed light machines use cutoff filters to selectively deliver the desired wavelengths. These wavelengths can be customized to reach the specific hair, blood vessel, or skin component being treated and can be modified with each pulse.

Pulsed light begins with all wavelengths of light, from 500 to 1,200 nm, including green, yellow, red, and infrared light. Various lower-range, shorter-wavelength (515 to 755 nm) cutoff filters block light shorter than the wavelength of the filter. Since longer wavelengths penetrate deeper into the target, longer wavelengths are used to treat deeper targets and to avoid and protect superficial parts of the skin. Shorter wavelengths are used to treat more superficial targets without damaging deeper areas of the skin.

Pulsed light can be delivered in pulses or bursts that vary from one to five pulses at a time. The duration of each pulse and the delay between

Term	Description
spot size	Size or width of laser beam
fluence	Measured in joules. Strength or intensity of the laser beam, spot size influences the amount of fluence needed for effective treatment. Stronger intensity with a longer pulse duration increases the damage to the surrounding tissue
wavelength	Measurement of light. Long wavelengths have deeper penetration than short wavelengths. The active medium determines wavelength
thermal storage coefficient	Storage of heat in the chromophore or target; surrounding tissue can be damaged when the thermal storage coefficient of the target is heated beyond its capacity
pulse duration	Time that the laser is on the skin, measured in milliseconds. Longer pulse widths have fewer side effects. The pulse should be longer than the thermal relaxation time
thermal relaxation time	The amount of time it takes for 50% of the heat energy to leave the target tissue. Measured in milliseconds. Skin has a thermal relaxation time between 600 and 800 milliseconds

Figure 27-9 Laser terms and their descriptions.

pulses can be modified for each treatment site. Longer durations are generally better for treating larger targets, and shorter pulse durations are generally better for treating smaller areas.

■ TYPES OF LASERS

There are two main types of lasers, and both are used in the esthetic field.

Ablative Lasers

This is a laser that ablates, or removes, skin. The **ablative** laser light is absorbed by the water, oxyhemoglobin, and melanin within the skin to accomplish this task. The more tissue to be removed, the higher the energy used and the more passes performed during treatment. The treatment is painful and requires topical anesthesia and some pain medication. Recovery time could last from a few days to a week or more.

This Type of Laser is Indicated For:

- Resurfacing (texture and wrinkling): Resurfacing is accomplished by targeting the water in the skin.
- Vascular lesions: Lasers destroy vascular lesions by targeting the oxyhemoglobin (red blood cells).
- Pigmented lesions: These are removed by the laser targeting the melanin in the skin.
- Loss of elasticity: This is treated with increased heat to target the dermal level. The ablative layer heats the dermis, which causes damage. This, in turn, stimulates the fibroblasts to create more collagen and elastin. This is the wound response.

Types of Ablative Lasers Used Are:

- Short and variable-pulsed erbium
- YAG (yttrium aluminium garnet)
- Fractional
- CO_2
- Titanyl phosphate (KTiOPO) lasers, also called KTP lasers
- Argon
- ND YAG (neodymium-doped [ND] yttrium aluminium garnet; $Nd:Y_3Al_5O_{12}$) ruby QS
- Alexandrite QS

Nonablative Lasers

Nonablative lasers do not remove the skin; the laser light heats the dermis, leaving the epidermis intact. The treatments require multiple sessions, usually in a series every three to four weeks. Treatments can be painful and can require topical anesthesia and some pain medication. New technology that creates minimal pain is being released. Recovery time is minimal.

This Type of Laser is Indicated For:

- Vascular lesions: Lasers destroy vascular lesions by targeting the oxyhemoglobin (red blood cells).
- Pigmented lesions: These are removed by targeting the melanin in the skin.
- Loss of elasticity: The increased heat wounds the dermal level.

Types of Nonablative Lasers Used Are:

- Intense pulsed light
- Pulsed dye

- ND
- YAG (normal mode and long pulse mode).

Hair Removal

Hair-removal lasers work by heating the melanin in the hair. Melanin is considered the primary chromophore for all hair-removal lasers currently on the market. Melanin occurs naturally in the skin and hair and gives them their color. There are two types of melanin in hair: **eumelanin,** which gives hair brown or black color, and **pheomelanin,** which gives hair a blonde or red color.

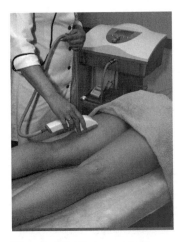

Figure 27-10 Laser hair removal is very popular.

Because of the selective absorption of photons of laser light, short-wavelength lasers (500 to 800 nm) are used to treat individuals with light skin and light brown or blond hair; lasers with a thin diameter and long wavelength (800 to 1,200 nm) are used for darker skin and coarse dark brown or black hair. Figure 27-10 shows an example of a hair-removal treatment.

The FDA permits the use of the phrase "permanent reduction", which describes what the machine will do. The use of the phrase "permanent removal" is not permitted for any laser. The intended meaning of "permanent" may be confusing to consumers, because most consumers understand it to mean that the hair will stop growing forever. However, the FDA permits the use of "permanent" as long as the laser reduces some visibly growing hairs for as short a time as one growth cycle—a matter of a few months for most body parts. In fact, many clinical studies have shown the rate of hair regrowth after laser epilation to be only slightly slower than regrowth after epilation by traditional methods.

Types of Lasers Used

- Ruby
- Alexandrite
- Diode
- ND, YAG (normal mode)
- IPL

See Figure 27-11 for a chart of lasers and the conditions indicated for their use.

■ NEW TECHNOLOGY

The search for new, nonablative antiaging technology is changing daily. What is considered "new" by the esthetician or consumer may actually be technology that has been in development for many years. The problem

Category of Laser	Used for	Types of Lasers Used
Ablative	Resurfacing, vascular lesions, pigmented lesions, loss of elasticity	Short and variable pulsed Erbium: YAG, Fractional lasers, CO_2 Laser, Titanyl Phosphate KTiOPO laser, (KTP), Argon, ND: YAG, Ruby QS, and Alexandrite QS
Nonablative	Vascular lesions, pigmented lesions, loss of elasticity	Intense Pulsed Light, Pulsed Dye, ND: YAG normal mode and long pulse
Hair Removal	Hair removal	Ruby, Alexandrite, Diode, ND: YAG normal mode, Intense Pulsed Light

Figure 27-11 Categories and types of lasers used.

with some of the new technology is that it does not have years of studies to guarantee the effectiveness of the treatment, like new drugs released on the market have. Without such studies, new technology may be used only to find out years later that it produces effects not anticipated. The section that follows provides an overview of technology currently being used and some indications for its use.

■ RADIOFREQUENCY

Radiofrequency (RF) technology uses electromagnetic radiation to heat up the dermal tissue, causing a wound process in the skin. RF is a form of electromagnetic energy between 300 MHz and 3 kHz. It is similar to lasers in that it creates a thermal change within the skin. Unlike lasers, RF does not target a chromophore; it is nonablative and generates heat through tissue resistance to the flow of electrons within the RF field. RF energy creates dermal heating to 149 degrees Fahrenheit. This causes collagen to shrink, which causes sagging skin to tighten as the dermis begins to heal. Within the skin, RF radiation will produce different thermal effects based on electrode configuration: monopolar RF will penetrate deeply into the dermis, but bipolar RF will provide only superficial penetration. Monopolar and bipolar RF are used together for more effective results, and RF is also combined with IPL to treat wrinkles and loss of elasticity. It has been found that the two technologies used together can have a better effect.

The results of RF are not immediate; it can take up to 12 weeks for the tightening effects to be visible. It is a painful treatment, and a mild sedative is given beforehand. Multiple treatments may be required.

■ PHOTOPNEUMATIC TECHNOLOGY

This technology is essentially a vacuum combined with IPL. The gentle vacuum is specifically designed to gently pull the target chromophore toward the light source in the attachment. The vacuum reduces the size of the blood vessel within the skin as the IPL is administered; this decreases the amount of competing chromophores, which allows four to five times more photons to impact the target. This technique also reduces the amount of input energy lost to reflection, scatter, and absorption. The claim is that this makes the IPL treatment five times more effective, providing a painless treatment for pigmentation problems, varicose veins, and hair removal. Results depend on the strength of the treatment, and multiple sessions may be required.

■ PLASMA

Plasma is inert nitrogen gas that is delivered into the skin. The skin starts to shed much like a chemical peel within a few days after application. The depth of treatment depends on the number of passes performed. Treatment is generally well-tolerated except for more aggressive treatments that require multiple passes.

This technology is used to treat fine to moderate wrinkles, pigmentation problems and skin lesions, and to tighten skin. Aggressive treatment requires topical anesthetic and oral sedatives, and may take multiple treatments; results are generally seen in 10 days.

■ FRACTIONAL RESURFACING

A **fractionated laser** utilizes the 1,550-nm wavelength and targets water in the skin, which leaves the stratum corneum attached. The laser beams are delivered in a randomized pattern, which creates columns of microscopic wounds within the dermis and epidermis. The healthy skin that surrounds the wounded tissue increases the wound healing process.

Fractional resurfacing treats moderate to severe wrinkles, acne scarring, and uneven skin texture. The skin may appear red and swollen for about three days after an aggressive treatment, which can be painful; oral pain medication may be indicated. A less aggressive treatment will not be as painful and posttreatment inflammation will be less apparent. It can take up to six treatments to visibly improve the skin, and results can be seen slowly.

Much more technology is under development, and it is important for an esthetician to be aware of the new technology being released. Estheticians need to know how to treat the skin after treatment to make the client more comfortable and maximize the results. For example, if a client receives fractional resurfacing but cannot take three days of downtime, it is important to demonstrate how to be compliant with proper wound-healing protocols, including the use of mineral-based makeup to cover redness and provide sun protection.

REFERENCES

1. D'Angelo, J., Dean, P., Dietz, S., Hinds, C., Lees, M., Miller, E., & Zani, A. (2003). *Milady's Standard Comprehensive Training for Estheticians.* New York: Thomson Delmar Learning.

2. Simmons, J. V. (1989, 1995). *Science and the Beauty Business: The Beauty Salon and Its Equipment* (2nd ed.). United Kingdom: Macmillan Press Ltd.

3. Lees, M. (2001). *Skin Care: Beyond the Basics.* New York: Thomson Delmar Learning.

4. Bickmore, H. (2004). *Milady's Hair Removal Techniques: A Comprehensive Manual.* New York: Thomson Delmar Learning.

5. Dover, J., Kamin, A. (2007). "Laser and Lights: A Technological Revolution." *Skin, Inc.* January 2007.

6. Pugliese, P. (2004). "Fundamentals of Laser Science, Part I." *Skin, Inc.* July 2004.

7. Hill, P., Bickmore, H. (2008). *Milady's Aesthetician Series: Advanced Hair Removal.* New York: Thomson Delmar Learning.

8. Nicholson, J., & Warfield, S. (2004). *Laser Safety for the Salon, Spa, and Small Medical Clinic.* New Jersey: Paramedical Consultants, Inc.

9. Friedman, D. J., & Gilead, L. T. (2007). "The Use of Hybrid Radiofrequency Device for the Treatment of Rhytids and Lax Skin." *Dermatology Surgery* 33: 543–551.

10. Hansen, I. (2007). "Fractional Resurfacing." *Medesthetics.* January/February: 28–35.

Body Equipment

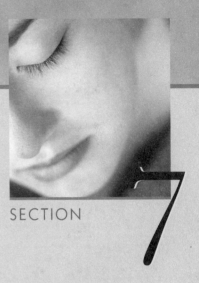

SECTION CONTENT

SECTION

7

Machine Treatments for the Body

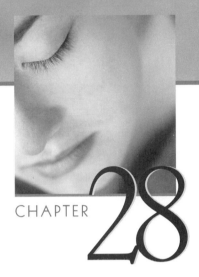

Body treatments are most often performed for exfoliation, skin conditioning, and metabolic stimulation. All of these effects can be created by machines that are generally used on the face. You will find that most of the technology used on the face is duplicated on the body. In this chapter we will look at the machines available for cellulite treatments, lymphatic drainage, and skin conditioning.

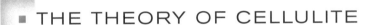

THE THEORY OF CELLULITE

Cellulite is the skin effect that first appears on a woman's thighs, then spreads to the stomach and buttock areas, giving skin a dimpled, orange-peel look. Cellulite is a controversial issue, and no one treatment is completely effective.

As elasticity decreases, cellulite will often spread to the chest, knees, and upper arms. The subcutaneous tissue located below the surface of the skin binds skin loosely to the underlying tissues or bone. Subcutaneous fat cells come in varying sizes and numbers in each individual. In women, the uppermost subcutaneous layer has large fat cell chambers separated by radial and arching dividing walls of connective tissue. These are held in place by the overlaying connective tissue of the dermis. In men, the uppermost part of the subcutaneous layer is thinner and has a crisscross network of connective tissue and a thicker dermis. See Figure 28-1 for an illustration of cellulite.

Estrogen plays a large role in the destruction of **collagen,** the building block of connective tissue. Cellulite is a multifaceted problem that relates to increased adipose cells, weakening of connective tissue, and poor circulation. As such, it requires treatment on multiple levels. Here are the options available with esthetic equipment, but keep in mind other modalities, such as diet and exercise, must be included.

315

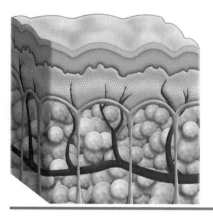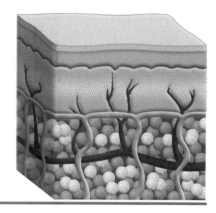

Figure 28-1 The left side is skin with cellulite; the right side is a normal view without cellulite.

■ VIBRATORY MASSAGE

Vibratory massage is an electrical massage treatment that produces a heating effect via friction on the skin's surface. It is used to create a slimming body treatment and provide a deep massage.

■ FUNCTIONS

Massage increases circulation, which helps cellular metabolism, increases blood and lymph movement to remove waste and toxins, provides gentle exfoliation, relaxes tense muscles, softens hard fatty deposits, stimulates nerve endings, and improves areas of cellulite. Figure 28-2 shows a massager.

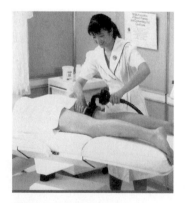

Figure 28-2 Vibratory massage equipment.

■ PREPARATION FOR TREATMENT

- Have your client fill out an assessment form.
- Check for contraindications.
- Have your client change into a robe and remove all jewelry and contact lenses.
- Analyze client concerns with the intake form.
- Explain the procedure.
- Make sure to test all equipment before applying treatment.
- Inspect all wires and electrodes.
- Follow manufacturer's instructions for the setup of your machine.

- Have the client lie on the bed and drape accordingly.
- Attach correct massager head. Figure 28-3 shows different heads.

■ HOW TO USE IT

Listed below are general descriptions of directions for use. Always check with your manufacturer or vendor for the protocols that are recommended for your equipment.

Step 1: After preparing and draping the client, apply treatment cream and turn on the machine.

Step 2: Start with the effleurage applicator on the arms in the direction of the lymphatic flow.

Step 3: Move over the abdomen, then the fronts of the legs.

Step 4: Have the client turn over; start at the legs and move upward.

Step 5: Apply four to six strokes to each treatment area. Figure 28-5 shows a diagram of movements.

Step 6: Change to the pétrissage applicator head and redrape the client.

Step 7: Repeat Step 2, moving downward; follow initial downward movement with circular movements.

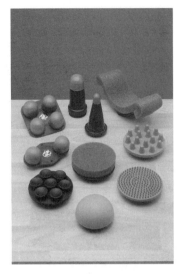

Figure 28-3 Vibratory massage attachments.

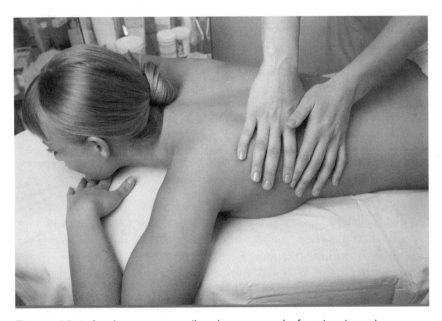

Figure 28-4 Apply massage oil, gel, or cream before treatment.

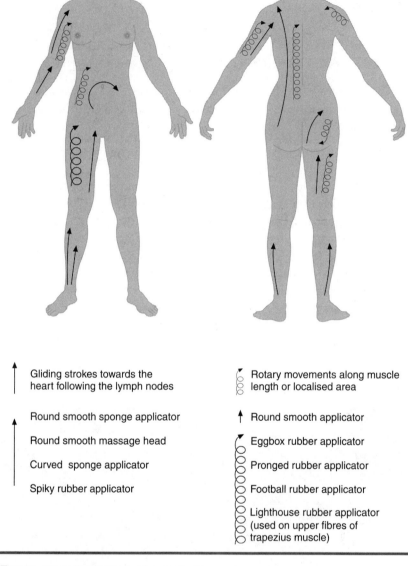

Figure 28-5 Illustration of massage movements.

↑	Gliding strokes towards the heart following the lymph nodes	⟨	Rotary movements along muscle length or localised area
↑	Round smooth sponge applicator	↑	Round smooth applicator
	Round smooth massage head		Eggbox rubber applicator
	Curved sponge applicator		Pronged rubber applicator
	Spiky rubber applicator		Football rubber applicator
			Lighthouse rubber applicator (used on upper fibres of trapezius muscle)

Step 8: Repeat again on the client's back. Lift and glide the skin under the applicator head with one hand.

Step 9: Continue treatment until a mild redness appears.

Step 10: Change to the friction applicator head, and apply small circular movements on treatment areas such as the trapezoids, either side of the spine, and around joints.

Step 11: Change to the percussion applicator head; move in one direction only, using one hand to lead or follow each stroke.

Step 12: Change back to effleurage treatment head, and complete treatment to soothe the skin.

Optional step: Manual massage can be used to complete the treatment and soothe the skin.

> **TIP** Bruising and skin irritation can be caused by too heavy an application or an incorrect choice of applicator head used in the wrong area and for too long.

■ GALVANIC CURRENT FOR THE BODY

Galvanic current is very effective as a body treatment for the penetration of active water-based ingredients. All of the facial benefits can be associated with the body application as well.

■ FUNCTIONS

Galvanic current increases the absorption of water-soluble products into the skin, reduces superficial swelling and puffiness, increases microcirculation in the cells, and improves skin texture.

■ PREPARATION FOR TREATMENT

- Have your client fill out an assessment form.
- Check for contraindications.
- Have your client change into a robe and remove all jewelry and contact lenses.
- Analyze client concerns on the intake form.
- Explain the procedure.
- Make sure to test all equipment before applying treatment.
- Inspect all wires and electrodes.
- Follow manufacturer's instructions for the setup of your machine.
- Set up your bed for a body wrap.

Step 1: Place heated pad on bed.

Step 2: Place a fitted sheet over the top.

Step 3: Place the blanket horizontally on the bed (this accommodates larger clients). If you have a king size blanket, place as usual.

Step 4: Place a flat sheet over the top.

Step 5: Place a plastic body wrap over the flat sheet. Make sure there is enough to completely wrap the client's body.

Step 6: Place a long bath towel on top for the client to lie under.

■ HOW TO USE IT

Step 1: Place electrodes on the bed in the proper positions. See Figure 28-6 for body electrode placement.

Step 2: Exfoliate skin with a dry brush using light circular movements. Follow lymphatic and blood flow towards the heart, and have the client sit up for the back application. When working on the legs, lift each one to work underneath.

Step 3: Use a sponge to saturate electrode sleeves with distilled water, and secure all electrodes to electrical leads.

Step 4: Apply active solution under negative electrodes (usually for cellulite). Always follow the manufacturer's directions.

Step 5: Apply conducting gel under positive electrodes.

Step 6: Firmly strap electrodes in place. Wrap the client for warmth.

Step 7: Turn the machine on, and turn on the negative pole.

TIP Always make sure that the body electrodes are fully saturated and in firm contact with the skin. They must not touch each other, or treatment will be ineffective.

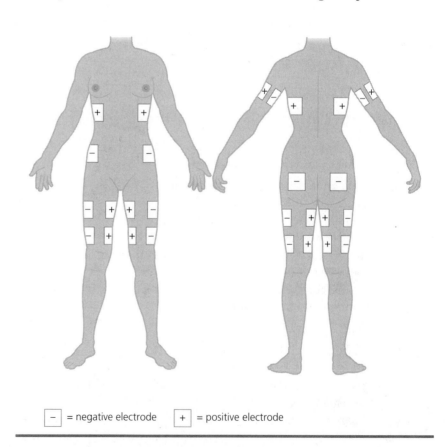

$\boxed{-}$ = negative electrode $\boxed{+}$ = positive electrode

Figure 28-6 Diagram of electrode placement.

Step 8: Proceed to turn the dial up until the client feels a slight tingling sensation.

Step 9: Increase amperage up to 4.25 mA max for 10 minutes. Subsequent treatments should last 20 minutes.

Step 10: Reverse polarity for 2 to 3 minutes to neutralize chemical reactions and soothe the skin.

Step 11: Slowly reduce the current and turn the machine off. A slight redness to the skin is normal.

Step 12: Remove electrodes and solution residue.

Step 13: Apply an appropriate mask to the body:

- Seaweed mask for detoxification and remineralizing
- Specific slimming mask for cellulite reduction
- Mud mask for retexturizing and remineralizing

Step 14: Wrap the client for 10 to 15 minutes, depending on manufacturer's instructions.

Step 15: Unwrap the client and remove product with warm towels or have the client shower.

Step 16: Apply slimming body cream and massage it in for 5 to 10 minutes.

■ MICROCURRENT FOR THE BODY

Microcurrent is another useful technology for body firming and cellulite treatment. It is often combined with vibratory massage and LED therapy for increased effectiveness. Figure 28-7 shows an example of equipment available.

■ FUNCTIONS

Microcurrent body treatments rejuvenate muscles, increase cellular functioning, improve skin texture, assist penetration of water-based products into the skin, improve lymphatic circulation, and increase blood circulation.

■ PREPARATION FOR TREATMENT

- Have your client fill out an assessment form.
- Check for contraindications.

TIP This treatment is not indicated for a wet room.

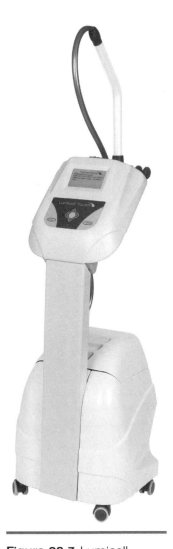

Figure 28-7 Lumicell.

- Have your client change into a robe and remove all jewelry and contact lenses.
- Analyze client concerns with the intake form.
- Explain the procedure.
- Make sure to test all equipment before applying treatment.
- Inspect all wires and electrodes.
- Follow manufacturer's instructions for the setup of your machine.
- Have your client drink eight ounces of water before treatment. Hydrated clients will have better conductivity.

HOW TO USE IT

Step 1: Use correct current and waveform for a body treatment application based on your manufacturer's instructions.

Step 2: Apply conductive gel to the skin. You must use an electrotherapy treatment gel; basic skin care products will not be as effective.

Step 3: Apply probes or gloves over the area that you are treating.

Step 4: If using gloves, use gliding movements toward the heart. When using probes, follow the manufacturer's directions. Here is a basic movement: place one probe stationary on the origin of the muscle you are working; slowly move the other probe toward the stationary probe. Repeat three to four times over each area.

Step 5: Remove unabsorbed conductive gel with warm towels.

Step 6: Follow with an appropriate treatment cream.

VACUUM SUCTIONING FOR THE BODY

Vacuum suctioning used on the body helps primarily with the movement of lymphatic fluid. This helps with nonmedical edema and is sometimes combined with other technology such as microcurrent, vibratory massage, and LED therapy.

FUNCTIONS

Vacuum suction improves blood and lymphatic flow, reduces swelling and puffiness, and provides gentle exfoliation. Figure 28-8 shows an example of vacuum suction for the body.

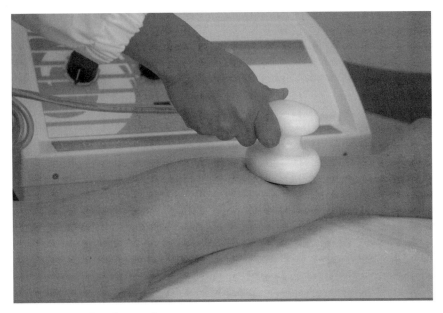

Figure 28-8 Bio-Dermology.

■ PREPARATION FOR TREATMENT

- Have your client fill out an assessment form.
- Check for contraindications.
- Have your client change into a robe and remove all jewelry and contact lenses.
- Analyze client concerns with the intake form.
- Explain the procedure.
- Make sure to test all equipment before applying treatment.
- Inspect all wires and electrodes.
- Follow manufacturer's instructions for the setup of your machine.

■ HOW TO USE IT

Step 1: Exfoliate skin with a dry brush with light circular movements; follow lymphatic and blood flow toward the heart. Have the client sit up for the back application. When working on the legs, lift each one to work underneath.

Step 2: Pick appropriate cream or oil for condition being treated, applying cream in an even layer on the skin.

Step 3: Pick the appropriate suction attachment for the body, and turn the machine on.

Step 4: Place the vacuum cup on the border of the area to be treated, and turn up the vacuum intensity until about an eighth of an inch of skin fills the bottom of the suction attachment.

Step 5: Gently lift the suction attachment, and let it glide gently toward the nearest lymph node. See Figure 28-9 for an example of the appropriate movements.

Step 6: At the end of each movement, break the vacuum seal by removing your finger from the hole at the top of the suction attachment or by gently placing a hand under the attachment.

Step 7: Repeat movements on the area again, up to six times.

Step 8: Move on to the next area to be treated, and adjust the vacuum level as needed.

Step 9: At the end of treatment, gently effleurage the remaining product into skin to enhance further lymphatic drainage.

TIP It is a good idea to have your clients drink as much water as they can after treatment. This will assist with the removal of toxins. Vacuum suction is a great treatment for clients on a detoxification program.

■ CONTRAINDICATIONS AND CAUTIONS

These contraindications and cautions will encompass all aspects of using machines for the body. It is important to have a specific consultation for a body treatment that is separate from your facial treatment. It is

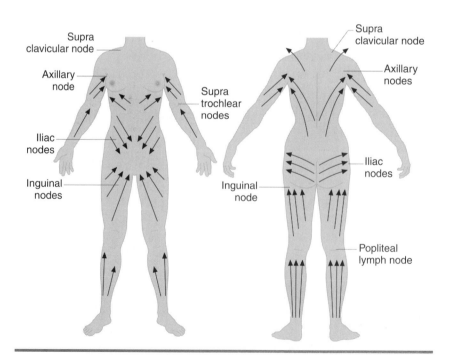

Figure 28-9 Application movements.

extremely important to determine contraindications or special needs that your client may have. Do not rely exclusively on the intake form; it is also important to verbally get information and clarification from your client.

- Metal implements in the body and pacemakers: Electricity concentrates in areas with a conductor, and pacemakers will be interrupted. IUDs are considered a metal implement for the purpose of galvanic body treatments.
- Pregnancy: Use caution when working on pregnant clients. They can be very sensitive. Get a doctor's approval before performing a body treatment with electricity.
- Heart problems: A heart in a compromised condition is unable to cope with an increased constriction or dilation of blood vessels. This can lead to fainting or a heart attack.
- Blood vessel disorders: Arteriosclerosis, or hardening of the arteries, affects the arteries' ability to handle increased blood flow. Fainting can occur when increased dilation of the blood vessels results from heat treatments.
- Skin inflammation: Most electrical treatments increase circulation, which can make inflammation worse.
- Skin disorders or diseases: These may be aggravated by treatment.
- Very sensitive skin: Treatment may be very uncomfortable for the client.
- Migraines or severe headaches: Treatment may cause worsening of existing headaches but is not known to cause them.
- Lack of tactile sensation (e.g., numbness due to stroke): A client with impaired sensation will not be able to gauge the intensity of the current, which could cause injury.
- Nervous clients: Treatment will be ineffective if the client cannot relax.
- Excessive metal dental work: Current will concentrate around metal. Porcelain veneers are not an issue, but clients with braces will be very uncomfortable.
- Metal piercings: Current will concentrate around the metal. Ask the client to remove jewelry.
- Epilepsy.
- Cuts and abrasions: Electrical current will concentrate in the area, because body fluids act as conductors.
- Severe bruising: Treatment will be uncomfortable for a bruised client.
- High or low blood pressure: These conditions could be made worse due to the increase in circulation. Even if these are treated and under control, use caution. Never leave such clients alone, and help them on and off the treatment bed.

- Recent scar tissue: Scarred skin is very sensitive and less resistant. Use caution when using electrotherapy and vacuum massage.
- HIV.
- History of blood clots (thrombosis) or embolism: Treatment could aggravate these conditions and cause a heart attack or stroke.
- Malignant melanoma: Cancer treatment must be completed, and client must be in remission. Obtain physician approval. Do not apply treatment when in doubt about a possible abnormality; instead, refer the client to a dermatologist.

Q & A

What are the pros and cons of using body treatment equipment?

Pros

Effectiveness: These modalities have been used for many years in the esthetic profession and have safe track records with visible benefits.
Safety: These are very safe machines; shocks come from poorly maintained machines or operator misuse. Bruising is only caused by operator misuse.

Cons

Ease of use: These machines are easy to use with minimal training, although there is a learning curve.
Cost: Machines are expensive. New combination modalities can cost as much as $16,000.
Training: In-depth training in electrotherapy, lymphatic drainage, and contraindications is required. This is an advanced technical class.
Maintenance: Consistent and thorough cleaning is required after every treatment to avoid errant shocks and attachment breakage.

Can I achieve results without body treatment equipment?

Yes and no. Body treatments can be performed without equipment. Treatment for cellulite is enhanced with equipment, and you get better results with a combination of machines, lifestyle changes, and a correct homecare regimen.

Should I buy or lease?

This decision must be based on your financial situation. This equipment has a high enough cost that it may warrant using a lease. It is a good idea to get professional financial advice before making major purchases. See Chapters 1 and 2 for additional information.

REFERENCES

1. D'Angelo, J., Dean, P., Dietz, S., Hinds, C., Lees, M., Miller, E., & Zani, A. (2003). *Milady's Standard Comprehensive Training for Estheticians*. New York: Thomson Delmar Learning.
2. Simmons, J. V. (1989, 1995). *Science and the Beauty Business: The Beauty Salon and Its Equipment* (2nd ed.). United Kingdom: Macmillan Press Ltd.
3. Lees, M. (2001). *Skin Care: Beyond the Basics*. New York: Thomson Delmar Learning.
4. Nordman, L. (2005). *Professional Beauty Therapy: The Official Guide to Level 3* (2nd ed.). London: Thomson Learning.
5. Pugliese, P. (2001). *Physiology of the Skin II*. Carol Stream, IL: Allured Publishing.

Appendix A

▪ STATE-BY-STATE LICENSING INFORMATION

Each state has its own laws, and listed here is a state-by-state listing with medical board contact information. Many states have no guidelines for machine usage, so it is important for you to verify your own state's requirements. You will notice a disturbing trend throughout this list: some states have taken away the ability to use noninvasive techniques, like microdermabrasion, except under the supervision of a physician.

Common Scope of Practice

As more technology becomes available in the esthetics market, many of our procedures can start to push beyond our licensed scope of practice. It is important to know what your legal scope is lest you lose your license if something happens. The general description that many state cosmetology boards and insurance carriers use is this: An esthetician may cleanse, exercise, massage, stimulate, or perform any other similar procedure on the skin or scalp by electrical, mechanical, or any other means. An esthetician may apply to the face an alcohol, cream, lotion, astringent, or cosmetic preparation or remove superfluous hair by the use of a depilatory, tweezers, or cosmetic preparation.

State Boards and Requirements

Esthetics is a dynamic industry that changes as technology changes, so what we know today is quickly outdated. The most current information may be found on each state's Web site. Verify your state's requirements regularly.

TIP State boards are trying to catch up with changes taking place in the esthetics industry. The requirements listed in this chapter may have changed.

ALABAMA

Alabama Board of Cosmetology
100 North Union Street #320
Montgomery, AL 36130
(334) 242-1918
http://www.aboc.state.al.us

Requirements

ESTHETICIAN: 1,500 clock hours or 1,200 credit hours

Machine Scope of Use

Class I devices only

Reciprocity

Must meet the hour requirements at the time of licensure. Must present proof of five years of licensed experience.

Continuing Education

Masters and instructors: 16 hours every two years

Medical Board Contact Information

Alabama Medical Board
P.O. Box 946 Montgomery, AL 36101-0946
(334) 242-4116
http://www.albme.org

ALASKA

Alaska Division of Occupational Licensing
P.O. Box 110806
Juneau, AK 99811-0806
(907) 465-2547
Susan_karlslyst@commerce.state.ak.us
http://www.commerce.state.ak.us

Machine Scope of Use

If you work in a medical office under the supervision of a physician, you may use this equipment. Otherwise, there is no regulation on equipment. An esthetician may do laser hair removal (cold only).

Requirements

COSMETICIAN: 350 hours
ESTHETICIAN: 350 hours or apprenticeship are required for licensing

Reciprocity

Must have completed 1,650 hours. Alaska will grant credit for work experience (500 hours for each year in the field). Note: A *cosmetologist* in Alaska may only do facials, hair removal, and makeup. A *hairdresser* only works with the hair; *two* licenses are required to do all these procedures.

Continuing Education
Not required
Medical Board Contact Information
Alaska Medical Board
Attn: Executive Administrator
Leslie A. Gallant
550 West 7th Avenue, Suite 1500
Anchorage, AK 99501-3567
(907) 269-8163
Leslie_Gallant@commerce.state.ak.us

ARIZONA
Arizona Board of Cosmetology
1721 East Broadway
Tempe, AZ 85282-1611
(480) 784-4539 EXT 227
Cheryl.adams@cb.state.az.us
http://www.cosmetology.state.az.us

Machine Scope of Use
From A.A.C. R-4-10-112(p): "derma plane procedures, blades, knives, lancets, and any tool that invades the skin shall not be used in a salon or school. A nipper . . . chemical peels . . . 2% phenol and 37 to 40% neutralized glycolic acid may be used. (Any machine or appliance which penetrates the dermis layer of the skin is considered invasive and is therefore prohibited [i.e., lasers]."

Further, Arizona has no such thing as a medical esthetician. In other words, an esthetician, cosmetologist, or nail technician working in a licensed salon may only do what their scope of practice definition allows. However, if the licensee is working in a licensed salon in a doctor's office, they can provide services within the scope of their own license while not under the doctor's direct supervision. When under the doctor's direct supervision—meaning while the doctor is in the building—and with a notice posted that services are not regulated by the board of cosmetology, additional services may be performed. But the services performed under the direct supervision of a doctor are most likely regulated by the medical board. If a complaint were to be received under the latter conditions, the board of cosmetology would certainly investigate but would reserve the right to refer to or work with the medical board. And while practicing as a licensed esthetician, cosmetologist, or nail technician and doing procedures covered by the board of cosmetology, the licensee must be working in a licensed salon. Specifically, if a licensee is advertising or holding oneself out as being licensed by the board, the licensee must be working in a licensed salon within the defined scope of practice.

Requirements

ESTHETICIAN: 600 hours

Reciprocity

In you come from another state, licensure in Arizona may be accomplished through license-for-license or by taking an examination. This requires an application for reciprocity and an explanation of licensure requirements. According to the state board, a person is entitled to receive a cosmetologist, esthetician, or nail technician license under the following conditions:

They submit to the board an application for a cosmetologist, esthetician, or nail technician license on a form supplied by the board.

They pay the prescribed fees.

They submit to the board satisfactory evidence of either of the following:

- Licensure in another state or country.
- Graduation from a school that offers a cosmetology, esthetics, or nail technology course substantially similar to the requirements of Arizona and passage of the board-approved cosmetology, esthetician, or nail technician examination.

Continuing Education

Not required

Medical Board Contact Information

Arizona Medical Board
9545 East Doubletree Ranch Road
Scottsdale, AZ 85258
(480) 551-2700
(877) 255-2212
questions@azmd.gov

ARKANSAS

Arkansas State Board of Cosmetology
101 East Capitol, Suite 108
Little Rock, AR 72201
(501) 682-2168
cosmo@arkansas.gov
http://www.arkansas.gov

Machine Scope of Use

A licensed electrologist may operate lasers and other equipment, but this is currently under review.

Requirements

ESTHETICIAN: 600 hours

Reciprocity
Granted to all those who hold a valid license who have passed *both* a written and a practical exam.

Continuing Education
Instructors: Eight hours every two years

Medical Board Contact Information
Arkansas State Medical Board
2100 Riverfront Drive
Little Rock, AR 72202
(501) 296-1802
http://www.armedicalboard.org

CALIFORNIA
California State Board of Barbering and Cosmetology
P.O. Box 944226
Sacramento, CA 94244-2260
(916) 445-0713
barbercosmo@dca.ca.gov
http://www.barbercosmo.ca.gov

Machine Scope of Use
The State of California prohibits the use of lasers, IPL, and ultrasound by licensed estheticians. These treatments are considered not within the scope of esthetic practice.

Requirements
ESTHETICIAN: 600 hours

Reciprocity
Not available. Applicants must take a written and practical exam. Barbers have to take both a written and a practical examination; however, barber instructors require only a written exam.

Continuing Education
Not required

Medical Board Contact Information
1426 Howe Avenue #54
Sacramento, CA 95825
(916) 263-2382
webmaster@mbc.ca.gov

COLORADO
Colorado Office of Barber and Cosmetologist Licensing
1560 Broadway #1340
Denver, CO 80202
(303) 894-7772

Barber-cosmetology@dora.state.co.us
http://www.dora.state.co.us

Machine Scope of Use

FDA Class I equipment may be used. Class II and Class III devices can be used only under the supervision of a physician and only within their scope of practice. Devices must be FDA-registered.

Requirements

COSMETICIAN: 550 hours

Reciprocity

Colorado does not have reciprocity, they have *endorsement;* everyone who holds an active license in another state may apply for endorsement, and everyone is reviewed on an individual basis.

Continuing Education

Not required

Medical Board Contact Information

Board of Medical Examiners
1560 Broadway Suite 1350
Denver, CO 80202
Medical Rule 800 has been adopted by the medical board to address the issue of nonmedical personnel using medical equipment.
http://www.dora.state.co.us

CONNECTICUT

Connecticut Department of Public Health, Cosmetology, and Licensing
410 Capitol Avenue MS #12 APP
P.O. Box 340308
Hartford, CT 06134
(860) 509-7569
http://www.ct-clic.com
http://www.dph.state.ct.us

Machine Scope of Use

No defined scope of use

Requirements

BARBER/COSMETICIAN: 1,500 hours

Reciprocity

Will accept licensing from states that require the same hours.

Continuing Education

Not required

Medical Board Contact Information

410 Capitol Avenue
P.O. Box 340308

Hartford, CT 06134-0308
(860) 509-8000
http://www.dph.state.ct.us

DELAWARE

Delaware Board of Cosmetology and Barbering
Canon Building #203
P.O. Box 1401
Dover, DE 19903
(302) 739-4522
Margaret_foreit@state.de.us
http://www.dpr.delaware.gov

Machine Scope of Use

Microdermabrasion is acceptable. Class II Class III may
be used directly under physician supervision but not
under an esthetician's license, but as a medical assistant
to physician.

Requirements

ESTHETICIAN: 300 hours, apprenticeship 600 hours

Reciprocity

Extended to all states and the District of Columbia

Continuing Education

Not required

DISTRICT OF COLUMBIA

John A. Wilson Building
1350 Pennsylvania Avenue NW
Washington, DC 20004
(202) 727-1000
dcra@dc.gov
http://www.asisvcs.com

Machine Scope of Use

No scope of use defined

Requirements

SKIN CARE: 350 hours

Reciprocity

Granted to all individuals whose current license is from
a state whose requirements are equivalent to those of DC.
Credit for work experience may be granted.

Continuing Education

Check with state board

Medical Board Contact Information

Department of Health Board of Medicine
717 14th Street NW
Suite 600
Washington, DC 20005
(877) 672-2174

FLORIDA

Florida Department of Business and Professional Regulation
1940 N Monroe Street
Tallahassee, FL 32399
(850) 487-1395
callcenter@dbpr.state.fl.us
http://www.myflorida.com

Machine Scope of Use

No defined scope

Requirements

SKIN CARE: 260 hours

Reciprocity

Given to individuals holding a license from another state whose requirements are the same or more stringent. Hair braiding registration is available in Florida following a two-day, 16-hour course. Home salons are allowed.

Continuing Education

16 hours every two years

Medical Board Contact Information

Medical Quality Assurance
4052 Bald Cypress Way
Tallahassee, FL 32399-3250
(850) 245-4224

GEORGIA

Georgia State Board of Cosmetology
166 Pryor Street SW
Atlanta, GA 30303
(478) 207-1430
http://www.sos.georgia.gov

Machine Scope of Use

No defined use

Requirements

ESTHETICIAN: 1,000 hours, apprenticeship 2,000 hours

Reciprocity

The Georgia State Board of Barbers and Georgia State Board of Cosmetology reciprocity requirements are according to OCGA

43-10-9, which states that reciprocity may be extended to licensees from other states and countries that have similar training and licensing requirements and that will extend reciprocity to Georgia licensees. Out-of-country applicants' training will be reviewed by the board, and applicants may be required to take the written and practical examinations. The Georgia State Board of Cosmetology does not reciprocate with California, Florida, Hawaii, or New York. For all other states, reciprocity will be granted or denied on an individual basis in accordance with the law.

Continuing Education
Five hours every two years

Medical Board Contact Information
Composite State Board of Medical Examiners
2 Peachtree Street NW, 36th Floor
Atlanta, GA 30303-3465
(404) 656-3913
medbd@dch.ga.gov

HAWAII
Hawaii Department of Commerce and Consumer Affairs
1010 Richards Street
P.O. Box 3469
Honolulu, HI 96801
(808) 586-3000
barber_cosm@dcca.hawaii.gov
http://www.hawaii.gov

Machine Scope of Use
The statutes and rules of the Board of Barbering and Cosmetology do not directly address the question about the use of FDA-approved equipment by licensed estheticians. However, the rules do include electricity as a subject in the curriculum for a student or apprentice in esthetics. This would appear to indicate that usage of some type of electric equipment would be allowed; however, it would have to fall within the scope of practice of a licensed cosmetologist or esthetician. Anything that goes beyond that scope would be considered medical-grade, and only a physician would be permitted to engage in that type of activity. The same would apply to microdermabrasion.

Requirements
ESTHETICIAN: 600 hours, apprenticeship 1,100 hours

Reciprocity
Granted to all with a current license from a state with equal or greater requirements. Work experience is a consideration if you have less schooling than required. Home salons and mobile salons are allowed.

Continuing Education
Not required

Medical Board Contact Information
DCCA-PVL
Attn: BME
P.O. Box 3469
Honolulu, HI 96801
(808) 586-2708
medical@dcca.hawaii.gov

IDAHO

Idaho Board of Cosmetology
650 West State Street, Room 100
P.O. Box 83720
Boise, ID 83702
(208) 332-1824
http://www.adm.idaho.gov

Machine Scope of Use
Currently under review

Requirements
ESTHETICIAN: 600 hours, apprenticeship 1,200 hours

Reciprocity
Granted to licensed applicants who provide official documentation
that the requirements for license under which the license was issued
are of a standard not lower than Idaho, or who provide official documentation that they have practiced for at least three years immediately prior to making application. Home salons are allowed. Mobile
salons are not allowed.

Continuing Education
Not required

Medical Board Contact Information
1755 Westgate Drive
PO Box 83720
Boise, ID 83720
(208) 327-7000
info@bom.state.id.us

ILLINOIS

Illinois Department of Professional Regulation
320 West Washington Street, 3rd Floor
Springfield, IL 62786
(217) 782-0800
http://www.idfpr.com

Machine Scope of Use
No defined scope

Requirements
ESTHETICIAN: 750 hours

Reciprocity
Based on laws in the issuing state at the time the applicant was licensed, as compared to Illinois law. The state does credit the applicant for work experience. Home salons and mobile salons are allowed.

Continuing Education
Ten hours every two years for esthetics

Medical Board Contact Information
Professional Regulation
320 West Washington
Springfield, IL 62786
(217) 785-0800

INDIANA
Indiana Professional Licensing Agency
State Board of Cosmetology Examiners
402 West Washington Street, Room WO72
Indianapolis, IN 46204
(317) 234-3031
http://www.in.gov

Machine Scope of Use
No defined scope of use

Requirements
ESTHETICIAN: 700 hours

Reciprocity
Applicants licensed as cosmetologists in other states may be licensed in the state of Indiana as long as the state they are originally licensed in has requirements equal to those of Indiana. Where training has not met Indiana's requirements, the applicant will receive 100 hours of credit for each year of practical work experience. Regardless of length of time licensed in another state, all applicants must take an examination on the rules and regulations for Indiana that pertain to the profession for which they are applying for licensure. If the issuing state did not require the applicant to take a practical examination, such an examination must be taken to become licensed in Indiana.

Continuing Education
16 hours every four years

Medical Board Contact Information
Professional Licensing Agency
Attn: Medical Licensing Board of Indiana
402 West Washington Street, Room WO72
Indianapolis, IN 46204
(317) 234-2060
pla3@pla.IN.gov

IOWA
Iowa Department of Public Health
Board of Cosmetology Arts and Sciences
Lucas Building, 5th Floor
321 East 12th Street
Des Moines, IA 50319-0075
(515) 281-4416
http://www.idph.state.ia.us

Machine Scope of Use
No defined use

Requirements
ESTHETICIAN: 600 hours

Reciprocity
Iowa does not have reciprocity with any state. People from certain states can apply for licensure by *endorsement* only if they have taken a national exam. Not all states use a national exam; some only use a state exam.

Continuing Education
12 hours every two years

Medical Board Contact Information
400 SW 8th Street, Suite C
Des Moines, IA 50309-4686
(515) 281-5171

KANSAS
Kansas State Board of Cosmetology
714 SW Jackson
Topeka, KS 66617-1139
(785) 296-3155
Kboc@kboc.state.ks.us
http://www.kansas.gov

Machine Scope of Use
Any medical device, including Class II and Class III devices, are regulated by the Kansas Board of Healing Arts. Regulation KAR 28-24-14 prohibits skin-removal techniques, practices that affect the

living layers of the skin, and devices, tools, or instruments that remove calluses or skin blemishes. Microdermabrasion is not allowed.

Requirements
ESTHETICIAN: 650 hours

Reciprocity
Candidate must have 1,500 hours, have been working in the field for at least one year, and hold a current license. If you have less than 1,500 hours, you will have to take a practical exam. You may, however, obtain a temporary permit that allows you to work pending examination.

Continuing Education
Instructors: 20 hours every two years

Medical Board Contact Information
Kansas Board of Healing Arts
235 SW Topeka Boulevard
Topeka, KS 66603-3068
(785) 296-7413
(888) 886-7205
http://www.ksbha.org

KENTUCKY

Kentucky State Board of Hairdressers and Cosmetologists
111 St. James Court
Frankfort, KY 40601
(502) 564-4262
http://www.kentucky.gov

Machine Scope of Use
No defined use

Requirements
COSMETOLOGIST: 1,800 hours

Reciprocity
Any applicant from out of state who holds a valid license and can show proof of two years current experience can take the cosmetology practical examination for licensing in Kentucky. The applicant must also meet the minimum requirements.

Continuing Education
Six hours every year

Medical Board Contact Information
Kentucky Board of Medical Licensure
310 Whittington Parkway, Suite 1B
Louisville, KY 40222
(502) 429-7150
http://www.kbml.ky.gov

LOUISIANA

Louisiana State Board of Cosmetology
11622 Sunbelt Court
Baton Rouge, LA 70809
(225) 756-3404
weblegis@legis.state.la.us
http://www.legis.state.la.us

Machine Scope of Use
No defined use

Requirements
ESTHETICIAN: 750 hours

Reciprocity
Reciprocity with all states for all types of licenses

Continuing Education
Not required

Medical Board Contact Information
Louisiana State Board of Medical Examiners
630 Camp Street
New Orleans, LA 70130
(504) 568-6820

MAINE

Maine State Board of Barbering and Cosmetology
State House Station 35
Augusta, ME 04333
(207) 624-8579
Cathleen.abitz@maine.gov
http://www.maine.gov

Machine Scope of Use
No defined scope of use

Requirements
ESTHETICIAN: 750 hours, apprenticeship 1,250 hours

Reciprocity
The state board waives the exam to grant a license to any applicant who seeks reciprocity provided the applicant has a valid license from a state whose requirements are equal to or greater than Maine's.

Continuing Education
Required for instructors only

Medical Board Contact Information
Board of Licensure in Medicine
161 Capitol Street
137 State House Station

Augusta, ME 04333-0137
(207) 287-3601
http://www.docboard.org

MARYLAND

Maryland State Board of Cosmetologists
500 North Calvert Street, Room 307
Baltimore, MD 21202-3651
(410) 230-6320
cos@dllr.state.md.us
http://www.dllr.state.md.us

Machine Scope of Use
In Maryland an esthetician may not do microdermabrasion; it is a service that only a doctor may perform. An esthetician may not do laser procedures and may not perform services using a laser or IPL.

Requirements
ESTHETICIAN: 600 hours
MAKEUP ARTIST: Applicant must submit proof of having successfully completed a board-approved course or program in makeup artist services

Reciprocity
Maryland grants reciprocity to those individuals who hold a license from a state whose requirements are the same as or greater than Maryland's.

Continuing Education
Not required

Medical Board Contact Information
Maryland Board of Physicians
4201 Patterson Avenue
Baltimore, MD 21215
(410) 764-4777
(800) 492-6836
http://www.mbp.state.md.us

MASSACHUSETTS

Massachusetts Division of Professional Licensure
239 Causeway Street
Boston, MA 02114
(617) 727-3074
Helen.peveri@state.ma.us
http://www.mass.gov

Machine Scope of Use
Currently under review

Requirements

ESTHETICIAN: 300 hours

Continuing Education

Not required

Medical Board Contact Information

Commonwealth of Massachusetts
Board of Registration in Medicine
560 Harrison Avenue, Suite G-4
Boston, MA 02118
(617) 654-9800
http://www.massmedboard.org

MICHIGAN

Michigan Bureau of Commercial Services, Board
of Cosmetology
P.O. Box 30018
Lansing, MI 48909
(517) 241-9201
bcsinfo@michigan.gov
http://www.michigan.gov

Machine Scope of Use

The Department of Labor and Economic Growth, which
regulates the cosmetology profession, and the Department
of Community Health, which regulates the medical profession,
have deemed lasers, IPL, and ultrasound to be of a medical
nature. Therefore, a physician or somebody under the
supervision of a physician would be required to perform
these services.

Requirements

ESTHETICIAN: 400 hours

Reciprocity

All individuals licensed in another state may obtain their
license in the state of Michigan by making an application to
the board and meeting the requirements of being at least
17 years of age and possessing a ninth-grade education.
No examination is required. For those individuals whose
states have requirements less stringent than those in Michigan,
a credit of 100 hours per every six months work experience
will be awarded.

Continuing Education

Not required

Medical Board Contact Information
Bureau of Health Professions
PO Box 30670
Lansing, MI 48909
(517) 335-0918
http://www.michigan.gov

MINNESOTA

Minnesota Board of Barber and Cosmetology Examiners
2829 University Avenue SE, Suite 710
St. Paul, MN 55414
(651) 201-2742
bce.board@state.mn.us
http://www.bceboard.state.mn.us

Machine Scope of Use
No defined scope of use

Requirements
ESTHETICIAN: 600 hours

Continuing Education
Required for instructors only

Medical Board Contact Information
Minnesota Board of Medical Practice
University Park Plaza
2829 University Avenue SE, Suite 500
Minneapolis, MN 55414-3246
(612) 617-2130
http://www.state.mn.us

MISSISSIPPI

Mississippi State Board of Cosmetology
3000 Old Canton Road, Suite 112
P.O. Box 55689
Jackson, MS 39296-5689
(601) 987-6840
nleflore@msbc.state.ms.us
http://www.msbc.state.ms.us

Machine Scope of Use
Currently under review

Requirements
ESTHETICIAN: 600 hours

Reciprocity
Permitted with Arkansas, Kansas, Louisiana, Minnesota, Montana, Nevada, Rhode Island, South Carolina, Tennessee, Vermont, and West Virginia

Continuing Education
Instructors: 24 hours every two years

Medical Board Contact Information
1867 Crane Ridge Drive, Suite 200-B
Jackson, MS 39216
(601) 987-3079
http://www.msbml.state.ms.us

MISSOURI
Missouri State Board of Cosmetology
3605 Missouri Blvd
P.O. Box 1062
Jefferson City, MO 65102
(573) 751-1052
cosmo@pr.mo.gov
http://pr.mo.gov

Machine Scope of Use
Currently under review

Requirements
ESTHETICIAN: 750 hours

Continuing Education
Instructors: 12 hours every two years

Medical Board Contact Information
Board of Registration for the Healing Arts
3605 Missouri Boulevard
P.O. Box 4
Jefferson City, MO 65102
(573) 751-0098
http://www.pr.mo.gov

MONTANA
Montana Board of Barbers and Cosmetologists
301 South Park, 4th Floor
P.O. Box 200513
Helena, MT 59620-0513
(406) 841-2335
dilbsdcos@mt.gov
http://www.mt.gov

Machine Scope of Use
No defined use

Requirements
ESTHETICIAN: 650 hours

Reciprocity
Applicants who do not have the hours required by Montana must take the national practical and written exams. An applicant may take the additional hours from an approved school.

Continuing Education
Required for instructors only; check with the state board

Medical Board Contact Information
Health Care Licensing Bureau
301 South Park, Room 430
P.O. Box 200513
Helena, MT 59620-0513
(406) 841-2300
http://www.mt.gov

NEBRASKA
Nebraska Department of Health and Human Services
Regulation and Licensure Credentialing Division
P.O. Box 95007
Lincoln, NE 68509 5007
(402) 471-2117
kris.chiles@hhss.ne.gov
http://www.hhs.state.ne.us

Machine Scope of Use
The Board of Medicine and Surgery has gone on record to state that use of a laser, for whatever purpose, is the practice of medicine and surgery. As such, these devices can only be used by a physician or a physician assistant in accordance with regulations regarding duties for physician assistants. This applies to IPL devices, which are considered to be lasers. Ultrasound has not been considered.

Requirements
ESTHETICIAN: 600 hours

Continuing Education
Eight hours every two years

Medical Board Contact Information
Department of Health and Human Services
301 Centennial Mall South
Lincoln, NE 68509
(402) 471-3121
http://www.dhhs.ne.gov

NEVADA

Nevada State Board of Cosmetology
1785 East Sahara Avenue, #255
Las Vegas, NV 89104
(702) 486-6542
nvcosmbd@govmail.state.nv.us
http://www.cosmetology.nv.gov

Machine Scope of Use

No defined use, but these rules apply:
NAC 644.367 Restriction on removal of skin

1. A cosmetologist or an esthetician may remove the uppermost layers of the facial skin by any method or means if only the uppermost layers of skin are removed and the removal is for the purpose of beautification.
2. In removing the uppermost layers of skin pursuant to this section, a cosmetologist or an esthetician:
   (a) May only use products that are commercially available for the removal of facial skin for beautification: and (b) Shall not mix or combine any such products unless the mixing or combining is required pursuant to the manufacturer's instructions for the products being mixed or combined.
3. A cosmetologist or esthetician shall not use any techniques or practices for the removal of skin that affects anything other than the uppermost layers of the facial skin.

Prohibited invasive procedures
NAC 644.368

1. Except as otherwise provided in this section, a licensee shall not perform any invasive procedure that includes, without limitation:
   (a) The application of electricity for the sole purpose of contracting a muscle
   (b) The application of a topical lotion, cream, or other substance that affects anything other than the uppermost layers of the skin
   (c) The penetration of the skin by metal needles
   (d) The abrasion of the skin below the uppermost layer of the skin
2. The provisions of paragraph (c) of subsection 1 do not apply to the use of electrolysis needles by a licensed electrologist.
3. As used in this section, "invasive procedure" means an act that affects the structure or function of the skin other than the uppermost layers of the skin.

Requirements

ESTHETICIAN: 600 hours

Reciprocity

All applicants must apply to the board, enclose $100, be at least 18 years of age, and have the equivalent of a tenth-grade education. The applicant must have passed a nationally recognized written test in the state of licensure and must hold a current license.

Continuing Education
Not required

Medical Board Contact Information
Board of Medical Examiners
1105 Terminal Way, Suite 301
Reno, NV 89502
or
P.O. Box 7238
Reno, NV 89510
(775) 688-2559
http://www.medboard.nv.gov

NEW HAMPSHIRE
New Hampshire State Board of Barbering, Cosmetology, and Esthetics
2 Industrial Park Drive
Concord, NH 03301
(603) 271-3608
webmaster@nh.gov
http://www.nh.gov

Machine Scope of Use
An esthetician is required to complete additional training prior to performing services in the following:

(1) Cosmetic chemical substances for exfoliation
(2) Body therapies including manual or mechanical lymphatic drainage massage as it relates to skin beautification
(3) Microdermabrasion or mechanical equipment for cosmetic exfoliation
(4) Light therapy devices
(5) Ultrasonic devices
(6) Microcurrent devices
(7) FDA-registered Class I and Class II devices

An esthetician is required to attend technical, hands-on training for each of the procedures/equipment before performing such services. The hands-on training may be obtained anywhere but must be specific to the service performed.

Requirements
ESTHETICIAN: 600 hours

Continuing Education
Required for instructors only; check with state board

Medical Board Contact Information
2 Industrial Park Drive #8
Concord, NH 03301
(603) 271-1203
http://www.nh.gov

NEW JERSEY
New Jersey Board of Cosmetology and Hairstyling
124 Haley Street
Newark, NJ 07102
(973) 504-6200
askconsumeraffairs@lps.state.nj.us
http://www.state.nj.us

Machine Scope of Use
No defined scope of use

Requirements
ESTHETICIAN: 600 hours

Continuing Education
Not required

Medical Board Contact Information
New Jersey Board of Medical Examiners
140 East Front Street
Trenton, NJ 08608
(609) 826-7100
http://www.state.nj.us

NEW MEXICO
New Mexico Board of Barbers and Cosmetologists
2550 Cerrilos Road
Santa Fe, NM 87505
(505) 476-4690
http://www.rld.state.nm.us

Machine Scope of Use
No defined scope of use

Requirements
ESTHETICIAN: 600 hours

Reciprocity
Applicants who have not completed a course of study equal to the requirements of this state may receive credit for work experience (150 hours of training for every six full months of work). Applicants who have completed a course with requirements equal to the requirements of New Mexico must furnish a transcript of hours and a copy of a valid license.

Continuing Education
Instructors: 12 hours every year

Medical Board Contact Information
New Mexico Medical Board
2055 South Pacheco
Building 400
Santa Fe, NM 87505
(505) 476-7220
http://www.nmmb.state.nm.us

NEW YORK
New York Department of State, Division of Licensing Services
84 Holland Avenue
Albany, NY 12208-3490
(518) 474-4429
licensing@dos.state.ny.us
http://www.dos.state.ny.us

Machine Scope of Use
New York currently regulates the use of lasers and IPL as follows:

In general, lasers are classified as medical devices or nonmedical devices by the FDA. If a particular laser device has been classified as a medical device, the laser can be used only by an individual licensed to practice medicine. On the other hand, if the laser device has been classified as a nonmedical device, it can be used, within the scope of their licensed practice, by an esthetics or cosmetology licensee but cannot be used by that licensee to perform any service that constitutes a medical procedure

Finally, Section 482 of the General Business Law provides, in part, that no individual shall use a laser unless such person holds a valid certificate of competence issued by the New York State Department of Labor.

Requirements
ESTHETICIAN: 600 hours

Continuing Education
Not required

Medical Board Contact Information
New York State Education Department
Office of the Professions
State Education Building, 2nd Floor
89 Washington Avenue
Albany, NY 12234
(518) 474-3817
http://www.nysed.gov

NORTH CAROLINA

North Carolina Board of Cosmetology
1201 Front Street, #110
Raleigh, NC 27609-7533
(919) 733-4117
nccosmo@intrex.net
http://www.cosmetology.state.nc.us

Machine Scope of Use

Electrical equipment is okay, but no specific information could be found on Class I, II, and III devices.

Requirements

ESTHETICIAN: 600 hours

Reciprocity

Applicant must meet hourly criteria as set forth by North Carolina and must also have been working in the field for a period of at least one year within the previous three years prior to applying.

Continuing Education

Eight hours every year

Medical Board Contact Information

North Carolina Medical Board
1203 Front Street
Raleigh, NC 27609-7533
or
P.O. Box 20007
Raleigh, NC 27619-0007
(919) 326-1100
(800) 253-9653
info@ncmedboard.org

NORTH DAKOTA

North Dakota Board of Cosmetology
P.O. Box 2177
Bismarck, ND 58502
(701) 224-9800
cosmo@gcentral.com
http://www.governor.state.nd.us

Machine Scope of Use

No scope defined

Requirements

COSMETICIAN: 1,800 hours

Continuing Education

Instructors: Eight hours every year

Medical Board Contact Information
State Board of Medical Examiners
418 East Broadway Avenue, Suite 12
Bismarck, ND 58501
(701) 328-6500
http://www.ndbomex.com

OHIO
Ohio State Board of Cosmetology
101 Southland Mall
3700 High Street, Suite 101
Columbus, OH 43207-4041
(614) 466-3834
http://www.cos.ohio.gov

Machine Scope of Use
No defined scope of use

Requirements
ESTHETICIAN: 750 hours

Continuing Education
Eight hours every two years

Medical Board Contact Information
77 South High Street, 17th Floor
Columbus, OH 43215-6127
(614) 466-3934
http://med.ohio.gov

OKLAHOMA
State of Oklahoma Board of Cosmetology
2401 NW 23rd, Suite 84
Shepherd Mall
Oklahoma City, OK 73107
(405) 521-2441
bmoore@oklaosf.state.ok.us
http://www.cosmo.state.ok.us

Machine Scope of Use
Class I devices may be used, but no further rules are provided on
Class II and Class III devices.

Requirements
ESTHETICIAN: 600 hours

Reciprocity
All states with equal or better requirements

Continuing Education
Not required

Medical Board Contact Information
Oklahoma Board of Medical Licensure and Supervision
5104 North Francis Avenue, Suite C
Oklahoma City, OK 73118-6020
(405) 848-6841

OREGON
Oregon Board of Cosmetology
700 Summer Street NE, Suite 320
Salem, OR 97301-1287
(503) 378-8667
hlo.info@state.or.us
http://www.oregon.gov

Machine Scope of Use
Use of Class II devices must be supervised by a physician. Class I and Class II devices may be employed within their intended use and scope of practice with appropriate training. Electrical equipment is allowed.
        For more information, visit: http://www.oregon.gov

Requirements
ESTHETICIAN: 500 hours

Reciprocity
A current license qualifies an applicant for examination.

Continuing Education
Not required

Medical Board Contact Information
Oregon Board of Medical Examiners
1500 SW 1st Avenue, Suite 620
Portland, OR 97201-5847
(971) 673-2700
http://www.oregon.gov

PENNSYLVANIA
Pennsylvania State Board of Cosmetology
Penn Center
2601 North Third Street
Harrisburg, PA 17110
(717) 783-8503
st-cosmetology@state.pa.us
http://www.dos.state.pa.us

Machine Scope of Use
Laser use for hair removal is considered to be a medical procedure and not the practice of any license issued by the state board of cosmetology.

Electrology is not specifically regulated but must be performed by a licensed cosmetologist or esthetician trained in electrology.

Requirements
COSMETICIAN: 300 hours

Reciprocity
With all states except AL, CA, CT, CO, GA, HI, NJ, NM, RI, and UT

Continuing Education
Not required

Medical Board Contact Information
State Medical Board
P.O. Box 2649
Harrisburg, PA 17105
(717) 787-8503
http://www.dos.state.pa.us

RHODE ISLAND

Rhode Island Department of Health, Division of Hairdressing and Barbering
3 Capitol Hill, Room 105
Providence, RI 02908-5097
(401) 222-2827
library@doh.state.ri.us
http://www.health.ri.gov

Machine Scope of Use
The Rhode Island Cosmetology Act does not refer to specific machines that can or cannot be used by a cosmetologist or esthetician. However, Class I, II, and III devices are considered medical equipment and can only be used by a licensed physician or a person trained and working under the supervision of a licensed physician.

Requirements
ESTHETICIAN: 600 hours

Reciprocity
Considered on an individual basis

Continuing Education
Not required

Medical Board Contact Information
3 Capitol Hill, Room 205
Providence, RI 02908-5097
(401) 222-3855
http://www.health.ri.gov

SOUTH CAROLINA
South Carolina Board of Cosmetology
Kingstree Building
110 Center View Drive
Columbia, SC 29210
(803) 896-4568
jonese@mail.llr.state.sc.us
http://www.llr.state.sc.us

Machine Scope of Use
No scope defined

Requirements
ESTHETICIAN: 450 hours

Reciprocity
Granted to those applicants who have completed the same requirements as South Carolina. You may have to pass the national exam.

Continuing Education
12 hours every two years

Medical Board Contact Information
Board of Medical Examiners
Synergy Business Park
Kingstree Building
110 Centerview Drive, Suite 202
Columbia, SC 29210
(803) 896-4500
http://www.llr.state.sc.us

SOUTH DAKOTA
South Dakota Cosmetology Commission
500 East Capitol
Pierre, SD 57501
(605) 773-6193
cosmetology@state.sd.us
http://www.state.sd.us

Machine Scope of Use
South Dakota does not allow estheticians to use lasers, LED, IPL, or ultrasound even under the supervision of a physician due to a medical board ruling. Microdermabrasion is allowed if the technician has 16 hours of training in microdermabrasion.

Requirements
COSMETICIAN: 2,100 hours

Reciprocity

You may become a licensed cosmetologist, esthetician, or nail technician in South Dakota through reciprocity if your current state license has equal or greater requirements than South Dakota. If you do not have a current license, then you must apply as a student.

Continuing Education

Not required

Medical Board Contact Information

Department of Health
125 South Main Ave
Sioux Falls, SD 57104
(605) 367-7781
http://www.state.sd.us

TENNESSEE

Tennessee State Board of Cosmetology
500 James Robertson Parkway
Nashville, TN 37243-1147
(615) 741-2515
Beverly.waller@state.tn.us
http://www.state.tn.us

Machine Scope of Use

Electrical equipment may be used as a Class I device that is made specifically for estheticians, who must have a minimum of four hours training on the Class I device. Any machine with a floor pedal may not be used by estheticians; these are to be used only by doctors. Under the supervision of a physician, estheticians may use whatever equipment the doctor permits.

Requirements

ESTHETICIAN: 750 hours

Reciprocity

Applicant must hold a license in a state whose requirements are the same as Tennessee. This is true for all licenses except nail technology, for which the state board requires theoretical and practical exams.

Continuing Education

Instructors: 16 hours every two years

Medical Board Contact Information

Board of Medical Examiners
227 French Landing, Suite 300
Nashville, TN 37243
(615) 532-3202
www.state.tn.us

TEXAS

Department of Licensing and Regulation
P.O. Box 12157
Austin, TX 78711
(512) 463-6599
customerservice@license.state.tx.us
http://www.license.state.tx.us

Machine Scope of Use

Chairs and beds used by facialists and pedicurists must be disinfected prior to providing client services. No other defined machine scope of practice was found.

Requirements

ESTHETICIAN: 750 hours

Reciprocity

Granted to applicants with licenses from another state whose requirements are the same as or greater than those of Texas.

Continuing Education

Eight hours every two years

Medical Board Contact Information

333 Guadalupe Tower 3, Suite 610
Austin, TX 78701
(512) 305-7010
http://www.tmb.state.tx.us

UTAH

Utah Division of Occupational and Professional Licensing
Board of Cosmetology
160 East, 300 South
Salt Lake City, UT 84111
(801) 530-6628
http://www.dopl.utah.gov

Machine Scope of Use

Master level estheticians may use laser under physician supervision, microdermabrasion, and electrical equipment. Basic level estheticians may use electrical equipment.

Requirements

ESTHETICIAN: 600 hours, 1,200 hours

Reciprocity

Granted to applicants from states with requirements that are substantially equal to those of Utah

Continuing Education

Not required

Medical Board Contact Information
Utah Division of Occupational and Professional Licensing
P.O. Box 146741
Salt Lake City, UT 84114-6741
(801) 530-6628
http://www.dopl.utah.gov

VERMONT
Vermont Secretary of State
Board of Barbers and Cosmetologists
Redstone Building
26 Terrace Street, Drawer 09
Montpelier, VT 05609-1101
(802) 828-2363
cwinters@sec.state.vt.us
http://www.vtprofessionals.org

Machine Scope of Use
Electrical equipment is acceptable, which specifically addresses use of lasers. The rule clearly states that laser use is not part of licensed activities of cosmetologists or estheticians. Also, Part 13 states that no microdermabrasion machine may be used by a licensee unless the machine meets the following criteria:

(a) When used according to manufacturer's instructions, no removal of the epidermis beyond the stratum corneum occurs.
(b) Microdermabrasion machine models used must be closed systems only.

Part 13.2 states:

(a) Licensees must be appropriately trained by the manufacturer before using equipment.
(b) Licensees must post or have on file a copy of the Certificate of Training issued by the manufacturer.
(c) Microdermabrasion machines must be used only in accordance with specific manufacturer's directions.
(d) Microdermabrasion machines must be maintained and filters changed in accordance with manufacturer's requirements and any applicable laws.
(e) Microdermabrasion machines must be kept in a clean, sanitary, and safe manner at all times.

13.3 Single Use: Aluminum oxide crystals or manufacturer approved corundum used in microdermabrasion machines may not be reused or recycled. Aluminum oxide crystals or approved corundum are for single-use purposes and must be discarded after each use in accordance with federal, state, and local disposal regulations for such substances. All products employed for microdermabrasion shall be used in accordance with manufacturer's recommendations.

13.5 New Devices, New Procedures: Warning to Practitioners

(a) New devices for cosmetology or esthetics appear on the market all the time. It is not feasible for the board to adopt new rules governing the use of each new device. The board does not preapprove particular devices for use in any of the fields covered by these rules.

(b) Practitioners should not assume that because a particular device is available on the market and being offered to licensees that it is safe or appropriate for use by licensees. Some devices seen in the recent past offered for sale to cosmetologists and estheticians, for example laser hair-removal devices and some microdermabrasion units, are considered medical devices. Their use constitutes medical practice outside the scope of practice of esthetic professions.

13.6 Duty to Use Devices Safely

It is the responsibility of licensees to ensure that the devices or materials they use are safe and used correctly. Failure to do so can be grounds for disciplinary action.

Requirements
ESTHETICIAN: 600 hours

Reciprocity
Granted to applicants who hold a license in states whose requirements are equal to or greater than those of Vermont

Continuing Education
Required for instructors only; check with state board

Medical Board Contact Information
Vermont Department of Health
108 Cherry Street
Burlington, VT 05402
(802) 863-7200
http://healthvermont.gov

VIRGINIA
Virginia Department of Professional and Occupational Regulation
Board for Barbers and Cosmetology
3600 West Broad Street
Richmond, VA 23230-4917
(804) 367-8509
dpor@dpor.virginia.gov
http://www.state.va.us

Machine Scope of Use
A two-tier esthetics licensing program has been implemented. Check with the board of cosmetology for exact machine requirements.

Requirements
COSMETOLOGIST: 1,500 hours
ESTHETICIAN: 600 hours (Basic), 1,200 hours (Master)

Reciprocity
Granted to applicants who have completed the same number of hours as required by Virginia. Credit is given to those who have worked in the industry for a minimum of six months.

Continuing Education
Not required

Medical Board Contact Information
6603 West Broad Street, 5th Floor
Richmond, VA 23230-1712
(804) 662-9900
http://www.dhp.virginia.gov

WASHINGTON
State of Washington Department of Licensing
Cosmetology Licensing Program
P.O. Box 9026
Olympia, WA 98507-9026
(360) 664-6626
plssunit@dol.wa.gov
http://www.dol.wa.gov

Machine Scope of Use
The rules apply to devices defined by the FDA as "prescriptive de-vices." They include devices that use a laser, light, radio frequency, or plasma (LLRP) to penetrate the skin and alter human tissue. Such devices can only be used by a physician or licensed professional under the supervision of a physician whose licensure and scope of practice allows the use of such devices. Estheticians are considered licensed professionals, so they would be required to work under a physician's supervision if they are using prescriptive LLRP devices.

Requirements
ESTHETICIAN: 600 hours

Reciprocity
No reciprocity; however, if an applicant provides proof of a current license in good standing in another state, territory, or foreign coun-try, they are eligible for examination for a fee.

Continuing Education
Not required unless placed on inactive status

Medical Board Contact Information
Washington State Department of Health
101 Israel Road SE, MS: 47890
Tumwater, WA 98501
(360) 236-4085
http://www.doh.wa.gov

WEST VIRGINIA
West Virginia State Board of Barbers and Cosmetologists
1716 Pennsylvania Avenue, #7
Charleston, WV 25302
(304) 558-2924
larryabsten@wvdhhr.org
http://www.wvdhhr.org

Machine Scope of Use
The board does not have any rules relating to FDA Class I, Class II, or Class III devices. Based upon advice from the state attorney general's office, the board has adopted a policy that would permit the use of these devices under the direct supervision of a physician.

Requirements
ESTHETICIAN: 600 hours

Reciprocity
Granted to those applicants with the same or greater requirements as those of West Virginia. However, an applicant with fewer hours than required may receive a credit of 300 hours for every year of practical experience.

Continuing Education
Not required

Medical Board Contact Information
West Virginia Board of Medicine
101 Dee Drive, Suite 103
Charleston, WV 25311
(304) 558-2921
http://www.wvdhhr.org

WISCONSIN
Wisconsin Department of Regulations and Licensing
Barbering and Cosmetology Examining Board
P.O. Box 8935
Madison, WI 53708
(608) 266-2112
web@drl.state.wi.us
http://drl.wi.gov

Machine Scope of Use
No scope defined

Requirements
ESTHETICIAN: 450 hours

Reciprocity
All applicants must have at least 4,000 hours of experience in licensed practice and have never been disciplined by the licensing authority in their state of licensure. Anyone who does not meet these requirements must attend a school in Wisconsin and be licensed after graduation.

Continuing Education
Not required

Medical Board Contact Information
Department of Regulation and Licensing
P.O. Box 8935
Madison, WI 53708-8935
(608) 266-2112
http://www.drl.wi.gov

WYOMING
Wyoming Board of Cosmetology
Peter Hansen Building, East Entrance
2515 Warren Avenue, Suite 302
Cheyenne, WY 82002
(307) 777-3534
http://www.plboards.state.wy.us

Machine Scope of Use
No use of machines that penetrate to the dermis is allowed, but no specific rules have been written about physician supervision. No use of the term *medical esthetician* is applied, but electrical equipment is allowed.

Requirements
ESTHETICIAN: 600 hours

Reciprocity
Granted for all states with equal or more stringent requirements, written and practical exam, or at least one year work history

Continuing Education
Not required

Medical Board Contact Information
Wyoming Board of Medicine
Colony Building, 2nd Floor
211 West 19th Street
Cheyenne, WY 82002
(307) 778-7053
http://www.wyomedboard.state.wy.us

Appendix B

EQUIPMENT MANUFACTURERS

This list does not include every manufacturer and distributor in the esthetics industry. Check industry resources for updated information. The author makes no warranty on the quality of the equipment, so exercise due diligence before purchasing.

General equipment includes steamers, beds, hot cabinets, waxing, multifunction units, imaging, and sensors.

Advanced technology includes microdermabrasion, microcurrent, laser, and IPL.

For the purposes of not duplicating listings, those manufacturers that have both types of equipment will be listed under the general category only.

General Equipment

A1A Facial and Skin Care Equipment
(866) 203-2330
info@a1afacial.com
http://www.a1afacial.com

Aesthetics Complete
(610) 265-3535
http://www.acispa.com

Allegra M. France
(323) 957-2301
Fax: 323-957-1346
http://www.allegramf.com

Amber Products
(800) 821.9188
(724) 695.1882
education@amberproducts.com
http://www.amberproducts.com

American International Industries
(323) 728-2999
customer_service@aiibeauty.com
http://www.aiibeauty.com

General Equipment

Athena Beauty
(800) 283-2298
info@athenabeauty.com
http://www.athenabeauty.com

Beauties City Supplies
(800) 903-3550
bcs@beautiescs.com
http://www.beautiescs.com

Beauty USA
(877) 343-1983
beautybusa@aol.com
http://www.beautybeautyusa.com

Canfield Scientific
(973) 276-0336
(800) 815-4330
info@canfieldsci.com
http://www.canfieldsci.com

CosmoPro
(866) 698-6580
cosmopro@cosmopro.com
http://www.cosmopro.com

Custom Craftworks
(800) 627-2387
http://www.customcraftworks.com

Custom Esthetics
(800) 874-4788
http://www.customestheticsltd.com

Equipro Beauty
(802) 928-3522
(877) 324-2226
info@equipro-bty.com
http://www.equipro-bty.com

Moritex USA
(877) 261-2100
sales@moritexusa.com
http://www.moritexusa.com

Pibbs Industries
(800) 551-5020
info@pibbs.com
http://www.pibbs.com

Silhouet-Tone
800-552-0418
info@sihouet-tone.com
http://www.silhouet-tone.com

Spa Revolutions
(888) 827-4683
http://www.sparevolutions.com

Takara Belmont
(732) 469-5000
info@takarabelmont.com
http://www.takarabelmont.com

Ultronics
(800) 262-6262
Fax: 330-916-7080
http://www.ultronicsusa.com

Universal Companies Inc.
(888) 558-5571
info@universalcompanies.com
http://www.universalcompanies.com

Advanced Technology

Advanced Therapeutics
(800) 944-1523 or
(610) 688-3441
http://www.advanthera.com

Aesthetic Solutions
888-345-4569
info@dermaglow.com
http://www.dermaglow.com

Aesthetics Medical
(972) 243-6961
http://www.acispa.com

Ageless Aesthetics
(877) 721-7975
http://www.agelessaesthetics.com

Alderm Direct
800-254-8505
http://www.aldermdirect.com

Altair Instruments
805-388-8503
info@diamondtome.com
http://www.diamondtome.com

Arasys Perfector
(866) 259-6864
(808) 395-0656
info@araysperfector.com
http://www.arasyperfector.com

Beauty Tech
305- 652-8985
888- 818-8890
info@beautytec.com
http://www.beautytec.com

Bellaire Industry
(631) 924-2751
http://www.ultrabeautydevice.com

Bio-Therapeutic
(800) 976-2544
info@bio-therapeutic.com
http://www.bio-therapeutic.com

Candela Corporation
(508) 358-7637
http://www.candelalaser.com

Cynosure
(800) 886-2966
http://www.cynosure.com

Dermamed USA
(888) 789-6342
info@dermamedusa.com
http://www.dermamedusa.com

Dermavista/Onyx Medical
(800) 333-5773
info@onyxmedical.com
http://www.dermavista.com

Dermawave
888-704-5888
dermawave@aol.com
http://www.dermawave.com

Dynatronics
800-874-6251
khc@dynatron.com
http://www.dynatronics.com

$Echo_2$ Plus, The Oxygen Treatment
800-592-3246
sales@echo2plus.com
http://www.echo2plus.com

Edge Systems Corporation
800-603-4996
contact@edgesystem.net
http://www.edgesystem.net

Advanced Technology

Flip 4
(430) 649-4244
info@flip4.com
http://www.flip4.ca

Gensis Biosystems
(972) 315-7888
http://www.genesisbiosystems.com

GentleWaves/Light BioScience
(888) 647-6219
mail@lightbioscience.com
http://www.lightbioscience.com

Innovative Med
(949) 458-1897
http://www.imi-spa.com

Light BioScience
(888) 647-6219
mail@lightbioscience.com
http://www.lightbioscience.com

LPG-Techno Derm, LLC
10800 Biscayne Blvd, Ste. 850
Miami, FL 33161
(888) 892-4588
Fax: (305) 892-4589
http://www.techno-derm.com

Lumenis
(877) 586-3647
http://www.lumenis.com

Lumiere Light Therapie
(Raymond Anthony International)
(866) 724-8267
info@lumierelight.com
http://www.lumierelight.com

MP2 Cosmetiques
(800) 778-9850
http://www.mp2cosmetiques.com

Radiancy
845-398-1647
http://www.radiancy.com

Science Innovative Aesthetics
(201) 332-4100
info@scienceaesthetics.com
http://www.scienceaesthetics.com

Skin Care Consultants
Lam Probe
(877) 760-8722 (East coast)
(877) 560-7546 (West coast)
http://www.lamskin.com

Skin For Life
(866) 312-7546
sales@skinforlife.com
http://www.skinforlife.com

Skin Star Inc.–Carol Cole
(760) 230-1322
http://www.skinstarinc.com

Sybaritic
(800) 445-8418
info@sybaritic.com
http://www.skinsenseinfo.com

Viora
(201) 332-4100
info@vioramed.com
http://www.vioramed.com

Appendix C

Equipment Checklist

Manufacturer/distributor: _____   How long in business: _____

Address: _____

Phone: _____   E-mail: _____

Web site: _____

Type of equipment: _____   Price: _____

Lease available? _____ Terms: _____

❑   UL listed? _____

❑   FDA-registered manufacturer? _____   FDA Reg number: _____

❑   ISO listed? _____   ISO registration type: _____

❑   CE mark? _____

❑   Warranty: _____   Term length: _____   Loaner program? _____

❑   Warranty valid only with use of manufacturer products? _____

❑   Cost per use estimate: _____

❑   Education included in price? _____   If not, cost for education: _____

❑   Technical assistance available? _____   Cost: _____

❑   Replacement parts available for purchase? _____

❑   Delivery time: _____   Cost: _____

Equipment Use: _____

❑   Clinical trials: _____   White paper available? _____

❑   Demonstration available? _____   Date performed? _____

369

Results

- ❏ Easy to use? _____

- ❏ Instructions easy to understand? _____

- ❏ Performed as promised? _____

Estimated Profit:

a. Monthly lease: $ _____   b. Price of service: $ _____

c. Est. clients per day: _____   d. Days open per year: _____   e. Daily overhead cost: $ _____

f. Technician cost per treatment: $ _____   g. Cost of supplies per treatment: $ _____

Estimated annual revenue = b × c × d

Daily cost estimate = ((a × 12) / d) + e + (f × c) + (g × c)

Estimated annual revenue − (Daily cost estimate × d) = Estimated annual profit

Estimated daily revenue = b × c

Daily cost estimate = ((a × 12) / d) + e + (f × c) + (g × c)

Estimated daily revenue − Daily cost estimate = Estimated daily profit

Appendix D

EDUCATION RESOURCES

This is not a complete list. Many esthetic schools are adding advanced education classes, so check with resources in your area.

POST-GRADUATE EDUCATION

AMERICAN ACADEMY OF MEDICAL AESTHETICS

303B National Road
Exton, PA 19341-2647
(610) 363-0225
http://www.aaoma.org

ATELIER ESTHÉTIQUE INSTITUTE OF ESTHETICS

386 Park Avenue South
Suite 1409
New York, NY 10016
(212) 725-6130
AEInstitute@aol.com
http://www.AEInstitute.net

ATLANTA INSTITUTE OF AESTHETICS

2 Dunwoody Park
Atlanta, GA 30333
(678) 805-0119
jocelynash@atlantaschoolofmassage.com
http://www.atlantaschoolofmassage.com

COLORADO ADVANCED ESTHETICS

7009 South Potomac Street, Suite 100
Centennial, CO 80112
(303) 768-8811
info@lasertrainingcourse.com
http://www.coadvancedskin.com

ESTHETICS NW

1 Centennial Loop
Suite #3
Eugene, OR 97401
(541) 344-7789
http://www.estheticsnw.com

EURO INSTITUTE

10904 SE 176th Street
Renton, WA 98055
(425) 255-8100
Toll-free: (877) 655-7546
Fax: (425) 255-8143
schinfo@euroinstitute.com
http://www.euroinstitute.com

FLORIDA COLLEGE OF NATURAL HEALTH

2001 W. Sample Road, Suite 100
Pompano Beach, FL 33064
(954) 975-6400
Toll Free: (800) 541-9299
Fax: (954) 975-9633
staylor@fcnh.com
http://www.fcnh.com

IMAJ INSTITUTE

7120 East Indian School Road, Suite B
Scottsdale, AZ 85251
(480) 361-8581
(480) 383-6108
admissions@imajschool.org
http://www.imajschool.com

INSTITUT DERMED

5589 Peachtree Road
Atlanta, GA 30341
(770) 454-7788
lross@idermed.com
http://www.idermed.com

INSTITUTE OF ADVANCED MEDICAL ESTHETICS

8547 Mayland Drive
Richmond, VA 23294
laura@theinstituteofadvancedmedicalesthetics.com
http://www.theinstituteofadvancedmedicalesthetics.com

INTERNATIONAL DERMAL INSTITUTE

1535 Beachey Place
Carson, CA 90746
(888) 292-5277
Fax: (310) 900-4040
http://www.dermalinstitute.com

MEDICAL AESTHETIC TRAINING
OF CALIFORNIA

2901 West Coast Highway, Suite #200
Newport Beach, CA 92663
(800) 972-6422
dean@camedtraining.com
http://www.camedtraining.com

MEDICAL ESTHETICS INTERNATIONAL

www.medical-esthetics.com

NEW YORK INSTITUTE OF BEAUTY

11 Oval Drive, Suite #180
Islandia, NY 11749
(631) 582-4737
info@nyib.com
http://www.nyib.com

PACIFIC INSTITUTE OF ESTHETICS

644 7th Court, Suite A
Hammond, OR 97121
(503) 741-0106
info@instituteofesthetics.com
http://www.instituteofesthetics.com

SKIN CARE AND SPA INSTITUTE

8707 Skokie Boulevard, Suite 106
Skokie, IL 60077
http://www.skin-care-institute.com

SKIN SCIENCE INSTITUTE

28 East 2100 South, Suite 217
Salt Lake, City UT 84115
(801) 983-0619
http://www.skinscienceinstitute.com

THE INSTITUTE OF ADVANCED MEDICAL ESTHETICS

8547 Mayland Drive
Richmond, VA 23294
(804) 908-3223
laura-iame@hotmail.com
http://www.iame-edu.com

THE SKIN AND MAKEUP INSTITUTE OF ARIZONA

7547 West Greenway Road, Suite 500
Peoria, AZ 85381
(623) 334-6700
pspringer@smi-a.com
http://www.smi-a.com

VICTORIA RAYNER CENTER FOR APPEARANCE AND ESTEEM

(415) 398-6013 or (202) 236-8510
http://www.victoriarayner.com

YVONNE DE VILAR SCIENTIFIC SKIN CARE

305 Maple Avenue West, Suite D
Vienna, VA 22180
(703) 890-0369
school@scientificskincare.com
http://www.scientificskincare.com

WEB RESOURCES

ESTHETICS AMERICA

http://www.ncacares.org

NATIONAL COALITION OF ESTHETIC ASSOCIATIONS

http://www.ncea.tv

ESTHETICIAN RESOURCE

http://www.estheticianresource.com

SPATRADE

http://www.spatrade.com

ISPA

http://www.experienceispa.com

Glossary

510K submission application required by the FDA for medical devices

5-alpha reductase an enzyme that converts to DHT (dihydrotestosterone), which causes sebum to become thick and promote a follicular blockage

A

AIDS acquired immune deficiency syndrome, caused by any of several retroviruses, especially HIV-1, that infect and destroy helper T cells of the immune system and cause a marked reduction in their number; HIV is transmitted by bodily fluids but not by casual contact

A.M. Best Company a company that publishes an annual insurance report

ablative surgical removal

abrasion irritation to the skin

Accutane brand name for generic isotretinoin, a form of vitamin A that is available by prescription only

acid a chemical that has a pH of less than 7

acid mantle the surface protection of the skin created by sebum and sweat

acne an inflammatory disease of the skin

actual cost includes not only the actual price of the equipment but the cost per service, amount paid to the technician, and overhead costs

acupressure the application of pressure with the thumbs or fingertips to the same points on the body stimulated in acupuncture for therapeutic benefit

adenosine triphosphate (ATP) supplies energy for many biochemical cellular processes

alipidic referring to skin, dry with no sebaceous secretions

alkaline a product with a pH greater than 7

alternating current an electric current that reverses its direction at regularly recurring intervals

amortization the reduction of value of an asset by prorating the cost over a period of years

ampere the measurement of current flowing along the path of a circuit

Ampère, André-Marie (1775–1836) French physicist

amplitude the measurement of alternating current wave; the intensity or strength of the wavelength

anion a negatively charged ion

anode the positive electrode

antiseptic preventing or arresting the growth of microorganisms

Arndt/Schultz law electricity follows the path of least resistance, which means that electrical current will move around the area of trauma

aromatherapy the use of essential oils for therapeutic benefit and to enhance a feeling of well-being

arteriosclerosis a chronic disease characterized by abnormal thickening and hardening of the arterial walls

arthritis chronic inflammation of joints

aseptic procedure a procedure outlined for technicians to use that prevents infection

autoclave an apparatus used for sterilization using superheated steam under pressure

axis the outer ring of an atom

ayurveda a form of alternative medicine that is the traditional system of medicine of India, which preceded and evolved independently of Western medicine and seeks to treat and integrate body, mind, and spirit using a comprehensive holistic approach, especially by emphasizing diet, herbal remedies, exercise, meditation, breathing, and physical therapy

B

bacilli straight, rod-shaped bacteria

bases see *alkaline*

benzalkonium chloride towelette an antiseptic and germicidal towelette

Botox trademark name for botulinum toxin type A

C

CE mark a mandatory conformity mark on many products placed on the market in the European Union

CSA (or CE) certification product testing and certification services for electrical, mechanical, plumbing, gas, and a variety of other products

capacitance a measure of the amount of electric charge stored for a given electric potential

capacitor an electrical device that can store energy in the electric field between a pair of conductors or plates

carbolic acid a toxic, colorless, crystalline solid with a sweet, tarry odor and antiseptic properties; also known as phenol, it was originally used by Joseph Lister in his pioneering technique of antiseptic surgery

carbon a chemical element with the symbol C, atomic number 6, and the fourth most abundant element in the universe by mass after hydrogen, helium, and oxygen

cathode an electrode through which positive electric current flows

cation a positively charged ion

cavitation a general term used to describe the behavior of voids or bubbles in a liquid

chickenpox an acute, contagious disease marked by low-grade fever and formation of vesicles

chromophore the part of the molecule that absorbs or detects light energy

chromospheres the part of a molecule that absorbs and attract photons of light

circuit a conductor connected to components to form a consistent pathway for electricity to move through

Class I exempt exempt from having to file a 510K form for FDA approval

claustrophobia fear of being in closed or narrow spaces

clinical trials a controlled test of a new drug or invasive medical device on human subjects conducted under the direction of the FDA before it is made available for use

closed circuit an electrical current that follows a continuous path between positive and negative poles

coagulate to cause to become viscous or thickened

cocci bacteria having a spherical shape

collagen an insoluble, fibrous protein that is the chief constituent of the fibrils of connective tissue and of the organic substance of bones

combination (HF) machine an esthetic machine that has multiple modalities built into one unit

comedone blackhead

complete circuit the entire path an electrical current follows from its source, through a conductor, and back to the source again

condenser see *capacitor*

conduction the movement of charged particles through an electrical conductor

conductor a medium that attracts electricity and helps it move along a circuit

contraindication a symptom, disease, or condition that prevents a client from receiving treatment

cosmeceuticals products that bridge the gap between pharmaceuticals and cosmetics; typically, they have a higher percentage of active ingredients

cosmetic sensitivity skin irritation that can be caused by cosmetics

cytochromes generally membrane-bound proteins that contain heme groups and carry out electron transport

cytoplasm a gelatinous, semitransparent fluid that fills most cells

D

demographic a specific group of the population

deoxyribonucleic acid (DNA) a nucleic acid that contains the genetic instructions used in the development and functioning of all known living organisms

dermal absorption absorption of products into the dermis

desincrustation a process of liquefying sebum in the skin with a galvanic current machine

desquamation the shedding of the outer layers of the skin

dihydrotestosterone (DHT) a form of the hormone testosterone that belongs to the class of hormones called androgens, formed primarily in the prostate gland, testes, hair follicles, and adrenal glands by the enzyme 5a-reductase

diode a device that allows electricity to flow in one direction only

diplococci round paired bacteria that cause bacterial pneumonia, sinusitis, and inflammation in the lungs

direct (high-frequency) application applying a high-frequency electrode directly to the skin and moving it around the face in a specific pattern

direct current an electrical current that moves in one direction with a constant strength

disincrustation see *desincrustation*

disinfect to free from infection, especially by destroying harmful microorganisms

distilled water water that has all of its impurities removed through distillation

dyschromia any disorder of pigmentation within the skin or hair

E

electroencephalogram (EEG) a test to detect problems in the electrical activity of the brain

edema an abnormal excess accumulation of fluid in the body

Einstein, Albert (1879–1955) a physicist generally regarded as one of the greatest scientists in history

elastin a protein in connective tissue that is elastic and allows many tissues in the body to resume their shape after stretching or contracting

elastosis a condition marked by loss of elasticity of the skin due to degeneration of connective tissue

electricity the flow of negative electrons along a conductor which creates a chemical, thermal or mechanical action

electrocoagulation use of high-frequency electrical current to clot and destroy tissue

electrodes a conductor used to establish electrical contact with a nonmetallic part of a circuit

electrolysis the production of chemical changes by passage of an electrical current through an electrolyte

electrolytes chemical substances which, when dissolved in water, change into electrically charged particles called ions and become capable of conducting electricity; Electrolytes are essential to the healthy function of all cells

electromagnetic pollution unhealthy frequencies of electricity that can harm the body

electron a fundamental subatomic particle that carries a negative electrical charge

electrophysiology the study of the electrical properties of biological cells and tissues

electrotherapy the use of electrical energy in therapeutic treatment

embolism the sudden obstruction of a blood vessel by a blood clot

environmental protection agency (EPA) an agency of the federal government formed to safeguard human health and the environment

environmental sensitivity a sensitivity to wind, sun, and other environmental factors

epilation hair removal

epilepsy any of various disorders marked by abnormal electrical discharges in the brain; typical symptoms include convulsions and seizures

ergonomics an applied science concerned with designing things to be safe and effective for repetitive work

erythema abnormal redness of the skin due to capillary inflammation

essential oil any concentrated, hydrophobic liquid containing volatile aroma compounds from plants

eumelanin found in hair and skin; colors hair grey, black, yellow, and brown

experimental study a study under the direct control of the investigator

extrinsic aging aging that is caused by environmental factors, such as smoking, sun damage, diet, and lifestyle

F

fango Italian word for mud

faradic current an interrupted direct current with a low frequency, which causes muscles to contract

fascia a sheet of connective tissue covering or binding together body structures

Federal Communications Commission (FCC) the agency of the federal government that oversees all international and interstate communication

Federal Trade Commission (FTC) agency designed to oversee free enterprise to prevent restrictions of trade, such as those caused by monopolies

fever blisters a painful sore that occurs in or around the mouth caused by herpes simplex type 1

fibroblasts a type of cell that synthesizes and maintains the extracellular matrix of tissues to provide a structural framework that plays a critical role in wound healing

fibromas non-cancerous tumors made up of connective tissue

Fitzpatrick typing skin typing based on melanin response within the skin; used in the medical field

fluorescence spectroscopy a type of measurement that analyzes fluorescence within a cell

folliculitis inflamed and infected hair follicles

Food and Drug Administration (FDA) the agency of the federal government that regulates food, medicines, medical devices, and cosmetics to ensure their safety and efficacy

Food, Drug, and Cosmetic (FD&C) Act a law passed in 1938 by Congress to give the FDA the authority to oversee the safety of food, drugs and cosmetics

fractionated laser a type of laser that treats the skin by using small dots to treat a fraction of skin with each pass instead of burning the whole area

free electrons electrons that may be shared with other atoms

frequency see also *hertz;* the measurement of waves passing a corresponding point per second

fulguration the process of "flashing electricity" and destroying tissue with electricity; also known as *sparking,* it is used to treat papules and pustules

fungi organisms that develop from spores and can cause many diseases; fungal infections are called *mycoses*

G

GFCI see *ground fault circuit interrupter*

galvanic burn a burn resulting from a buildup of hydrochloric acid on the skin from improper use of galvanic current

galvanic current direct current used in electro-therapy treatments

genital herpes a viral infection transmitted through intimate contact with the moist mucous linings of the genitals; the herpes simplex type 2 virus settles in the nerve roots near the spinal cord and causes painful blisters during outbreaks

Glogau classification of aging aging classification system developed by Dr. Richard Glogau; the system classifies the severity of wrinkles

Golgi apparatus a cytoplasmic organelle that is active in the modification and transport of proteins

Golgi, Camillo (1843–1926) Italian physician and scientist who in 1898 identified the Golgi apparatus, the intracellular reticular apparatus that processes proteins and fats

ground fault circuit interrupter (GFCI) an electrical wiring device that disconnects a circuit whenever it detects that the flow of current is not balanced between the active conductor and the neutral conductor

ground state the lowest energy state of an atom

H

HIPAA the Health Insurance Portability and Accountability Act; Title II provides privacy rules that dictate how protected health information (PHI) is used. PHI relates to all aspects of client care, including payment information

HIV see *AIDS*

hemangioma a usually benign tumor made up of blood vessels that typically occurs as a purplish or reddish slightly elevated area of skin

hepatitis inflammation of the liver

herpes viruses that cause disease; herpes simplex causes watery blisters on the skin or mucous membranes of the lips, mouth, face, or genital region

hertz a unit of frequency equal to one cycle per second

homeostasis the maintenance of relatively stable internal physiological conditions, such as body temperature or the pH of blood, under fluctuating environmental conditions

hot cabinet an electrical cabinet that heats towels

hyaluronidase an enzyme that facilitates the spread of fluids through tissues by lowering the viscosity of hyaluronic acid

hyperbaric oxygen therapy the medical use of oxygen at higher-than-atmospheric pressure for the treatment of non-healing wounds, decompression sickness, virulent bacterial infection and carbon monoxide poisoning

hyperhydrosis excessive sweating

hyperkeratosis also known as *retention hyperkeratosis,* an abnormal buildup of dead skin cells in the stratum corneum

hyperpigmentation a condition that results in areas of discoloration on the face and body caused by overproduction of melanin

hypopigmentation loss of pigmentation in the skin

I

implements items used in a treatment (such as extractor tools)

in vitro relating to cells cultured and studied in a laboratory

in vivo relating to cells studied in the body

indications (for use) visual clues that direct the technician to the correct type of treatment to perform

indirect (high-frequency) application a esthetic treatment in which the client holds the electrode while the esthetician massages the client's skin

inductance a property of an electric circuit by which an electromotive force is induced in it by a variation of current either in the circuit itself or in a neighboring circuit

inductance coil see *Oudin coil*

inflammatory lesions cysts, papules, and pustules

inflammatory stage a stage of wound healing in which the tissues become inflamed

infrared electromagnetic radiation that cannot be seen with the naked eye; ranges from .8 micrometers to 1 millimeter

insulator a substance that does not allow electricity to flow through it

intended use a statement provided by the manufacturer to the FDA to determine the classification of a medical device

intense pulsed light (IPL) laser device that uses non-coherent light for hair removal and skin resurfacing

intensifier coil a long tube with a metal coil running through the middle; used in high-frequency electrodes

intensifier electrode known as a mushroom electrode, it is the electrode commonly used for high fractionated laser frequency application

International Organization for Standardization (ISO) international standard-setting body composed of representatives from various national standards organizations; founded in 1947 and headquartered in Geneva, Switzerland, the organization promulgates worldwide industrial and commercial standards

interpolar effect the movement of ions within the body

intrinsic aging aging caused by genetic factors, such as heredity, general physical health, and the natural aging process

ion channels proteins that help to establish and control the small voltage gradient across the membrane of all living cells

ionized solution also called electrolytes, this water-based solution is a conductor of electricity and contains salts and acids, which increase conductivity. When electrolytes are dissolved in water, they split and form ions that carry either a positive or negative charge. Ionized means an ionic compound separated into positive and negative ions

iontophoresis the process of propelling ions into the skin through water-based lotions and gels

IPL see *intense pulsed light*

J

joules in physics, the unit of measurement of work and energy

K

keloid a type of scar which is caused by an overgrowth of tissue around the site of injury

keratinized skin skin with a buildup of dead skin cells; usually has a rough texture

kilohertz 1,000 hertz

kilowatts 1,000 watts

L

lacunae a small cavity, pit, or discontinuity in an anatomical structure that can be caused by ultrasound application

laser light amplification by the stimulated emission of radiation

Laser Rider an insurance term which relates to additional coverage that includes laser procedures

leasing giving possession and use of equipment, property, or other items in return for periodic payments

LED light-emitting diode

libel the making of false statements in print that damage another's reputation

lice tiny bugs that live on other animals or on plants, sucking their blood or fluids

light visible electromagnetic radiation of various wavelengths that travels at approximately 186,282,397 miles per second in a vacuum

lipase an enzyme that causes the breakdown of fats and lipoproteins, usually into fatty acids and glycerol

lipid soluble a product that will dissolve in the presence of oil

Lister, Joseph (1827–1912) an English surgeon who promoted the idea of sterile surgery; he successfully introduced carbolic acid (phenol) to sterilize surgical instruments and to clean wounds

loupe a magnifying lamp

Lyme disease an acute inflammatory disease characterized initially by red skin lesions, fatigue, fever, and chills; caused by the bite of a tick

lymphatic flow the circulation of lymph fluid

lysosome saclike cellular organelle that contains various hydrolytic enzymes

luminous intensity the strength of light measured by a light meter

M

Macintyre violet ray tube a form of high frequency electrode that emits a violet color

magnifying lamp see *loupe*

Magnuson–Moss Warranty Act (1975) a United States federal law that governs warranties on consumer products

mains the source of an electrical charge

malignant melanoma an often deadly form of skin cancer

manual exfoliation exfoliation that is done with abrasive material

manufacturer registration required by the FDA when manufacturing medical devices

marine-based products that use algae and/or seawater as their main ingredients

medi-spa a spa that has a physician on staff and provides spa services as well

megahertz a unit of frequency equal to one million hertz

melanin the color produced in hair and skin that is an important part of the immune system, protecting against ultraviolet radiation and impairing the production of vitamin D when produced in excess; the two types of melanin are eumelanin and pheomelanin

melasma a dark pigmentation of the skin

metabolism the sum of the processes by which a particular substance is used in the living body

microcirculation blood circulation in the micro-vascular system

microcurrent a esthetic modality that uses micro- and nanocurrent to firm tissue and stimulate cell renewal

microdermabrasion an esthetic modality that uses aluminum oxide crystals or industrial diamond heads attached to a vacuum to exfoliate the skin

microorganisms an organism of microscopic or ultramicroscopic size

milia tiny white bumps or small cysts within the skin

milliamps (mA) one thousandth of an ampere

mitochondrion any of various round or long cellular organelles that are found outside the nucleus, produce energy for the cell through cellular respiration, and are rich in fats, proteins, and enzymes

modality products, protocols, or equipment used in a treatment

moisture meter a type of skin analysis tool that measures the amount of water and sebum within the skin

mononucleosis an acute infectious disease associated with Epstein-Barr virus and characterized by fever, swelling of lymph nodes, and fatigue

muscle reeducation the process of lengthening or shortening muscles

mushroom electrode see *intensifier electrode*

N

negative pole also known as the cathode, it is the negative electrical charge used in galvanic current

nonablative without removing live tissue

noninflammatory lesions comedones and milia

nonsteroidal anti-inflammatory drug (NSAID) drugs with an anti-inflammatory effect that reduce pain, fever, and inflammation without steroids

O

observational studies studies that are based on clinical observation, which is open to interpretation by the investigator

occlusion a shutting off or obstruction of something

ohm measurement of resistance that electrical current faces as it moves through a circuit

Ohm's law an equation that measures the relationship between volts and amps

open circuit when the flow of electricity is interrupted by a switch or device that breaks the connection

orbital area the area around the eyes

organelle a specialized subunit within a cell that has a specific function and is enclosed within its own lipid membrane

oscillation a flow of electricity changing periodically from a maximum to a minimum

Oudin coil high frequency current generator

oxyhemoglobin hemoglobin loosely combined with oxygen, which it releases to the tissues

P

pacemaker an electrical device for stimulating or steadying the heartbeat or reestablishing the rhythm of an arrested heart

papovirus a group of viruses that causes Common warts (*verruca vulgaris*) and Flat warts (*verucca plana*)

papules small, solid, usually conical elevations of the skin caused by inflammation and accumulated sebum secretion

parafango a mixture of paraffin and mud; used for facial treatment

parasites organisms that live in, with, or on another organism

pathogenic bacteria bacteria capable of causing disease

pathogenic factors factors capable of causing disease

pH a measure of acidity and alkalinity of a solution; a value of 7 represents neutrality, lower numbers indicate increasing acidity, and higher numbers increasing alkalinity; each unit of change represents a tenfold change in acidity or alkalinity

phagocytosis the engulfing and usually the destruction of particulate matter by phagocytes that serves as an important bodily defense mechanism against infection and foreign bodies

pheomelanin a form of melanin in hair and skin that is responsible for the red or pink color

photobiology a branch of biology that deals with the effects of light on living things

photodiode a type of photodetector that is capable of detecting the quantity of light and changing it into electricity, depending on the use

photon a measurement of light

piezoelectric effect ability of crystals and certain ceramics to generate an electric potential in response to applied mechanical stress

Planck, Max (1858–1947) a German physicist considered to be the founder of quantum theory, and therefore one of the most important physicists of the twentieth century

plasma the fluid part of blood and lymph

polar effect chemical effect that occurs at the site of the electrode when using galvanic current

positive pole see *anode*

postinflammatory pigmentation pigmentation that occurs after inflammation caused by injury to the skin

proliferative stage the stage in the cell renewal process in which the cells divide and grow

protein metabolism various biochemical processes responsible for the synthesis of proteins and amino acids and the breakdown of proteins

protein synthesis the creation of proteins using DNA and RNA

proteolytic enzyme peel protein-dissolving enzyme mask

pustules small, circumscribed elevations of the skin containing pus and having an inflamed base

Q

quality assurance program a program that a business creates to ensure that standards of manufacture and services are always consistent

R

radiofrequency a frequency or rate of oscillation within the range of about 3 Hz to 300 GHz

randomized controlled laboratory study a study done strictly in the lab that facilitates basic research; the results are not always applicable to the clinical study because they do not also consider the impact of the study on the group

randomized controlled trial (RCT) a study where the investigator has control over the conditions; considered the most effective type of study

rectifier a device for converting alternating current into direct current

reducing the current see *step-down*

refractive index the ratio of the speed of light in one medium to that in another medium

remodeling stage (or maturation) a wound healing stage in which cell proliferation speeds up

Retin A trade name used for a preparation of tretinoin

retrovirus single-stranded RNA virus

rheostat a resistor for regulating a current by means of variable resistances

ribosomes any of the RNA and cytoplasmic granules that are sites of protein synthesis

rosacea a chronic inflammatory disorder often involving the skin of the nose, forehead, and cheeks that is characterized by congestion, flushing, telangiectasia, and marked nodular swelling of tissues, especially of the nose

Rubin system aging classification system created by dermatologist Dr. Mark Rubin

S

saponification the hydrolysis of a fat by an alkali

saturator electrode a long tube with a metal coil running through the middle; this is the electrode the client holds as you perform a manual high-frequency massage

scabies contagious itch or mange caused by parasitic mites

scarred ostia scarred hair follicles

scope of practice a legal definition of services allowed by state regulating boards

sebaceous hyperplasia enlarged sebaceous glands; happens more commonly in older adults

sebaceous secretions sebum secreted from sebaceous glands

seborrhea abnormally increased secretion and discharge of sebum that produces an oily appearance of the skin and dead skin cell buildup

selective photothermolysis a process in which laser wavelengths heat the skin and are absorbed by the target chromophore, which is the part of the molecule that absorbs or detects light energy

shiatsu acupressure massage that originated in Japan

short circuit a break in the insulator

singlet oxygen a form of reactive oxygen species, which is linked to oxidation of LDL cholesterol and resultant cardiovascular effects

sinusoidal current the most common AC waveform

skin sensor new technology that allows estheticians to analyze the elasticity of the skin and the sebum within it

skin tag a small, soft, pendulous growth on the skin, especially around the eyes or on the neck, armpits, or groin

slander false statements made about someone

smallpox a contagious disease caused by a poxvirus, it is characterized by skin eruption with pustules, sloughing, and scar formation

sodium bicarbonate baking soda

sodium chloride salt

solar lentigines freckles

sonophoresis a process that exponentially increases the absorption of topical compounds into the epidermis and dermis

sparking a technique used in high-frequency applications to treat pustules and papules

spirilla bacteria with a cell body that twists like a spiral

Standard and Poor's publishes an annual insurance report

staphylococci also known as staph, bacteria that are pus-forming and grow in clusters

static electricity created when a large number of atoms gain or lose electrons, giving an object an electrical charge

step-down reducing the current by a transformer

step-up increasing the current by a transformer

sterilization the elimination of microbiological organisms

stratum corneum first layer of skin

streptococci bacteria that resemble a string of beads and are pus-forming

support equipment any equipment used to facilitate business; for example, a washer and dryer

syphilis a curable sexually transmitted disease

T

tactile sensitivity skin's sensitivity to texture, touch, and temperature

target market the market segment to which a particular product is marketed, often defined by age, gender, geography, and socioeconomic grouping

telangiectasia an abnormal dilation of red, blue, or purple superficial capillaries

Tesla, Nikola (1856-1943) inventor and engineer who discovered and patented the rotating magnetic field, the basis of most alternating-current machinery, and claimed more than 700 inventions; the tesla, a unit of magnetic induction, was named in his honor

thrombosis the formation or presence of a blood clot within a blood vessel

toxin a poisonous substance that is a specific by-product of the metabolic activities of a living organism capable of inducing antibody formation

trade associations professional organizations that a licensed professional can join to enhance their knowledge and networking skills. These organizations can help an esthetician represent their industry with government officials

transepidermal water loss (TEWL) the measurement of the quantity of water that passes from inside the body through the skin to the surrounding atmosphere via diffusion and evaporation processes

transformer a device that transfers electrical energy from one circuit to another

U

ultraviolet (UV) radiation from the sun; it comes in UVA (320-400 nm), UVB (290-320 nm), and UVC (100-290 nm)

UVC a shortwave ultraviolet light at about 100-290 nm, mostly absorbed by the ozone; can be found in germicidal lamps

Underwriters Laboratories (UL) a U.S. not-for-profit, privately owned and operated product safety testing and certification organization

V

valence shell the outermost shell of an atom, which contains the electrons most likely to account for the nature of any reactions involving the atom and the bonding it has with other atoms

vaporization the process of converting into vapor

varicose veins veins that have become enlarged and twisted

vasoconstrictor any substance that acts to cause narrowing of the blood vessels

vasodilator any substance that acts to cause the opening of blood vessels

ventouse a glass attachment that is used with the vacuum machine

Viennese massage see *indirect (high-frequency) application*

virus any of a large group of submicroscopic infective agents that are regarded either as extremely simple microorganisms or as extremely complex molecules; typically a virus contains a protein coat surrounding an RNA or DNA core of genetic material but no semipermeable membrane, and they are capable of growth and multiplication only in living cells to cause various important diseases in humans, animals, and plants

voltage the force or measured push rate that the electrical current delivers along a conductor

W

warranty an obligation that an article or service sold is as factually stated or legally implied by the seller and that often provides for a specific remedy, such as repair or replacement, in the event the article or service fails to meet the warranty

watt the unit of measurement for electrical power used by a machine

wave theory in physics, a theory concerned with the properties of wave processes independent of their physical origin

wavelength the distance between repeating units of a propagating wave of a given frequency

X

xanthoma a fatty, irregular yellow patch or nodule containing lipid-filled foam cells; occurs in the skin or in internal tissue; xanthelasma is the name for the xanthoma found specifically on the eyelid

Index